Longitudinal Models
in the
Behavioral and Related Sciences

European Association of Methodology Series

The purpose of the European Association of Methodology (EAM) book series is to encourage the development and application of methodological and statistical techniques in social and behavioral research. Sponsored by the European Association of Methodology, the series is open to contributions from Behavioral, Social, Educational, Health, and Economic Sciences. The goal of the EAM book series is to advance fundamental research in Methodology & Statistics by providing a platform for publishing books that focus on state-of-the-art methods and techniques in applied research at an accessible level.

Books in the EAM series can be authored or edited. Proposals should include the following: (1) Title; (2) authors/editors; (3) a brief description of the volume's focus and intended audience; (4) a table of contents; (5) a timeline including planned completion date. Proposals should be sent to one of the members of the EAM book series editorial board noted on the website at http://www.eam-online.org. Members of the EAM editorial board are Joop Hox (Utrecht University), Michael Eid (Free University Berlin), Edith de Leeuw (Utrecht University), and Vasja Vehovar (University of Ljubljana).

van Montfort/Oud/Satorra: Longitudinal Models in the Behavioral and Related Sciences, 2007

Books in the series published by Lawrence Erlbaum Associates, Publishers
(www.erlbaum.com <http://www.erlbaum.com>).

Longitudinal Models
in the
Behavioral and Related Sciences

Edited by

Kees van Montfort
*Free University Amsterdam and Business University Nyenrode,
The Netherlands*

Johan Oud
Radboud University Nijmegen, The Netherlands

Albert Satorra
Universitat Pompeu Fabre, Spain

 LAWRENCE ERLBAUM ASSOCIATES, PUBLISHERS
2007   Mahwah, New Jersey   London

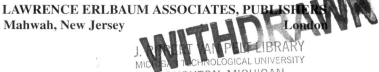

Camera ready copy for this book was provided by the editors.

Lawrence Erlbaum Associates, Inc., Publishers
10 Industrial Avenue
Mahwah, New Jersey 07430
www.erlbaum.com

Cover design by Tomai Maridou

Library of Congress Cataloging-in-Publication Data

Longitudinal models in the behavioral and related sciences / edited by Kees van Montfort, Johan Oud, Albert Satorra.
    p. cm.

Includes bibliographical references and index.

ISBN 0-8058-5913-6 (cloth : alk. paper)
1. Psychology—Mathematical models. I. Montfort, Kees van. II. Oud, Johan. III. Satorra, Albert.
BF39.L58   2007
300.1'1—dc22   2006017399
                                                               CIP

Printed in the United States of America
10 9 8 7 6 5 4 3 2 1

Contents

PART 1: THEORETICAL DEVELOPMENTS

PART 2: APPLICATIONS

Contributors

Shelley A. Blozis
University of California, Department of Psychology,
One Shields Avenue, Davis, CA 95616
United States of America
Email: sablozis@ucdavis.edu

Juan-Carlos Bou
Universitat Jauma I, Business Administration and Marketing,
Avda. Sos Baynat, S/N, Castellon 12071
Spain
Email: bou@emp.uji.es

Sy-Miin Chow
University of Notre Dame, Department of Psychology,
108 Haggar Hall, 46656 Notre Dame
United States of America
Email: schow@nd.edu

Eldad Davidov
University of Basel, Department of Sociology,
Petersgraben 27, 4051 Basel
Switzerland
Email: eldad.davidov@unibas.ch

Uwe Engel
Univeristy of Bremen, Social Statistics and Research Group,
Department of Social Sciences, Celsiusstrasse, Bremen 28359
Germany
Email: uwe.h.engel@t-online.de

Alexander Gattig
Univeristy of Bremen, Social Statistics and Research Group,
Department of Social Sciences, Celsiusstrasse, Bremen 28359
Germany
Email: gattig@empas.uni-bremen.de

Kevin J. Grimm
University of Virginia, Department of Psychology,
PO Box 400871, Charlottesville, VA 22904-4871
United States of America
Email: kjg5c@cms.mail.virginia.edu

Fumiaki Hamagami
University of Virginia, Department of Psychology,
Charlottesville, Virginia
United States of America
fh3s@virginia.edu

Nicholas T. Longford
SNTL, Leicester, UK, and Department d'Economia I Empresa
Universitat Pompeu Fabra, Ramon Trias Farga 25-27, 08005 Barcelona
Spain
Email: nick.longford@upf.edu

John J. McArdle
University of Soutern California, Department of Psychology,
Los Angeles, CA 90089
United States of America
jmcardle@usc.edu

Kees van Montfort
Free University Amsterdam and Business University Nyenrode,
Department of Econometrics, De Boelelaan 1105, 1081 HV Amsterdam
The Netherlands
Email: kvmontfort@feweb.vu.nl

Ab Mooijaart
Leiden University, Department of Psychology,
Chair section Method and Statistics, Wassenaarseweg 52,
PO Box 9555, 2300 RB Leiden
The Netherlands
Email: mooijaart@fsw.leidenuniv.nl

Johan Oud
Radboud University Nijmegen, Behavioral Science Insititute,
Gerrit van Durenstraat 4, 6525 DT Nijmegen
The Netherlands
Email: j.oud@pwo.ru.nl

Maartje E.J. Raijmakers
University of Amsterdam, Department of Psychology,
Roetersstraat 15, 1018 WB Amsterdam
The Netherlands
m.e.j.raijmakers@uva.nl

Jost Reinecke
University of Bielefeld, Faculty of Sociology,
PO Box 100131, 33501 Bieleveld
Germany
Email: reinecke@uni-trier.de

Mark de Rooij
Leiden University, Methods and Statistics Group,
Department of Psychology, Wassenaarseweg 52, Leiden 2333AK
The Netherlands
Email: rooijm@fsw.leidenuniv.nl

Willem Saris
University of Amsterdam, Sociology Department,
Kloveniersburgwal 48, Amsterdam 1012 CX
The Netherlands
Email: saris030@planet.nl

Albert Satorra
Universitat Pompeu Fabra, Department d'Economia I Empresa,
Ramon Trias Fargas 25-27, 08005 – Barcelona
Spain
Email: albert.satorra@upf.edu

Annette Scherpenzeel
University of Amsterdam, Sociology Department,
Kloveniersburgwal 48, Amsterdam 1012 CX,
The Netherlands
Email: a.scherpenzeel@planet.nl

Elmar Schlueter
University of Marburg, Department of Psychology,
Gutenbergstrasse 18, 35032 Marburg,
Germany
Email: e_schluet@gmx.de

Peter Schmidt
Justus-Liebig-Universitaet, Department of Political Sciences,
Giessen
Germany
Email: Schmidt.braunfels@t-online.de

Verena Schmittmann
University of Amsterdam, Department of Developmental Psychology,
Roetersstraat 15, Amsterdam 1018 WB
The Netherlands
Email: v.d.schmittmann@uva.nl

Julia Simonson
University of Bremen, Social Statistics and Research Group,
Department of Social Sciences, Celsiusstrasse, Bremen 28359
Germany
Email: simonson@uni-bremen.de

Herman Singer
Fern Universitaet in Hagen,
Department of Statistics and Methods of Social Research,
Universitaetsstr. 41, D- 58084 Hagen
Germany
Email: hermann.singer@fernuni-hagen.de

Tom Snijders
University of Groningen, ICS/Department of Sociology,
Grote Rozenstraat 31, 9721 JL Groningen
The Netherlands
Email: t.a.b.snijders@ppsw.rug.nl

Christian Steglich
University of Groningen, ICS/Department of Sociology,
Grote Rozenstraat 31, 9721 JL Groningen
The Netherlands
Email: c.e.g.steglich@rug.nl

Jeroen Vermunt
Tilburg University, Department of Methodlogy and Statistics,
Warandalaan 2, 5037AB Tilburg
The Netherlands
Email: j.k.vermunt@uvt.nl

Ingmar Visser
University of Amsterdam, Department of Psychology,
Roetersstraat 15, Amsterdam 1018 WB
The Netherlands
Email: i.visser@uva.nl

Preface

Over the past decade there has become widespread agreement that serious causal analysis should be based on longitudinal data. The longitudinal models and analysis procedures in this book are written by experts in the field and represent current longitudinal approaches in the behavioral and related sciences. Divided into two parts, Theoretical Developments and Applications, the book is intended for methodologists and statisticians who use longitudinal analysis. The book reviews various models that are used in the behavioral and related sciences (psychology, sociology, education, economics, management, and medical sciences) and the technical problems involved in their formulations. In addition, the contents offer researchers new ideas about the use of longitudinal analysis in solving problems that arise due to the specific nature of the design and data available.

The first part of the book demonstrates the latest theoretical developments. Chapters 1 and 6 address problems that arise due to the categorical nature of the data available. Chapters 2, 4, and 5 deal with issues related to continuous observation processes such as the damped differential oscillator, stochastic differential equations, and nonlinear dynamic systems. Chapter 3 considers problems arising when network analysis is extended to longitudinal data and Chapter 7 considers statistical modeling problems associated with grown-curve data.

The second part of the book, the applied chapters, demonstrates how specific problems of empirical research with longitudinal data can be solved. Chapter 9 deals with heterogeneity on the patterns of a firm's profit; Chapter 17, patterns of house prices; Chapter 10 discusses delinquent behavior of adolescents; Chapter 11, nonlinearity in growth in assessing cognitive aging; Chapter 13 is concerned with cross-lagged effects in authoritarianism;

Chapter 16, measurement error issues in longitudinal research; and Chapter 15 addresses distance association for the analysis of change. The second part demonstrates that applying longitudinal modeling should be done with great caution, not only on the statistical side, such as the use of new methods for finite mixture modeling, but also regarding the interpretation of the results.

We thank the authors for their willingness to contribute to the book, the reviewers for their expertise and time invested, and Lawrence Erlbaum for their decision to publish the book and giving it a place in the European Association of Methodology (EAM) book series.

Kees van Montfort, Han Oud and Albert Satorra

Chapter 1

Latent Markov Models for Categorical Variables and Time-Dependent Covariates

Ab Mooijaart

Leiden University, The Netherlands

Kees van Montfort

Free University Amsterdam, The Netherlands

1.1 INTRODUCTION

Poulsen (1982), Van De Pol and De Leeuw (1986), Langeheine (1988), Van De Pol and Langeheine (1989), Langeheine and van de Pol (1990), Collins and Wugalter (1992) and Vermunt (1996) discuss Latent Markov (LM) models in which the state and output variables are categorical and there are no input variables. The main issue of this chapter is the role of time-dependent input variables for Latent Markov models. The LM models are closely related to latent class models. These latter models have their origin in the 1950s (see Lazarsfeld, 1950) and a general framework of these models was given by Lazarsfeld and Henry (1968). The main breakthroughs of the latent class model was in the 1970s (see the work of Goodman, 1974a, 1974b; and Haberman, 1979). The main issue for our model in comparison to the latent class models are the latent class models for multiple groups. In these models the whole population is divided in several subpopulations, where each subpopulation may have different model parameters. In such a setup, it is possible to test whether some parameters are invariant or not over the several groups. This approach is analogous to the simultaneous factor analysis in several groups of Jöreskog (1971) and, for categorical variables, to the simultaneous analysis of several subpopulations (see Clogg & Goodman, 1984, 1985, 1986; Hagenaars, 1990). The groups might correspond to gender or different time periods. However, in latent class models and also in the latent Markov models of van de Pol and Langeheine, the samples do not change over time. In the model we propose here, the input may be dependent on time, that is, after some period, some subsamples may have different treatments (input). This approach can be important in experimental designs, in which, after some period, different groups of persons get different treatments.

Our model is a generalization of latent class models for just one time point. For instance, Dayton and Macready (1988a,1988b) and Clogg (1993) formulated latent class models with concomitant variables. These concomitant variables, or covariates, may be categorical (grouping variables) or continuous. Other papers related to these latent class models with covariates include De-Sarbo and Wedel (1994), Formann (1992), and Van Der Heijden, Dessens, and Bockenholt (1996). Although, in this chapter we discuss categorical variables only, their models are a special case of the model we propose here, because we have more than one time point.

Vermunt, Langeheine and Bockenholt (1999) and Vermunt and Magidson (2005) already presented a logit regression approach that allows to regress the latent states occupied at the various points in time on time-varying covariates. In fact, dealing with categorical variables, their model is a parameterized version of our model. Our approach is more straightforward and the estimation results are easier to interpret.

The model of this chapter is closely related to growth models (see Agresti, 2002; Hedeker, 2004). Nevertheless, we concentrate on changes between consecutive time points whereas growth models study developments of individuals over time. The research goal and the dependency between the repeated measures are different for our approach and that of the growth model approach.

In section two of this chapter we formulate our model in detail. An EM estimator of the model parameters is derived in the next section. Finally, we discuss an empirical example.

1.2 FORMULATION OF THE MODEL

Define y_t as an output variable at time point t, x_t as an input variable at time point t, and z_t as a latent state variable at time point t. All variables are random variables. We start with one input and one output variable. In Figure 1-1, an example of the model for 4 time points, from t-2 to t+1, is given. We see in this figure that the time is channeled only through the state variables z. Furthermore, there are no direct effects from the input variables, x, on the output variables y. It is possible to introduce a state variable, called z_0, that influences z_1.

So z_1 is influenced by the first input variable x_1, and a previous state variable that is completely unknown because it has no input and output variable. Although this state variable z_0 may be important, we assume, just as Langeheine and van de Pol did, that it is equal to zero. The letters F, G, and H are matrices that will contain model parameters. For instance, matrix F will contain the transition parameters of the state variables from time point $t-1$ to t. Note that the matrices F, G, and H are assumed to be invariant over time. This assumption is not crucial for our discussion of the model and can be easily relaxed.

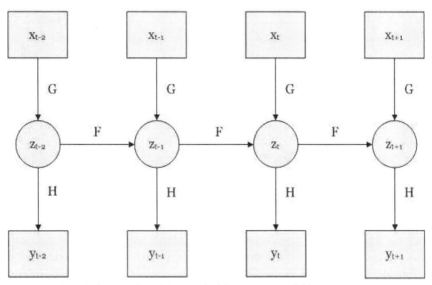

Figure 1-1. Graphical description of the model with one output variable.

In Figure 1-1 there is only one input and output variable at each time categorical and because the input variables are exogenous variables, it is sufficient to create one new input variable as the Cartesian product of all input variables. For the output variables, such a trick is not possible, because the output variables are non-fixed endogenous variables. In Figure 1-2, we see a method for dealing with two output variables at each time point. At each time point, we have two state variables (in general, as much as there are output variables, indicators, at each time point). These state variables are equal to each other for each time point. This can be formulated by restricting the transition matrix between the state variables at each time to the identity matrix. Furthermore, each output variable is an indicator of one state variable. So in general, the case of multiple indicators is a restricted case of the case with just one output variable for each time point and so it is not necessary to discuss the case with multiple indicators in detail. Note that by this formulation, the number of output variables may be different from the actual number of state variables.

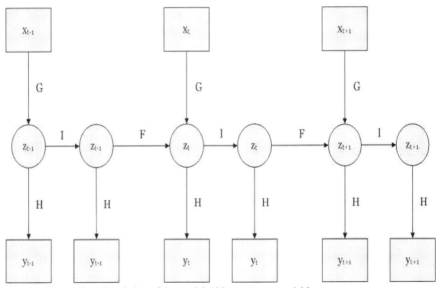

Figure 1-2. Graphical description of the model with two output variables.

We first derive for three time points the joint probability of the state variables and the output variables conditional upon the input variables. This joint probability is a crucial part of the complete likelihood function that is needed for the EM algorithm presented in this chapter.

Let **J** be the set consisting of all variables, that is the input, output, and state variables. Then the joint probability of these variables can be written as

$$P[J] \equiv P[y_1,y_2,y_3,z_1,z_2,z_3,x_1,x_2,x_3]$$

$$= P[y_3|y_1,y_2,z_1,z_2,z_3,x_1,x_2,x_3]P[y_1,y_2,z_1,z_2,z_3,x_1,x_2,x_3]. \tag{1}$$

The output variable depends on the latent variable only, so the first term in Equation 1 can be written as $P[y_3|z_3]$. Now the first equation can be rewritten as

$$P[J] = P[y_3|z_3]P[z_3|y_1,y_2,z_1,z_2,x_1,x_2,x_3]P[y_1,y_2,z_1,z_2,x_1,x_2,x_3]. \tag{2}$$

The state variable at time point t depends only directly on the state variables at time point $t-1$ and the input variables at time point t. It depends indirectly, that is through the state variables at time point $t-1$, on all previous state and input variables. So the second term in Equation 2 can be written as $P[z_3|z_2,x_3]$. Now define $Q_t \equiv P[y_t|z_t]\,P[z_t|z_{t-1},x_t]$, then we have

$$P[J] = Q_3\,P[y_1,y_2,z_1,z_2,x_1,x_2,x_3].\qquad\qquad(3)$$

In the same way we can continue to elaborate the second term in the third equation. This gives

$$P[J] = Q_3\,P[y_2|y_1,z_1,z_2,x_1,x_2,x_3]\,P[y_1,z_1,z_2,x_1,x_2,x_3]$$

$$= Q_3\,P[y_2|z_2]\,P[y_1,z_1,z_2,x_1,x_2,x_3]$$

$$= Q_3\,P[y_2|z_2]\,P[z_2|y_1,z_1,x_1,x_2,x_3]\,P[y_1,z_1,x_1,x_2,x_3]$$

$$= Q_3\,P[y_2|z_2]\,P[z_2|z_1,x_2]\,P[y_1,z_1,x_1,x_2,x_3]$$

$$= Q_3\,Q_2\,P[y_1,z_1,x_1,x_2,x_3].$$

Repeating this process for y_1 and z_1 gives the result

$$P[J] = Q_3 Q_2 Q_1 P[x_1,x_2,x_3].\qquad\qquad(4)$$

From Equation 4 it follows for the joint distribution of the output and state variables, conditional the input variables

$$P[y_1,y_2,y_3,z_1,z_2,z_3|x_1,x_2,x_3] = Q_1 Q_2 Q_3 .$$

Obviously, the generalization to T time points becomes

$$P[\,y\,,z\,|\,x\,] = \prod_{t=1}^{T} P[\,y_t\,|\,z_t\,]\,P[\,z_t\,|\,z_{t-1}\,,x_t\,],\qquad\qquad(5)$$

where y, z, and x are vectors with elements y_t, z_t and x_t, for $t=1,...,T$.

Special Case I: No Input Variables

Because our model, in which there are input variables, is closely related to the model without input variables, we briefly discuss this latter model first and at the same time, some notations are introduced.

With no input variables, all x vectors can be eliminated in Equation 5. This gives

$$P[\,y,z] = \prod_{t=1}^{T} P[y_t \mid z_t] P[z_t \mid z_{t-1}],$$

(6)

This defines the likelihood function of the dynamic factor analysis model, but now for categorical variables only (see Molenaar, 1985). We start with the simple case for $T=3$, again. According to Equation 6 we can write

$$P[y_1=i,\ y_2=j,\ y_3=k,\ z_1=\alpha,\ z_2=\beta,\ z_3=\gamma] =$$

$$P[z_1=\alpha]\ P[y_1=i|z_1=\alpha]\ P[z_2=\beta|z_1=\alpha]$$

$$\cdot P[y_2=j|z_2=\beta]\ P[z_3=\gamma|z_2=\beta]\ P[y_3=k|z_3=\gamma].$$

Assume the state variables have r categories, and define F_t as the $(r \times r)$ transition matrix of the state variables of time $t-1$ to time point t. Furthermore, assuming stationarity, then it holds $F_t = F$. So, for instance, we can write

$$P[z_2 = \beta|z_1 = \alpha] = f_{\beta\alpha}.$$

Obviously, it holds

$$\sum_{\beta=1}^{r} f_{\beta\alpha} = 1$$

The conditional probabilities of the output variables given a latent state at time point t, are collected in a $(k \times r)$ matrix H_t, where k is the number of categories of variable y. Again, we assume a stationary process, which means that it holds that $H_t = H$. So we can write, for instance,

$$P[y_1 = i|z_1 = \alpha] = h_{i\alpha}.$$

Furthermore

$$\sum_{i=1}^{k} h_{i\alpha} = 1.$$

It follows that

$$P[y_1=i,\ y_2=j,\ y_3=k,\ z_1=\alpha,\ z_2=\beta,\ z_3=\gamma] = \mu_\alpha h_{i\alpha} f_{\beta\alpha}\, h_{j\beta}\, f_{\gamma\beta}\, h_{k\gamma},$$

where μ_α is the proportion of subjects in category α of the first state variable. Obviously, it holds

$$\sum_{\alpha=1}^{r} \mu_\alpha = 1.$$

Define now the sample size n and the probability $\theta_{\alpha\beta\gamma ijk}$ of a respondent being in cell $(\alpha,\ \beta,\ \gamma,\ i,\ j,\ k)$. Then under the multinomial distribution, $n\theta_{\alpha\beta\gamma ijk}$ are the expected frequencies. So, the logarithm of the complete likelihood function, that is for all output and state variables, can be written as

$$\ln L(\mathbf{y},\mathbf{z};\mathbf{U}) = \sum_{\alpha\beta\gamma ijk} n_s\, \theta_{\alpha\beta\gamma ijk}\, \ln\left(\mu_\alpha\, h_{i\alpha}\, f_{\beta\alpha}\, h_{j\beta}\, f_{\gamma\beta}\, h_{k\gamma}\right),$$

where $\mathbf{U}$ is a vector consisting of all unknown parameters, that is r parameters μ_α, kr parameters $h_{i\alpha}$, and r^2 parameters $f_{\beta\alpha}$. Note that the θ's play the role of the observations, although they are unknown because the z variables are not observed. This principle of unobserved observations plays a crucial role in the EM algorithm discussed later.

For several subpopulations, the logarithm of the complete likelihood function can be written as

$$\ln L(\mathbf{y},\mathbf{z};\mathbf{U}) = \sum_s \ln L(\mathbf{y}_s, \mathbf{z}_s; \mathbf{U}_s) =$$

$$= \sum_s \sum_{\alpha\beta\gamma ijk} n_s\, \theta_{\alpha\beta\gamma ijk;s}\, \ln\left(\mu_{\alpha;s}\, h_{i\alpha;s}\, f_{\beta\alpha;s}\, h_{j\beta;s}\, f_{\gamma\beta;s}\, h_{k\gamma;s}\right). \qquad (7)$$

where $s = 1,...,S$ is the index for subpopulation s. Note that all parameters are now defined for each subpopulation.

Special Case II: Input Variables

We start with the simple case for $T = 3$, again. According to Equation 6 we can write

$$P[y_1=i, y_2=j, y_3=k, z_1=\alpha, z_2=\beta, z_3=\gamma | x_1=a, x_2=b, x_3=c]$$

$$= P[z_1=\alpha|x_1=a]\, P[y_1=i|z_1=\alpha]\, P[z_2=\beta|z_1=\alpha, x_2=b]$$

$$\cdot P[y_2=j|z_2=\beta]\, P[z_3=\gamma|z_2=\beta, x_3=c]\, P[y_3=k|z_3=\gamma].$$

Obviously, it follows

$$P[y_1=i, y_2=j, y_3=k, z_1=\alpha, z_2=\beta, z_3=\gamma] =$$

$$\sum_{abc} p_{abc}\, P[y_1=i, y_2=j, y_3=k, z_1=\alpha, z_2=\beta, z_3=\gamma|$$

$$x_1=a, x_2=b, x_3=c].$$

$$(8)$$

where p_{abc} is the proportion of sample elements with input scores a, b, c on time points 1, 2, and 3, respectively. Because 8 can be written as

$$P[y_1=i, y_2=j, y_3=k, z_1=\alpha, z_2=\beta, z_3=\gamma] =$$

$$\sum_{abc} p_{abc}\, \mu_{\alpha;a}\, h_{i\alpha}\, f_{\beta\alpha;b}\, h_{j\beta}\, f_{\gamma\beta;c}\, h_{k\gamma}.$$

So the logarithm of the complete likelihood function can be written as

$$\ln L(\mathbf{x}, \mathbf{y}, \mathbf{z}; \mathbf{U}) = \sum_{abc} p_{abc} \sum_{\alpha\beta\gamma} \sum_{ijk} n\,\theta_{\alpha\beta\gamma ijk;abc} \ln(\mu_{\alpha;a}\, h_{i\alpha}\, f_{\beta\alpha;b}\, h_{j\beta}\, f_{\gamma\beta;c}\, h_{k\gamma}).$$

$$(9)$$

where $\theta_{\alpha\beta\gamma ijk;abc}$ is the probability of a respondent with input scores $a, b,$ and c on time 1, 2, and 3, respectively, being in cell $(\alpha, \beta, \gamma, i, j, k)$.

Let us compare this likelihood function with the likelihood function in the case of no input variables and several subpopulations (see Equation 7). Suppose all the input scores are equal for all time points, and suppose this score is s, then it holds $a = b = c = s$, and $p_{abc}n = p_s n = n_s$. Furthermore, in the case of no input variables, suppose that the factor loadings in matrix H are invariant in the subpopulations, i.e. $h_{ia;s} = h_{ia}$, then the likelihood functions in Case I and II are equal. This shows that the case with no input variables and with subpopulations is a special case of the general case with input variables if the factor loadings are invariant over the subpopulations.

1.3 EM ALGORITHM IN THE LATENT MARKOV MODEL WITH TIME-DEPENDENT COVARIATES

In this section, we discuss how to estimate the model parameters in the general model. We assume that for all models stationarity holds, that is we assume $F_t = F$, $G_t = G$, and $H_t = H$. In the EM algorithm two steps are defined: the E (Expectation) - step and the M (Maximization) - step.

E-step.
In the E-step, the expectation of the sufficient statistics of the complete multinomial distribution, conditional the observed frequencies and the model parameters is formulated. Define

$$\varsigma_{\alpha\beta\gamma ijk;abc} \equiv \mu_{\alpha;a}\, h_{ia} f_{\beta\alpha;b}\, h_{j\beta} f_{\gamma\beta;c}\, h_{k\gamma,}$$

then the conditional expectation of the sufficient statistics can be written as

$$\theta_{\alpha\beta\gamma ijk;abc} = (p_{ijk;abc}\, /\, \varsigma_{+++ijk;abc})\, \varsigma_{\alpha\beta\gamma ijk;abc},$$

where $p_{ijk;abc}$ are observed proportions denoting the proportions of subjects in category i, j, and k of the three output variables with, at the same time input scores a, b, and c on the three input variables. Furthermore, the $"+"$ symbols in $\varsigma_{+++ijk;abc}$ denotes the summation over the indices α, β, and γ. For analogous formulations in the latent Markov model, see Van de Pol and de Leeuw (1986).

M-step.
In the M-step, the logarithm of the complete likelihood function in Equation 9 is maximized as a function of the unknown parameters. For instance, for estimating $\mu_{\alpha,a}$ we define

$$L^* = \ln L(\,\mathbf{x}, \mathbf{y}, \mathbf{z}; \mathbf{U}\,) - m\,(\sum_{\alpha} \mu_{\alpha;a} - 1),$$

where m is a Lagrange multiplier and the side condition is

$$\sum_\alpha \mu_{\alpha;a} = 1.$$

The derivative of L^* with respect to $\mu_{\alpha;a}$ is

$$\frac{dL^*}{d\mu_{\alpha;a}} = \sum_{bc} P_{abc} \sum_{\beta\gamma}\sum_{ijk} \frac{n\,\theta_{\alpha\beta\gamma ijk;abc}}{\mu_{\alpha;a}} - m. \qquad (10)$$

Equating this derivative equal to zero and summing over α, gives

$$\sum_{bc} P_{abc} \sum_{\alpha\beta\gamma ijk} n\,\theta_{\alpha\beta\gamma ijk;abc} = m\sum_\alpha \mu_{\alpha;a} = m.$$

Now substituting m into Equation 10 gives

$$\mu_{\alpha;a} = \frac{\sum_{bc} P_{abc}\sum_{\beta\gamma ijk} n\,\theta_{\alpha\beta\gamma ijk;abc}}{\sum_{bc} P_{abc}\sum_{\alpha\beta\gamma ijk} n\,\theta_{\alpha\beta\gamma ijk;abc}}.$$

In shorter notation, this can be written as

$$\mu_{\alpha;a} = \frac{\sum_{bc} P_{abc}\,\theta_{\alpha+++++;abc}}{\sum_{bc} P_{abc}\,\theta_{++++++;abc}}.$$

In an analogous way we can estimate $h_{i\alpha}$ and $f_{\beta\alpha;b}$, assuming stationarity. This gives

$$h_{i\alpha} = \frac{\sum\limits_{abc} P_{abc} \left[\theta_{\alpha++i++;abc} + \theta_{+\alpha++i+;abc} + \theta_{++\alpha++i;abc} \right]}{\sum\limits_{abc} P_{abc} \left[\theta_{\alpha++++;abc} + \theta_{+\alpha++++;abc} + \theta_{++\alpha+++;abc} \right]},$$

$$f_{\beta\alpha;b} = \frac{\sum\limits_{ac} P_{abc}\, \theta_{\alpha\beta++++;abc} + \sum\limits_{ab} P_{abc}\, \theta_{+\alpha\beta+++;abc}}{\sum\limits_{ac} P_{abc}\, \theta_{\alpha+++++;abc} + \sum\limits_{ab} P_{abc}\, \theta_{+\alpha++++;abc}}.$$

So the EM algorithm runs as follows: First define some start values of the unknown parameters; then compute $\theta_{\alpha\beta\gamma ijk;abc}$ by the E-step; find new estimates for $\mu_{a;a}$, $h_{i\alpha}$, and $f_{\beta\alpha;b}$ as given in the M-step. Repeat the whole procedure as many times as necessary for reaching convergence.

1.4 AN EMPIRICAL EXAMPLE

This section applies the introduced method on panel data of consumer behaviour. These data are available from the research institute AGB (located in Dongen, The Netherlands) and contain about 300 panel-members (= households). During a year the purchasing behaviour with respect to several margarine brands is registered every four months for each panel member. For each panel member for each time period, among others, what is known is the district (two categories) and whether several margarine brands have been bought (two categories per brand: no purchase or purchase). We have restricted our analysis to the two brands with the largest market shares (together about 45%).

The author's research questions are:
1. To what extent do the two individual brands have the same buyers?
2. What is the size of the brand loyalty for each brand?
3. Is the factor District of importance in the first two questions?

In our analysis we consider a Latent Markov model with three time points of measurement ($T = 3$) and at each time point: two output variables (= indicators; the purchase of brand A and the purchase of brand B), one input variable (= District), and one state variable. All the variables are categorical with two categories. The transition matrix F of the state variables and the matrix H, with the conditional probabilities of the output variables given a latent state, have dimension (2×2).

To answer the first research question we use the relation between the output variables and the state variables, that is the matrix H. Question two can be answered by means of the dynamic part of the model (= the transition matrix F). For the last research question, the explanatory categorical input variable District can be used.

About five percent of the panel members moved to another district during the year. Therefore we have to deal with a model with time-dependent covariates (i.e., the variable District) instead of a multigroup analysis.

We create an observed frequency table of size $2^3 * 2^3 * 2^3$, which will be used to fit our Latent Markov model with time-dependent covariates. A PC-program using Pascal 7.0 is written to obtain EM-estimates. To be sure that the model is identified, we have to investigate whether the corresponding information matrix is of full rank (i.e., none of the eigen values of the information matrix is zero). It turned out that the identification of the considered model was guaranteed for our data.

In order to test the model against the data, one may look at the loglikelihood ratio statistic (twice the difference between the loglikelihood of the data and the model). This loglikelihood ratio statistic (G^2) is asymptotically chi-square distributed with degrees of freedom equal to the number of different response patterns of the observed input and output variables, minus the number of independent model parameters. However, the number of cells in the observed frequency table is 512 with most of the cells equal to zero, whereas the number of independent parameters is 10. Using such a large number of degrees of freedom means that every model will fit certainly. Furthermore, the sparseness of our frequency table makes this test very difficult (Haberman, 1977).

Nevertheless, it is also possible to compare the fit of two nested models by calculating two times the difference in the loglikelihood ratio statistics of the two nested models and using the difference in the number of independent parameters as the number of degrees of freedom. Therefore, in this empirical example, apart from the already mentioned Latent Markov model with input variable District (model M_4), we also fit some more restrictive models:
- a latent class or latent Markov model without latent change across time and without an input variable (M_1);
- a latent class or latent Markov model without latent change across time and with the input variable District (M_2);
- a Latent Markov model without input (M_3).

Table 1-1 gives for model M_2, M_3, and M_4 the G^2-difference with a more restrictive model (respectively model M_1, M_1, and M_2).

Of course, the most restrictive model M_1 has the largest value for G^2. When we introduce the input variable District (model M_2), the fit will increase significantly. Furthermore, models M_3 and M_4 are the dynamic versions of models M_1 and M_2. The former models fit significantly better than do the latter. So, the dynamic aspect of our model may not be dropped.

The EM-algorithm we use can be programmed easily, iterations are computationally attractive, and convergence is ensured. Otherwise, it may converge to a local maximum of the likelihood function. We should use different starting values for the unknown parameters to increase confidence that the maximum found is indeed the global maximum. In our empirical analysis, we indeed used several different starting values, which all converged to the same end values.

Another general handicap of the EM-algorithm is that it often requires much iterations. In our empirical example, we were not confronted with this problem. Apart from the different starting values for the parameters we needed at most about a hundred iterations.

Table 1-2 presents the estimates of the unknown parameters H, F, and μ of our model M_4. The factor loadings (matrix H for brand A and B) indicate that latent class 0 corresponds with no purchase of brand B, whereas brand A will be bought with probability 0.72. For latent class 1, there will be no purchase of brand A and a possible purchase of brand B (probability 0.53). We see that latent class 0 is the purchase of brand A and latent class 1 is the purchase of brand B. Additionally, the two brands have totally different buyers.

The transition matrix F indicates the change (or stability) between successive time points. For district 2, the transition matrix between two sequential time points is equal to the unity matrix. This indicates that the degree of brand loyalty for each of the two brands is high. In district 1, there is more change and the two brands have a smaller degree of loyalty. The values of the transition coefficients (in matrix F) show that between two successive time periods, the state can go from 0 to 1 with probability 0.09. A state-change in the opposite direction has a probability of 0.03. Therefore, the number of buyers of product A will decrease, whereas the number of buyers of product B will increase slightly with time.

Furthermore, the matrix μ indicates that district 1 contains more buyers of product B and less buyers of product A than district 2.

Once the EM estimates of the model parameters have been computed, their variances may be found from the information matrix. This is the inverse of the matrix of second order derivatives of the loglikelihood function toward all independent parameters. Fortunately, the second order derivatives of the multivariate loglikelihood function (see Equation 9) result in rather simple expressions. In our example, the variances of the parameter estimates are very small. All the empirical variances are smaller than 0.01.

From our investigations, it follows that the Latent Markov model with time-dependent covariates for categorical data can answer the research questions of our empirical example. Furthermore, the EM-algorithm is computationally easy and works rather quickly.

In our model, we assume that the transition matrix and the factor loading matrices do not depend on time. Maybe we can get a significantly better model fit by relaxing this assumption (see Fahrmeir & Kaufmann, 1987, who deal with regression models for non-stationary categorical time series). However, if we allow for both F and H to change, it may be very difficult to interpret results.

Note. The AGB data used in this example are available upon request.

TABLE 1-1
The Fit of the Models

Model	G^2	Compared To	G^2-Difference	df
M_1, no dyn., no input	126.8	-	-	-
M_2, no dyn., D as input	123.1	M_1	3.7	1
M_3, dyn., no input	119.8	M_1	7.0	2
M_4, dyn., D as input	113.0	M_2	10.1	4

TABLE 1-2

The Parameter Estimates H, F, and μ

Separate factor-loading matrices H (parameters h_{ia}) for brand A and B:

	no purchase brand A	purchase brand A
state category 0	0.28	0.72
state category 1	0.97	0.03

	no purchase brand B	purchase brand B
state category 0	1.00	0
state category 1	0.47	0.53

Separate transition matrices F (parameters $f_{\beta a}$) for district 1 and district 2:

	district 1	
	state category 0	state category 1
state category 0	0.91	0.09
state category 1	0.03	0.97

	district 2	
	state category 0	state category 1
state category 0	1.00	0
state category 1	0	1.00

Conditional probability $\mu_{\alpha,a}$ in time point $t = 1$
for state category α given district a:

	state category 0	state category 1
district 1	0.39	0.61
district 2	0.57	0.43

REFERENCES

Agresti, A. (2002). *Categorical data analysis*. New York: Wiley.

Clogg, C. C. (1993). Latent class models: Recent developments and prospects for the future. In G. Arminger, C. C. Clogg, M. E. Sobel (Eds.), *Handbook of statistical modeling in the social sciences* (pp. 311–359).New York: Plenum.

Clogg, C. C., & Goodman, L. A. (1984). Latent structure analysis of a set of multidimensional contingency tables. *Journal of the American Statistical Association*, *79*, 762–771.

Clogg, C. C., & Goodman, L. A. (1985). Simultaneous latent structure analysis in several groups. In N.B. Tuma (Ed.), *Sociological methodology*, (pp. 81–110), San Francisco: Jossey-Bass.

Clogg, C. C., & Goodman, L. A. (1986). On scaling models applied to data from several groups. *Psychometrika*, *51*, 123–135.

Collins, L. M., & Wugalter, S.E. (1992). Latent class models for stage-sequential dynamic latent variables. *Multivariate Behaviorial Research*, *27*, 131–157.

Dayton, C. M., & Macready, G.B. (1988a). Concomittant-variable latent class models. *Journal of the American Statistical Association*, *83*, 173–178.

Dayton, C. M., & Macready, G.B. (1988b). A latent class covariate model with applications to criterion referenced testing. In R. Langeheine and J. Rost (Eds.). *Latent trait and latent class models*, (122–167). New York: Plenum.

DeSarbo, W. S., & Wedel, M. (1994). A review of recent developments in latent class regression models. In R. Bagozzi (Ed.), *Handbook of marketing research* (435–466). Blackwell, UK: Oxford.

Fahrmeir, L., & Kaufmann, H. (1987). Regression models for non-stationary categorical time series. *Journal of Time Series Analysis*, *8*, 2, 147–160.

Formann, A. K. (1992). Linear logistic latent class analysis for polytomous data. *Journal of the American Statistical Association*, *87*, 476–486.

Goodman, L. A. (1974a). The analysis of systems of qualitative variableswhen some of the variables are unobservable. *American Journal of Sociology*, *79*, 1179–1259.

Goodman, L. A. (1974b). Exploratory latent structure analysis using both identifiable and unidentifiable models. *Biometrika*, *61*, 215–231.

Haberman, S. J. (1977). Log-linear models and frequency tables with small expected cell counts. *Annals of Statistics*, 5, 1148–1169.

Haberman, S. J. (1979). *Analysis of qualitative data. Vol 2. New developments*. New York: Academic Press.

Hagenaars, J. A. (1990). *Categorical longitudinal data: Log-linear, panel, trend and cohort analysis*. London: Sage.

Hedeker, D. (2004). Introduction to growth modeling. In D. Kaplan (Ed.), *The Sage handbook of quantitative methodology for the social sciences* (pp. 215–234). Thousand Oakes: Sage Publications.

Jöreskog, K. G. (1971). Simultaneous factor analysis in several groups. *Psychometrika, 36*, 409–426.

Langeheine, R. (1988). Manifest and latent Markov chain models for categorical panel data. *Journal of Educational Statistics, 13*, 299–312.

Langeheine, R., & Van De Pol, F. (1990). A unifying framework for Markov modeling in discrete space and discrete time. *Sociological Methods & Research, 18*, 416–441.

Lazarsfeld, P. F. (1950). The logical and mathematical foundation of latent structure analysis. In E.A. Suchman, P.F. Lazarsfeld, S.A. Starr, and J.A. Clausen (Eds.), *Studies in social psychology in world war II, Vol 4, Measurement and prediction* (pp. 362–412). Princeton, N.J.: Princeton University Press.

Lazarsfeld, P. F., & Henry, N. W. (1968). *Latent structure analysis.* Boston: Houghton-Mifflin.

Molenaar, P. C. M. (1985). A dynamic factor model for the analysis of multivariate time series. *Psychometrika, 50*, 181–202.

Poulsen, C.S. (1982). *Latent structure analysis with choice modeling applications*, Unpublished doctoral dissertation, University of Pennsylvania.

Van De Pol, F., & De Leeuw, J. (1986). A latent Markov model to correct for measurement error. *Sociological Methods and Research, 15*, 118–141.

Van De Pol, F., & Langeheine, R. (1989). Mixed Markov models, mover-stayer models, and the EM algorithm, with an application to labour market data from the Netherlands Sociometric panel. In R. Coppi , S. Bolasco (Eds), *Multiway data analysis* (pp. 58–73). Amsterdam: North-Holland.

Van Der Heijden, P. G. M., Dessens, J., & Bockenholt, U. (1996). Estimating the concomitant variable latent class model with EM algorithm. *Journal of Educational and Behavioral Statistics. 21*, 215–229.

Vermunt, J. K. (1996). Log-linear event history analysis, Unpublished doctoral dissertation, Tilburg University, The Netherlands.

Vermunt, J. K., Langeheine, R., & Bockenholt, U. (1999). Latent Markov models with time-constant and time-varying covariates. *Journal of Educational and Behavioral Statistics, 24*, 178–205.

Vermunt, J. K., & Magidson, J. (2005). *Technical guide to GOLD 4.0: basic and advanced.* Belmont, MA: Statistical Innovations Inc.

Chapter 2

Comparison of Four Procedures to Estimate the Damped Linear Differential Oscillator for Panel Data

Johan Oud

Radboud University Nijmegen, The Netherlands

2.1 INTRODUCTION

In several publications, Boker and colleagues (Boker, 2002; Boker & Graham, 1998; Boker & Nesselroade, 2002; Boker, Neale, & Rausch, 2004) have drawn attention to oscillating movements and the importance of oscillating movements in psychology. Different ways to describe and estimate such oscillating movements were proposed by them. Most recently, Boker et al. (2004) introduced the multivariate latent differential equation (MLDE) approach, which is a model as well as an estimation procedure. The model formulates a differential equation model on the latent variable level. The estimation procedure uses structural equation modeling (SEM), in particular the program Mx (Neale, Boker, Xie, & Maes, 1999), to simultaneously estimate the parameters of the differential equation model and the measurement model. In the estimation procedure, the differential equation model is approximated.

From 1990 onward, Singer and colleagues (Singer, 1990, 1993, 1995, 1998; Hamerle, Nagl, & Singer, 1991; Hamerle, Singer, & Nagl, 1993) worked on the estimation of continuous-time state space models by means of panel data. The MLDE and other oscillating and nonoscillating behavior models are special cases of the continuous-time state space model. The program LSDE (Linear Stochastic Differential Equations), written by Singer (1991), performs the maximum likelihood estimation of the model for panel data on the basis of the so-called exact discrete model (EDM). The EDM makes sure that the

19

parameters estimated are exactly equal to the parameters of the underlying differential equation model.

Hamerle, Nagl, and Singer (1991) heavily criticized the use of structural equation modeling (SEM) in estimating the differential equation model, because the nonlinear restrictions implied by the EDM could not be imposed during estimation. However, Oud and Jansen (2000) showed how more recent nonlinear SEM software packages such as Mx (Neale et al., 1999) can also be employed for maximum likelihood estimation of the continuous-time state space model parameters by means of the EDM, applying the nonlinear constraints of the EDM directly during estimation. This constitutes a third procedure to estimate the differential equation model for oscillating movements.

Finally, Oud (2006) developed an additional approximate procedure, which like MLDE uses SEM but is based on the approximate discrete model (ADM) instead of the EDM. Like the EDM, the ADM originated with Bergstrom (1966, 1984). A big advantage of the ADM-SEM procedure is that less nonlinearly oriented SEM programs like LISREL, that lack the exponential function, can also be used. In fact, the ADM utilizes only simple linear restrictions to approximate the differential equation model.

With so many and so different procedures available, it seems appropriate to compare them and find out their similarities and differences, especially possible differences in quality. This will be done in a Monte Carlo simulation study. The contribution starts with a precise description of the oscillator in deterministic and stochastic form. Then the four estimation procedures are presented. Whereas the MLDE directly models the oscillator and does not accommodate for random subject effects, the other procedures indeed model the oscillator as a special case of the general state space model and admit random subject effects as special state variables. In all four procedures, the model provides a measurement part, allowing the oscillating variables to be latent. Also in the measurement-model part of all four procedures, measurement invariance over time may be implemented and tested. Finally, the simulation study and its results are discussed and conclusions for the application of the procedures in practice drawn.

2.2 THE DAMPED LINEAR DIFFERENTIAL OSCILLATOR IN DETERMINISTIC AND STOCHASTIC FORM

For more than three centuries in most fields of science, the standard approach of dynamic phenomena is continuous time modeling by means of differential equations. An example is the differential equation

$$\frac{d^2y(t)}{dt^2} = \alpha\frac{dy(t)}{dt} + \beta y(t) \, , \tag{1}$$

that can be used to describe oscillating movements with the pendulum motion as a well-known example. In the model, acceleration $d^2y(t)/dt^2$ is made dependent on velocity $dy(t)/dt$ as well as on location $y(t)$. For reasons explained later, α is called the damping parameter and β the frequency parameter. Important dynamic properties of the model can be found by writing Equation 1 as a state model with state variables $x_1(t) = y(t)$, $x_2(t) = dy(t)/dt$ in state vector $\mathbf{x}(t) = [x_1(t) \ x_2(t)]'$:

$$\frac{d\mathbf{x}(t)}{dt} = \mathbf{A}\mathbf{x}(t) \qquad \text{with} \qquad \mathbf{A} = \begin{bmatrix} 0 & 1 \\ \beta & \alpha \end{bmatrix}, \qquad (2)$$

and looking to the eigenvalues $\lambda_{1,2}$ of the so-called drift matrix $\mathbf{A}$:

$$\lambda_{1,2} = a \pm bj = \alpha/2 \pm j\sqrt{-\alpha^2/4 - \beta}. \qquad (3)$$

The eigenvalues first distinguish oscillatory from nonoscillatory movements. For $-\alpha^2/4 > \beta$ the eigenvalues $\lambda_{1,2} = a \pm bj$ (j the imaginary number $\sqrt{-1}$) become complex, which implies oscillation. As in physics, economics, and other fields (Singer, 1991, 1992a, 1999), examples of continuous time oscillating behavior patterns abound in psychology as well. Mood (Gottschalk, Bauer, & Whybrow, 1995), feelings of depression (Bisconti, 2001; Sarrias, Artigas, Martinez, & Gelpi, 1989), and anxiety (Cummings & Davies, 2002), for example, are oscillating phenomena to be modeled accordingly (Boker, 2002; Boker & Graham, 1998; Boker & Nesselroade, 2002; Boker, Neale, & Rausch, 2004). Some groups of people show higher oscillation frequency than other ones, whereas the amplitude (strength) as well as the phase of the oscillations, determined by initial conditions, may differ in different people.

The eigenvalues also define stability or damping as it is usually called in the case of oscillatory movements. The condition of all eigenvalues of $\mathbf{A}$ having nonpositive real part ($a \leq 0$ and thus $\alpha \leq 0$ in Equations 2–3) implies a stable movement. For $a < 0$ and thus $\alpha < 0$, the movement described is asymptotically stable, meaning that it goes oscillating or nonoscillating toward an equilibrium position. The asymptotic stability requirement (all eigenvalues of $\mathbf{A}$ having negative real part) is the direct continuous time analog of the well-known discrete time requirement (all eigenvalues located within the unit circle). In both cases, it means that the trajectory converges to the equilibrium trajectory. Stability analysis is of prime importance in judging the plausibility of a model. Instability or diverging behavior means that the system would more or less quickly explode according to the model. In most cases this is not realistic, so that a new and better model has to be found, or not desirable, so that control measures should be taken to prevent the system from diverging.

An important property of oscillating movements is the time period, that is, the time elapsed before the oscillation starts repeating its motion. This also depends on the eigenvalues. Based on the angular frequency b (imaginary part of the eigenvalue), the time period is $Tp = 2\pi/b$ and the frequency $Fr = 1/Tp$. For zero damping ($\alpha = 0$), the negative of the frequency parameter $-\beta = (2\pi Fr)^2$ becomes proportional to the squared frequency and this explains the name of frequency parameter.

Typically, however, the description of oscillating and non-oscillating behavior patterns by Equation 2 turns out to be less than perfect in fields like economics and psychology as well as in special fields of physics. Continuous time noise is needed and found in the famous Wiener process $W(t)$, limiting form of the discrete time random walk process (Arnold, 1974, p. 46; Jazwinski, 1970, pp. 70–74; Wiener, 1923). Added in the following way to Equation 2, it results in stochastic differential equation

$$\frac{d\mathbf{x}(t)}{dt} = \mathbf{A}\mathbf{x}(t) + \mathbf{G}\frac{d\mathbf{W}(t)}{dt}. \tag{4}$$

The transformation matrix $\mathbf{G}$ transforms the standard Wiener (vector) process $\mathbf{W}(t)$ with covariance matrix $\mathrm{cov}[\mathbf{W}(t)] = t\,\mathbf{I}$ to more general Wiener process $\mathbf{G}\mathbf{W}(t)$ with covariance matrix $t\mathbf{Q}$ for $\mathbf{Q} = \mathbf{G}\mathbf{G}'$. Thanks to the work of the Japanese mathematician Itô (1944, 1951), stochastic differential equations can be solved in a quite general fashion and the effect of continuous time noise computed over arbitrary discrete time intervals. Whereas Itô's solution is valid for stochastic time-varying matrices $\mathbf{G}(t)$, Ruymgaard and Soong (1985, pp. 70–75) consider the simpler case of fixed time-varying matrices $\mathbf{G}(t)$, defining general Wiener process $\int_0^t \mathbf{G}(s)d\mathbf{W}(s)$ with covariance matrix $\int_0^t \mathbf{Q}(s)ds$ for $\mathbf{Q}(t) = \mathbf{G}(t)\mathbf{G}'(t)$. In the state space form

$$\frac{d\mathbf{x}(t)}{dt} = \begin{bmatrix} 0 & 1 \\ \beta & \alpha \end{bmatrix}\mathbf{x}(t) + \begin{bmatrix} 0 & 0 \\ 0 & \gamma \end{bmatrix}\frac{d\mathbf{W}(t)}{dt} \tag{5}$$

of the simple stochastic oscillator considered here,

$$\frac{d^2y(t)}{dt^2} = \alpha\frac{dy(t)}{dt} + \beta y(t) + \epsilon(t) \quad \text{with} \quad \epsilon(t) = \gamma\frac{dW(t)}{dt}, \tag{6}$$

the special case of a fixed time-invariant matrix $\mathbf{G} = \begin{bmatrix} 0 & 0 \\ 0 & \gamma \end{bmatrix}$ is used.

2.3 ESTIMATING THE OSCILLATOR BY MEANS OF A MULTIPLE SUBJECT SAMPLE

To estimate a stochastic differential equation model like Equations 4–5 in the case of a sample of multiple subjects (panel data), Arminger (1986) employed the so-called "indirect" method, which consists of first estimating discrete time parameters by means of an SEM program and then in a second step deriving the continuous time parameter values using the exact discrete model (EDM). The EDM, introduced in 1961–1962 by Bergstrom (1988), links in an exact way the discrete time model parameters to the underlying continuous time model parameters by means of nonlinear restrictions. Hamerle, Nagl, and Singer (1991) argued that the nonlinear constraints between the continuous time and discrete time parameters in the EDM should be directly imposed during estimation and therefore criticized the indirect method. The use of SEM programs like LISREL (Jöreskog & Sörbom, 1996) was criticized by them, because such programs do not provide the necessary matrix exponential nonlinear constraints and therefore cannot apply the direct method. A simple example where the indirect method breaks down is in the case of unequal observation intervals, because then the imposition of simple equality constraints in the SEM program does not work.

2.3.1 LSDE Procedure. As an alternative, Singer (1991) wrote the LSDE (linear stochastic differential equations) program. This program performs maximum likelihood estimation of the parameters of the following stochastic differential equation:

$$\frac{d\mathbf{x}(t)}{dt} = \mathbf{A}\mathbf{x}(t) + \boldsymbol{\kappa} + \mathbf{B}\mathbf{u}(t) + \mathbf{G}\frac{d\mathbf{W}(t)}{dt} , \tag{7}$$

which has Equations 4 and 5 as special cases. To avoid misunderstanding about the nature of $\frac{d\mathbf{W}(t)}{dt}$ (Hamerle et al., 1991, pp. 204–205), it is often written as

$$d\mathbf{x}(t) = [\mathbf{A}\mathbf{x}(t) + \boldsymbol{\kappa} + \mathbf{B}\mathbf{u}(t)]dt + \mathbf{G}d\mathbf{W}(t) . \tag{8}$$

It contains additional input effects $\mathbf{B}\mathbf{u}(t)$ and random subject effects $\boldsymbol{\kappa}$. For convenience, the random subject effects will be called trait variables in the sequel. Effects $\mathbf{B}\mathbf{u}(t)$ of fixed input variables in $\mathbf{u}(t)$ accommodate for nonzero and nonconstant mean trajectories $E[\mathbf{x}(t)]$. By the specification of trait variables $\boldsymbol{\kappa}$ subject-specific conditional mean trajectories are obtained, keeping a subject-specific distance from $E[\mathbf{x}(t)]$.

Estimating the continuous time parameters in Equation 7 on the basis of discrete time panel data requires the EDM to be derived first. The EDM relates the discrete time parameters and trait variables in the discrete time state Equation 9,

$$\mathbf{x}_t = \mathbf{A}_{\Delta t}\mathbf{x}_{t-\Delta t} + \boldsymbol{\kappa}_{\Delta t} + \mathbf{B}_{\Delta t}\mathbf{u}_{t-\Delta t} + \mathbf{w}_{t-\Delta t}$$
$$\text{with } \text{cov}(\mathbf{w}_{t-\Delta t}) = \mathbf{Q}_{\Delta t}, \qquad (9)$$

for successive observation time points $t, t - \Delta t, \dots$, to their continuous time counterparts in Equation 7 via exact expressions:

$$
\begin{aligned}
\mathbf{A}_{\Delta t} &= e^{\mathbf{A}\Delta t}, \\
\boldsymbol{\kappa}_{\Delta t} &= \mathbf{A}^{-1}(\mathbf{A}_{\Delta t} - \mathbf{I})\,\boldsymbol{\kappa}, \\
\mathbf{B}_{\Delta t} &= \mathbf{A}^{-1}(\mathbf{A}_{\Delta t} - \mathbf{I})\,\mathbf{B}, \\
\mathbf{Q}_{\Delta t} &= \text{irow}[(\mathbf{A} \otimes \mathbf{I} + \mathbf{I} \otimes \mathbf{A})^{-1}(\mathbf{A}_{\Delta t} \otimes \mathbf{A}_{\Delta t} - \mathbf{I} \otimes \mathbf{I})\,\text{row}(\mathbf{G}\mathbf{G}')], \\
\boldsymbol{\Phi}_{\kappa_{\Delta t}} &= \mathbf{A}^{-1}(\mathbf{A}_{\Delta t} - \mathbf{I})\boldsymbol{\Phi}_{\kappa}\,(\mathbf{A}'_{\Delta t} - \mathbf{I})\mathbf{A}'^{-1}, \\
\boldsymbol{\Phi}_{\kappa_{\Delta t}, x_{t_0}} &= \mathbf{A}^{-1}(\mathbf{A}_{\Delta t} - \mathbf{I})\boldsymbol{\Phi}_{\kappa, x_{t_0}}.
\end{aligned}
\qquad (10)
$$

Here, $\otimes$ is the Kronecker product, "row" is the rowvec operation, putting the elements of a matrix rowwise in a column vector, "irow" the inverse operation. The expression for $\mathbf{B}_{\Delta t}$ assumes the input variables to be piecewise constant between measurements. More complicated paths of the input variables are considered by Hamerle et al. (1991), Oud and Jansen (2000), and Singer (1992b, 1995). The matrices $\boldsymbol{\Phi}_{\kappa_{\Delta t}}, \boldsymbol{\Phi}_{\kappa}, \boldsymbol{\Phi}_{\kappa_{\Delta t}, x_{t_0}}, \boldsymbol{\Phi}_{\kappa, x_{t_0}}$ are the covariance matrices of the variables indicated in the subscripts, respectively. It should be noted that all expressions of the EDM involve the highly nonlinear matrix exponential

$$
\begin{aligned}
e^{\mathbf{A}\Delta t} &= \sum_{k=0}^{\infty}(\mathbf{A}\Delta t)^k/k! \\
&= \mathbf{I} + \mathbf{A}\Delta t + \frac{1}{2}\mathbf{A}^2\Delta t^2 + \frac{1}{6}\mathbf{A}^3\Delta t^3 + \dots .
\end{aligned}
\qquad (11)
$$

The matrix exponential solves the differential equation's homogeneous part $\frac{d\mathbf{x}(t)}{dt} = \mathbf{A}\mathbf{x}(t)$.

If the state variables in vector $\mathbf{x}(t)$, written $\mathbf{x}_t$ on the discrete observation time points, cannot be directly observed (latent variables), a measurement equation in terms of observed variables $\mathbf{z}_t$ is added to the EDM:

$$\mathbf{z}_t = \mathbf{C}_t\mathbf{x}_t + \mathbf{D}_t\mathbf{u}_t + \mathbf{v}_t \quad \text{with} \quad \text{cov}(\mathbf{v}_t) = \mathbf{R}_t. \qquad (12)$$

Because the oscillator with $x_1(t) = y(t)$ and $x_2(t) = dy(t)/dt$ has $x_2(t)$ defined in terms of $x_1(t)$, there are no observed variables for $x_2(t)$ and the second column of $\mathbf{C}_t$ equals $\mathbf{0}$.

Details about the LSDE procedure can be found in Singer (1991, 1993). The likelihood is directly maximized with respect to the continuous time parameters in Equation 7. The latent variables case is treated by means of EM and quasi-Newton algorithms with the E-step of the EM algorithm implemented by means of the Kalman smoother. The program LSDE (Singer, 1991) is written in SAS/IML with its source accessible and easily adaptable by the user.

2.3.2 EDM-Mx Procedure. Oud and Jansen (2000) showed how more recent nonlinear SEM software packages like Mx (Neale, Boker, Xie, & Maes, 1999) can also be employed for maximum likelihood estimation of the continuous-time state space model parameters, using the direct method, applying the non-linear constraints of the EDM directly during estimation. Oud and Jansen (2000) also generalized the EDM to cover not only time-invariant parameter matrices $\mathbf{A}, \mathbf{B}, \mathbf{G}$, but also matrices $\mathbf{A}(t), \mathbf{B}(t), \mathbf{G}(t)$ with parameters varying continuously over time according to a general polynomial scheme.

Although for a time-invariant model, both Singer's LSDE procedure and Oud and Jansen's EDM-Mx procedure aimed at the same exactly specified differential equation model and at one and the same maximum likelihood solution for the differential and measurement parameters in Equations 7 and 12, the procedures follow quite different roads to attain that common goal. As explained in Oud (2004), a major difference between the two procedures is that the LSDE procedure involves repeated calculation of the latent state vector for all subjects in the E-step of the EM algorithm by means of the Kalman smoother, whereas in the EDM-Mx procedure, the latent state vector is derived out of the loglikelihood function. It seems worthwhile to find out whether these different roads and the quality of the results produced by both programs are able to end up with the same solution.

Computation of the matrix exponential $e^{\mathbf{A}\Delta t}$ in both LSDE and Mx is done by diagonalization of $\mathbf{A} = \mathbf{F}\mathbf{\Lambda}\mathbf{F}^{-1}$ ($\mathbf{\Lambda}$ the diagonal eigenvalue matrix and $\mathbf{F}$ the eigenvector matrix) and computing scalar exponentials in $e^{\mathbf{A}\Delta t} = \mathbf{F}e^{\mathbf{\Lambda}\Delta t}\mathbf{F}^{-1}$. A problem in the use of Mx is that it does not allow manipulation of the imaginary parts of the eigenvalues and eigenvectors in further calculations. Fortunately, the exponentials of the imaginary parts can be expressed in terms of sine and cosine functions (Euler's formula: $e^{\pm\delta j} = \cos\delta \pm j\sin\delta$), which are offered by the Mx program. Using these functions, real $\mathbf{A}$ with complex eigenvalues can be directly transformed into real $e^{\mathbf{A}\Delta t}$ in terms of sine and cosine function values as follows. If

$$\mathbf{A} = \mathbf{F}\mathbf{\Lambda}\mathbf{F}^{-1}$$

$$= \begin{bmatrix} a+\alpha j & a-\alpha j \\ b+\beta j & b-\beta j \end{bmatrix} \begin{bmatrix} c+\delta j & 0 \\ 0 & c-\delta j \end{bmatrix} \begin{bmatrix} a+\alpha j & a-\alpha j \\ b+\beta j & b-\beta j \end{bmatrix}^{-1},$$

then

$$
e^{\mathbf{A}\Delta t} = e^{c\Delta t}
\begin{bmatrix}
\cos(\delta\Delta t) + \frac{ab+\alpha\beta}{\alpha b-a\beta}\sin(\delta\Delta t) & \frac{a^2+\alpha^2}{a\beta-\alpha b}\sin(\delta\Delta t) \\[2mm]
\frac{b^2+\beta^2}{\alpha b-a\beta}\sin(\delta\Delta t) & \cos(\delta\Delta t) + \frac{ab+\alpha\beta}{a\beta-\alpha b}\sin(\delta\Delta t)
\end{bmatrix}.
$$

2.3.3 ADM-SEM Procedure. The applicability of the EDM and the exact LSDE and EDM-Mx procedures is much more general than is perhaps inferred from the word "exact." The solution in the EDM may be numerical in case no analytic solution exists. In fact, Singer (1998) and Oud and Jansen (2000) give many examples of numerical solutions in the EDM. Crucial for the EDM is the exact solution or the possibility of coming arbitrarily close to the exact solution by sufficiently decreasing the time interval. The approximate models, used in the two remaining procedures, ADM-SEM (approximate discrete model via SEM) procedure and MLDE (multivariate latent differential equation) procedure, miss this property. In both, the degree of approximation is determined by the actual time interval between measurements, which cannot be made arbitrarily small.

Instead of on Equation 9 in the EDM, which is in reduced form, the ADM is based on structural form

$$
\mathbf{x}_t = \mathbf{A}_0\mathbf{x}_t + \mathbf{A}_\ell\mathbf{x}_{t-\Delta t} + \boldsymbol{\kappa}_\ell + \mathbf{B}_\ell\mathbf{u}_{t-\Delta t} + \mathbf{w}_{\ell,t-\Delta t}\,. \tag{13}
$$

The structural form is recognized by the appearance of the state vector $\mathbf{x}_t$ on both sides of the equation. It simultaneously contains two kinds of effect coefficients between the state variables, matrix $\mathbf{A}_0$ with instantaneous effects from "current endogenous" $\mathbf{x}_t$ and matrix $\mathbf{A}_\ell$ with lagged effects from "lagged endogenous" $\mathbf{x}_{t-\Delta t}$. Transforming the structural form to the reduced form in Equation 9, one finds

$$
\mathbf{x}_t = [(\mathbf{I}-\mathbf{A}_0)^{-1}\mathbf{A}_\ell]\,\mathbf{x}_{t-\Delta t} + \boldsymbol{\kappa} + [(\mathbf{I}-\mathbf{A}_0)^{-1}\mathbf{B}_\ell]\,\mathbf{u}_{t-\Delta t} + \mathbf{w}_{t-\Delta t} \tag{14}
$$

and for the EDM parameter matrices $\mathbf{A}_{\Delta t}$ and $\mathbf{B}_{\Delta t}$ in Equation 9

$$
\begin{aligned}
\mathbf{A}_{\Delta t} &= (\mathbf{I}-\mathbf{A}_0)^{-1}\mathbf{A}_\ell = e^{\mathbf{A}\Delta t}\,, \\
\mathbf{B}_{\Delta t} &= (\mathbf{I}-\mathbf{A}_0)^{-1}\mathbf{B}_\ell = \mathbf{A}^{-1}(e^{\mathbf{A}\Delta t}-\mathbf{I})\mathbf{B}\,.
\end{aligned} \tag{15}
$$

This shows that there are clear relationships between the coefficients in the reduced form matrices $\mathbf{A}_{\Delta t}, \mathbf{B}_{\Delta t}$ and the structural form matrices $\mathbf{A}_0, \mathbf{A}_\ell, \mathbf{B}_\ell$ on the one hand, and those in the underlying differential equation matrices $\mathbf{A}, \mathbf{B}$ on the other hand. However, in the EDM there is no need to put the constraints explicitly on the structural form (Equation 13), because they are put directly and exactly on the reduced form (Equation 9).

Nevertheless, Bergstrom (1966, 1984, pp. 1172–1173) provided a rationale for using the structural form. It allows for replacement of the EDM's nonlinear constraints (between reduced form equation and differential equation) by the ADM's linear constraints (between structural form equation and differential equation). Replacing the nonlinear constraints in the EDM by the simple linear constraints

$$
\begin{aligned}
\mathbf{A}_0 &= \tfrac{1}{2}\tilde{\mathbf{A}}\Delta t \,, \\
\mathbf{A}_\ell &= \mathbf{I} + \tfrac{1}{2}\tilde{\mathbf{A}}\Delta t \,, \\
\mathbf{B}_\ell &= \tilde{\mathbf{B}}\Delta t \,, \\
\mathbf{Q}_\ell &= \tilde{\mathbf{Q}}\Delta t \quad \text{for } \mathbf{Q}_\ell = \mathrm{cov}(\mathbf{w}_{\ell, t-\Delta t})
\end{aligned} \tag{16}
$$

on the structural form matrices leads to quite reasonable "trapezoid" (Gard, 1988, p. 192) approximations $\tilde{\mathbf{A}}$, $\tilde{\mathbf{B}}$, and $\tilde{\mathbf{G}}$ ($\tilde{\mathbf{G}}$ Cholesky factor of $\tilde{\mathbf{Q}}$) of the differential equation matrices $\mathbf{A}$, $\mathbf{B}$, and $\mathbf{G}$. In fact, the ADM is viewed by Bergstrom as a justification for nonrecursive structural equation modeling in econometrics (Bergstrom, 1966).

The trapezoid approximation compares favorably with the popular but relatively crude "rectangle" approximation. In the approximation of the homogeneous part $\frac{d\mathbf{x}(t)}{dt} = \mathbf{A}\mathbf{x}(t)$ of the differential equation, the rectangle approximation uses only the value $\mathbf{x}_{t-\Delta t}$ at the starting point of the interval: $\frac{\Delta \mathbf{x}_t}{\Delta t} = \tilde{\tilde{\mathbf{A}}}\mathbf{x}_{t-\Delta t}$ or $\mathbf{x}_t = (\mathbf{I} + \tilde{\tilde{\mathbf{A}}}\Delta t)\mathbf{x}_{t-\Delta t}$, whereas the trapezoid approximation averages the values at the starting and endpoint of the interval: $\frac{\Delta \mathbf{x}_t}{\Delta t} = \tilde{\mathbf{A}}(\mathbf{x}_t + \mathbf{x}_{t-\Delta t})/2$ or $\mathbf{x}_t = \mathbf{A}_0\mathbf{x}_t + \mathbf{A}_\ell\mathbf{x}_{t-\Delta t}$ (see $\mathbf{A}_0$ and $\mathbf{A}_\ell$ in Equation 16). This improvement is easily seen by putting both the exact nonlinear matrix exponential form of $\mathbf{A}_\Delta$ and the approximate linear constraint forms in power series expansion:

$$
\begin{aligned}
\mathbf{A}_\Delta &= e^{\mathbf{A}\Delta t} \\
&= \mathbf{I} + \mathbf{A}\Delta t + \tfrac{1}{2}\mathbf{A}^2\Delta t^2 + \tfrac{1}{6}\mathbf{A}^3\Delta t^3 + \tfrac{1}{24}\mathbf{A}^4\Delta t^4 + \dots \text{ (exact)} \\
\mathbf{A}_\Delta &= (\mathbf{I} - \tfrac{1}{2}\tilde{\mathbf{A}}\Delta t)^{-1}(\mathbf{I} + \tfrac{1}{2}\tilde{\mathbf{A}}\Delta t) \\
&= \mathbf{I} + \tilde{\mathbf{A}}\Delta t + \tfrac{1}{2}\tilde{\mathbf{A}}^2\Delta t^2 + \tfrac{1}{4}\tilde{\mathbf{A}}^3\Delta t^3 + \tfrac{1}{8}\tilde{\mathbf{A}}^4\Delta t^4 + \dots \text{ (trapezoid)} \\
\mathbf{A}_\Delta &= \mathbf{I} + \tilde{\tilde{\mathbf{A}}}\Delta t \text{ (rectangle)} \,.
\end{aligned} \tag{17}
$$

Whereas the rectangle approximation truncates the exact series, the weights in the trapezoid approximation are seen to go down only less quickly than in the exact series. This fundamental difference between trapezoid-based approximations and rectangle-based approximations clearly proves the superiority of the former, being particularly important in the case of large observation intervals.

For the implementation of the ADM constraints in SEM, two cases should be distinguished. In the first and simpler case, the observation intervals Δt

are equal and can be set at $\Delta t = 1$. Then according to Equation 16, one needs only to constrain the off-diagonal elements in $\mathbf{A}_0$ and $\mathbf{A}_\ell$ to be equal and each diagonal element in $\mathbf{A}_\ell$ to be 1 plus the corresponding diagonal element in $\mathbf{A}_0$. Then one computes $\tilde{\mathbf{A}}$ as $2\mathbf{A}_0$ and $\tilde{\mathbf{B}}$ and $\tilde{\mathbf{Q}}$ are immediately given. The second case applies when successive observation intervals Δt are unequal, $\Delta t \neq 1$, or both. Then the linear constraints in Equation 16 need a specification with a $\Delta t \neq 1$ for each interval and additionally defined parameters in $\tilde{\mathbf{A}}$, $\tilde{\mathbf{B}}$, and $\tilde{\mathbf{Q}}$ (Jöreskog & Sörbom, 1996, pp. 345–348, explain how to define new parameters in LISREL). Finally, in this case, the latent variables in $\boldsymbol{\kappa}_\ell$ in Equation 13 do not themselves represent the continuous-time trait variables $\boldsymbol{\kappa}$, but, by writing $\boldsymbol{\kappa}_\ell = (\mathbf{I}\Delta t)\boldsymbol{\kappa}$ and fixing the diagonal elements of successive trait effect-matrices $\mathbf{I}\Delta t$ at the appropriate Δt in the SEM model, the SEM program estimates the correct trait covariance matrix $\tilde{\boldsymbol{\Phi}}_\kappa$ and trait-state covariance matrix $\tilde{\boldsymbol{\Phi}}_{\kappa, x_{t_0}}$.

Although the exact nonlinear constraints of the EDM can be implemented in SEM programs such as Mx and in general should be preferred, in less nonlinearly oriented SEM programs like LISREL, that lack the exponential function, only the ADM can be used. Details about the ADM and the ADM-SEM procedure are given in Oud (2006). An appendix gives a LISREL script to implement the ADM. The chapter also evaluated the results of the ADM-SEM procedure in comparison with the EDM-Mx procedure but not yet for the oscillator.

2.3.4 MLDE Procedure. In contrast to the previous procedures that all estimate the oscillator as a special case of the state space model, the MLDE (multivariate latent differential equation) procedure (Boker et al., 2004) directly models the oscillator in Equation 6 by means of SEM. In addition, a particularly simple approximation is chosen. Whereas the previous procedures exactly or approximately specify the variables $y(t)$, $\frac{dy(t)}{dt}$, $\frac{d^2y(t)}{dt^2}$ at each of the time points as they develop over time, in the MLDE they are approximated only once, at time point t_m in the middle of the observed time range. So, in a sense, the longitudinal model is reduced to a cross-sectional model with three latent variables $y(t)$, $\frac{dy(t)}{dt}$, $\frac{d^2y(t)}{dt^2}$ located at a single time point t_m. It is clear that the MLDE approximation will be worse, the longer the observed time range, and this independently of the frequency of observation time points.

The approximation is specified in the measurement part $\mathbf{z} = \boldsymbol{\Lambda}\boldsymbol{\eta} + \boldsymbol{\varepsilon}$ of the SEM model. The latent vector $\boldsymbol{\eta}$ contains the three approximated latent variables $\widetilde{y(t)}$, $\widetilde{\frac{dy(t)}{dt}}$, $\widetilde{\frac{d^2y(t)}{dt^2}}$ and $\mathbf{z}$ the Tk observed variables: T the number of observation time points $(t_0, \ldots, t_{T-1})$, k the number of observed measures

$(i = 1, \ldots k)$ for $y(t)$. A particular row of $\mathbf{z} = \boldsymbol{\Lambda}\boldsymbol{\eta} + \boldsymbol{\varepsilon}$ reads

$$
z_i(t) = \begin{bmatrix} c_i & c_i\Delta t & c_i\frac{\Delta t^2}{2} \end{bmatrix} \begin{bmatrix} \widetilde{y(t)} \\ \widetilde{\frac{dy(t)}{dt}} \\ \widetilde{\frac{d^2y(t)}{dt^2}} \end{bmatrix} + v_i(t) \tag{18}
$$

with c_i as the loading of the particular measure z_i on $y(t)$,
$\Delta t = t - t_m = \ldots, -2\tau, -\tau, 0, \tau, 2\tau, \ldots,$
if the number of observation time points T is uneven (τ the interval between observation time points), and
$\Delta t = t - t_m = \ldots, -1.5\tau, -0.5\tau, 0.5\tau, 1.5\tau, \ldots,$
if the number of observation time points T is even. The authors (Boker et al., p. 160) explained the remaining loadings $c_i\Delta t$ and $c_i\frac{\Delta t^2}{2}$ by noting that "since $\int 1 d\tau = \tau$ and $\int \tau d\tau = \tau^2/2$, we can construct the first and second derivatives using these weights."

Although the approximations

$$
\begin{aligned}
F &= \widetilde{y(t)} = y(t_m)\,, \\
dF &= \widetilde{\frac{dy(t)}{dt}} = \frac{y(t) - y(t - 2\Delta t)}{2\Delta t}\,, \\
d2F &= \widetilde{\frac{d^2y(t)}{dt^2}} = \frac{[y(t) - y(t_m)] - [y(t_m) - y(t - 2\Delta t)]}{\Delta t^2}
\end{aligned}
$$

lead indeed to

$$
z_i(t) = c_i y(t) + v_i(t)\,, \tag{19}
$$

it is seen that the precision of the approximations decreases as the observed time range increases, thus yielding larger Δts in the procedure.

The SEM model is completed with the latent variable covariance matrix

$$
\Psi = \begin{bmatrix} \sigma_F^2 & \sigma_{F,dF} & 0 \\ \sigma_{dF,F} & \sigma_{dF}^2 & 0 \\ 0 & 0 & \sigma_{\epsilon_{d2F}}^2 \end{bmatrix}\,,
$$

latent variable effects matrix

$$
\boldsymbol{B} = \begin{bmatrix} 0 & 0 & 0 \\ 0 & 0 & 0 \\ \tilde{\beta} & \tilde{\alpha} & 0 \end{bmatrix}\,,
$$

and measurement error covariance matrix $\boldsymbol{\Theta}$, which together with $\boldsymbol{\Lambda}$ define the SEM model as a whole. It should be noted that for comparison with the previous procedures, one should compute $\tilde{\gamma} = \sqrt{\sigma_{\epsilon_{d2F}}^2}$. Because the approximations σ_F^2, σ_{dF}^2, and $\sigma_{dF,F}$ only refer to the time point t_m in the middle of the observed time range, the model lacks the initial variance and covariance parameters of the previous procedures. The model also does not contain trait variance and covariance parameters as is possible in the previous procedures.

2.4 SIMULATION STUDY

2.4.1 Design of the Simulation Study. To evaluate the effectiveness of the procedures in recovering parameter values of the oscillator, two Monte Carlo simulations were performed. Because it was expected that the addition of a trait variable (random subject effects) could considerably deteriorate the quality of the estimators, the simulated model in Simulation I was without trait variable. The trait variable was added to the simulation model in Simulation II. Apart from the trait variable, both models were identical. True parameter values for the model in Simulation I are given in Tables 2–1 and 2–2, for the model in Simulation II and Tables 2–3 to 2–4. In Simulation I the differential equation reads as follows:

$$\frac{d^2y(t)}{dt^2} = -0.04\frac{dy(t)}{dt} - 0.20y(t) + 2.0\frac{dW(t)}{dt} , \qquad (20)$$

and in Simulation II:

$$\frac{d^2y(t)}{dt^2} = -0.04\frac{dy(t)}{dt} - 0.20y(t) + \kappa + 2.0\frac{dW(t)}{dt} . \qquad (21)$$

In both simulations, the combination of $\alpha = -0.04$ and $\beta = -0.20$ implies an oscillating movement, because $-\alpha^2/4 = -0.0004$ is greater than $\beta = -0.20$, and a damped oscillation, because α is negative. Because $\sqrt{-\alpha^2/4 - \beta} = 0.4468$, a time period of $Tp = 2\pi/0.4468 = 14.1$ is implied.

In both simulations, 500 samples of size $N = 700$ were generated with measurements of the oscillating variable $y(t)$ at four observation time points t_i having observation interval 1: $t_0 = 0, t_1 = 1, t_2 = 2, t_3 = 3$. Often in behavioral science, latent variables are the subject of interest, measured in a nontrivial measurement model. Therefore, the oscillating latent variable $y(t)$ was made part of a measurement model in four observed variables that was identical at each of the measurement time points t_i:

$$\begin{bmatrix} z_{1,t_i} \\ z_{2,t_i} \\ z_{3,t_i} \\ z_{4,t_i} \end{bmatrix} = \begin{bmatrix} 1 \\ 0.5 \\ 0.7 \\ 0.9 \end{bmatrix} y(t_i) + \begin{bmatrix} 0 \\ 2 \\ 3 \\ 4 \end{bmatrix} + \begin{bmatrix} v_{1,t_i} \\ v_{2,t_i} \\ v_{3,t_i} \\ v_{4,t_i} \end{bmatrix}$$
$$\quad \mathbf{z}_{t_i} \qquad\qquad \mathbf{c} \qquad\quad \mathbf{d} \qquad\quad \mathbf{v}_{t_i}$$

$$(22)$$

$$\text{with } \mathbf{R} = \text{cov}(\mathbf{v}_{t_i}) = \begin{bmatrix} 7 & 0 & 0 & 0 \\ 0 & 8 & 0 & 0 \\ 0 & 0 & 9 & 0 \\ 0 & 0 & 0 & 10 \end{bmatrix}.$$

Loading 1 and measurement origin 0 for observed variable z_{1,t_i} are fixed in the usual way for identification reasons. Because the quality results for the parameters of the remaining measures were almost identical, Tables 2–1 to 2–4 provide only information about the measurement parameters of observed variable z_{2,t_i}.

Subtracting the loading 1 and the measurement origin 0, the measurement model contains 10 parameters to be estimated (3 loadings in **c**, 3 measurement origins in **d**, and 4 measurement error variances in **R**). Together with the differential equation model parameters α, β, γ and the initial variance and covariance parameters $\sigma^2_{x_{1,t_0}}, \sigma^2_{x_{2,t_0}}, \sigma_{x_{1,t_0},x_{2,t_0}}$ (see true values in Tables 2–1 and 2–2), for convenience expressed in terms of $x_1(t) = y(t)$ and $x_2(t) = dy(t)/dt$, the total number of parameters to be estimated in the model of Simulation I equals 16. As this has to be done by using 16 observed means and $(16 \times 17)/2 = 136$ nonidentical elements in the data covariance matrix, the model for Simulation I has $df = 136$. Additional parameters in the model of Simulation II are the trait variance and covariance parameters $\sigma^2_\kappa, \sigma^2_{\kappa,x_{1,t_0}}, \sigma_{\kappa,x_{2,t_0}}$ (see true values in Tables 2–3 and 2–4), the total number of parameters to be estimated in the model of Simulation II becoming 19 and $df = 133$.

Steps in both simulations were that first, the exact model implied moment matrix of the true model was calculated by the Mx program on the basis of the EDM. This was done by letting the Mx script for estimating the EDM fix the parameter values of the EDM at the simulated true values. Next, the samples were generated by the PRELIS program, using the procedure explained in Jöreskog & Sörbom (1996, pp. 189–194). Then all parameters (16 in Simulation I and 19 in Simulation II) were estimated for each of the 500 samples by each of the four procedures. Two programs were used. The LSDE program (Singer, 1991) was used in the LSDE procedure. In the three remaining procedures, the Mx program (Neale et al., 1999) was used with the ML option. The ADM-SEM and MLDE procedures could also have been implemented by other SEM program packages but nothing is lost by using the same program that makes the design of the simulation study and the comparison of results easier. Finally, the results were summarized in two measures; bias $\bar{\hat{\theta}} - \theta$, which is the mean estimate over the 500 samples minus the true parameter value θ, and the root mean squared error RMSE $= \sqrt{\overline{(\hat{\theta} - \theta)^2}}$. Because RMSE can

TABLE 2–1

The Oscillator without Trait Variable in Simulation I: Bias of the Four Estimation Procedures

Parameter	True value	LSDE	EDM-Mx	ADM-SEM	MLDE
Oscillator					
α	-0.04	-0.00003	-0.00003	-0.00334	0.02140
β	-0.20	0.00013	0.00013	-0.00785	0.00635
γ	2.00	-0.01433	-0.01433	0.16352	-0.80410
Initial var/cov					
$\sigma^2_{x_1,t_0}$	180	-0.60787	-0.60829	0.73794	
$\sigma^2_{x_2,t_0}$	120	-0.03323	-0.03335	4.34717	
σ_{x_1,t_0,x_2,t_0}	-40	0.29496	0.29459	-0.43566	
Measurement					
c_2	0.50	0.00014	0.00014	0.00014	0.00020
d_2	2.00	0.00212	0.00212	0.00214	0.00215
$\sigma^2_{v_2,t_i}$	8.00	-0.01076	-0.01076	-0.00737	0.01080
χ^2	df=136	3.09922	3.09921	3.56903	46.40518

TABLE 2–2

The Oscillator without Trait Variable in Simulation I: RMSE of the Four Estimation Procedures

Parameter	True value	LSDE	EDM-Mx	ADM-SEM	MLDE
Oscillator					
α	-0.04	0.00950	0.00950	0.01059	0.02337
β	-0.20	0.00585	0.00585	0.01005	0.00844
γ	2.00	0.15479	0.15479	0.23764	0.80962
Initial var/cov					
$\sigma^2_{x_1,t_0}$	180	9.87160	9.87129	9.99994	
$\sigma^2_{x_2,t_0}$	120	6.75111	6.75113	8.21163	
σ_{x_1,t_0,x_2,t_0}	-40	5.91874	5.91878	5.98624	
Measurement					
c_2	0.50	0.00345	0.00345	0.00348	0.00349
d_2	2.00	0.06186	0.06186	0.06195	0.06195
$\sigma^2_{v_2,t_i}$	8.00	0.21838	0.21838	0.21726	0.21852
χ^2	df=136	16.68283	16.68285	16.79551	51.3428

be written as RMSE $= \sqrt{\text{bias}^2 + \text{variance}}$, it equals the standard error of the parameter estimates for zero bias; for nonzero bias it is a measure of the combined effect of bias and sampling variability. In the case of χ^2, bias and RMSE are given with regard to the expected value in large samples which is equal to df. So, 3.09922 in the first column of Table 2–1 means that the mean χ^2 was 3.09922 greater than $df = 136$.

2.4.2 Results of Simulation I: Oscillator without Trait Variable. The simulation results for the oscillator without trait variable are shown in Tables 2–1 and 2–2 and will be summarized as follows.

• Almost no differences are found between the four procedures in the quality of the measurement parameter estimates. Although for the MLDE procedure, the bias in these parameter estimates is slightly higher, it does not lead to higher RMSE values than in the other procedures.

• Although computationally quite different, the LSDE and EDM-Mx procedures, both constructed to give the exact maximum likelihood solution, indeed result in the same estimates. The extremely small differences in bias and RMSE occurring at a few places are clearly caused by differences in computing precision. Virtually zero bias in both exact procedures is found for the damping parameter α and frequency parmeter β. Slightly higher biases are found in the variance parameters γ, $\sigma^2_{x_{1,t_0}}$, and $\sigma^2_{x_{2,t_0}}$ and still a little bit higher in covariance parameter $\sigma_{x_{1,t_0},x_{2,t_0}}$. The same pattern applies for RMSE.

• The bias in the ADM-SEM procedure is clearly bigger than in the exact procedures for all parameters except the measurement parameters. However, this does hardly lead to higher RMSE values than in the exact procedures. So, the bias of the ADM-SEM procedure is partly compensated by lower standard errors. In terms of RMSE, the quality of the approximate ADM-SEM procedure is not much worse than of the exact procedures.

• The approximate MLDE procedure does not give estimates of the initial variances and covariance, because the variables are specified only once in the middle of the observation time range. However, where the parameters are the same, the approximate MLDE procedure gives considerably higher biases (bias in α and γ is about 50% of the true value) as well as higher RMSE values than the exact procedures. The MLDE procedure also gives higher biases and RMSE values than the ADM-SEM procedure except for the frequency parameter β.

• As in other simulation studies (Marsh & Hau, 1999; Oud, Jansen, & Haughton, 1999), under the correct model, small positive biases are found for the χ^2-values (from their expected value or model's df) using exact procedures. It is in agreement with the quite reasonable behavior of the approximate ADM-SEM procedure that its χ^2-bias is only slightly higher than for the exact procedures. The much bigger χ^2-bias for the MLDE procedure proves that its approximate model does not fit the data. A major reason for the misfit could

TABLE 2–3

The Oscillator with Trait Variable in Simulation II: Bias of Three Estimation Procedures

Parameter	True	LSDE	EDM-Mx	ADM-SEM
Oscillator				
α	-0.04	-0.00454	-0.00454	-0.03312
β	-0.20	0.00113	0.00113	0.00427
γ	2.00	-0.19933	-0.20026	0.60489
Initial var/cov				
$\sigma^2_{x_1,t_0}$	180	-0.57936	-0.57930	-0.76202
$\sigma^2_{x_2,t_0}$	120	0.22370	0.22379	5.52694
σ_{x_1,t_0,x_2,t_0}	-40	0.25372	0.25368	-0.53126
Trait				
σ^2_κ	130	1.96893	1.96926	15.19194
$\sigma^2_{\kappa,x_1,t_0}$	25	-0.36483	-0.36492	-1.75022
$\sigma^2_{\kappa,x_2,t_0}$	45	0.22638	0.22653	5.03443
Measurement				
c_2	0.50	0.00005	0.00005	0.00005
d_2	2.00	0.00200	0.00200	0.00200
$\sigma^2_{v_2,t_i}$	8.00	-0.01100	-0.01100	-0.01080
χ^2	df=133	3.12724	3.12721	3.13941

be that only a single set of values $y(t)$, $\frac{dy(t)}{dt}$, $\frac{d^2y(t)}{dt^2}$ is fitted to different observation time points.

2.4.3 Results of Simulation II: Oscillator with Trait Variable. The simulation results for the oscillator with trait variable are shown in Tables 2–3 and 2–4. Because the MLDE procedure (Boker et al., 2004) does not accommodate for trait variables, the tables compare only three procedures; the two exact procedures, LSDE and EDM-Mx, and the approximate ADM-SEM procedure.

• Again, almost no differences between the procedures are found in the quality of the measurement parameter estimates. Also, the addition of the trait variable does not deteriorate the quality of the measurement parameter estimates. At some places, one even observes a slight improvement.

• In general, although the bias for parameters other than the measurement parameters is also limited, the estimates nevertheless suffer considerably from the introduction of the trait variable. It leads even to the RMSE of α exceeding α itself. One would conclude for most samples that $\alpha = 0$ cannot be rejected and therefore that the oscillatory movement might be frictionless or infinite.

TABLE 2–4

The Oscillator with Trait Variable in Simulation II: RMSE of Three Estimation Procedures

Parameter	True	LSDE	EDM-Mx	ADM-SEM
Oscillator				
α	-0.04	0.06612	0.06612	0.08588
β	-0.20	0.02449	0.02449	0.03015
γ	2.00	1.03541	1.03720	1.62536
Initial var/cov				
$\sigma^2_{x_{1,t_0}}$	180	9.84669	9.84669	9.84630
$\sigma^2_{x_{2,t_0}}$	120	8.24447	8.24460	10.12866
$\sigma_{x_{1,t_0},x_{2,t_0}}$	-40	6.03110	6.03098	6.21571
Trait				
σ^2_{κ}	130	19.81746	19.81727	26.98867
$\sigma^2_{\kappa,x_{1,t_0}}$	25	8.30507	8.30507	9.41319
$\sigma^2_{\kappa,x_{2,t_0}}$	45	7.16881	7.16893	10.07245
Measurement				
c_2	0.50	0.00173	0.00173	0.00173
d_2	2.00	0.06191	0.06191	0.06191
$\sigma^2_{v_{2,t_i}}$	8.00	0.22006	0.22006	0.22001
χ^2	df=133	16.60604	16.60604	16.61406

• Compared to the initial variances and covariances, the trait variable (unobserved heterogeneity) has parameters with relatively high bias as well as high RMSE.

• Again, there can be no doubt that the two exact procedures give the same solution.

• The results of the ADM-SEM procedure conform to those of the oscillator without trait variable: The ADM-SEM procedure has higher bias than the exact procedures but these differences tend to be mitigated in terms of the RMSE values.

• There is virtually no difference between the procedures with regard to the χ^2 fit measure, in bias nor in RMSE.

2.5 CONCLUSIONS

In this contribution, it was first observed that oscillating movements abound in psychology as in many other sciences and are in need of appropriate estimation procedures in the case of panel data. At least four quite different estimation procedures have been developed in recent years: Singer's linear stochastic differential equation (LSDE) procedure, Oud and Jansen's exact discrete model via Mx (EDM-Mx) procedure, Oud's approximate discrete model via SEM (ADM-SEM) procedure, and Boker, Neale, and Rausch's multivariate latent differential equation (MLDE) procedure. The four procedures had not previously been compared in a systematical way. Whereas MLDE directly models the oscillator and does not accommodate for trait variables, the other procedures model the oscillator as a special case of the general state space model and admit trait variables as special state variables. An advantage of the ADM-SEM procedure is that it can be used by means of the less nonlinearly oriented SEM-programs like LISREL. Input files for the four procedures can be obtained from the author's website *www.socsci.ru.nl/ hano/.*

Most important results from the simulation study are first, that the exact procedures, LSDE and EDM-Mx, lead indeed to the same results as they should. So, for big samples with N larger than the total number of variables, it does not make any difference whether one uses the LSDE or EDM-Mx procedure. In contrast to the EDM-Mx procedure, LSDE may be used in cases of N less than the total number of variables, particularly in the case $N = 1$ (time series case). Second, the addition of trait variables (random subject effects) to the model can have a detrimental effect on the quality of the estimation results, even in the case of the exact procedures. In fact, the inclusion of a trait variable requires a big sample. Even $N = 700$ as used in this simulation study may not be large enough in some cases.

The approximate procedures, ADM-SEM and MLDE, lag considerably behind the exact procedures in quality of estimation results. In general, their use cannot be recommended. In the case of MLDE, crucial parameters in the oscillator show biases around 50% of the true parameter value. The ADM-SEM procedure has a tendency to compensate for the biases with smaller standard errors of the parameters.

REFERENCES

Arminger, G. (1986). Linear stochastic differential equations for panel data with unobserved variables. In N. B. Tuma (Ed.), *Sociological methodology* (pp. 187-212). San Francisco, CA: Jossey-Bass.

Arnold, L. (1974). *Stochastic differential equations.* New York: Wiley.

Bergstrom, A. R. (1966). Nonrecursive models as discrete approximations to systems of stochastic differential equations. *Econometrica, 34,* 173–182.

Bergstrom, A. R. (1984). Continuous time stochastic models and issues of aggregation over time. In Z. Griliches & M. D. Intriligator (Eds.),

Handbook of econometrics (Vol. 2, pp. 1145–1212). Amsterdam: North-Holland.

Bergstrom, A. R. (1988). The history of continuous-time econometric models. *Econometric Theory, 4*, 365–383.

Bisconti, T. L. (2001). *Widowhood in later life: A dynamical systems approach to emotion regulation.* Unpublished doctoral dissertation, University of Notre Dame, IN.

Boker, S. M. (2002). Consequences of continuity: The hunt for intrinsic properties within parameters of dynamics in psychological processes. *Multivariate Behavioral Research, 37*, 405–422.

Boker, S. M., & Graham, J. (1998). A dynamical systems analysis of adolescent substance abuse. *Multivariate Behavioral Research, 33*, 479–507.

Boker, S. M., & Nesselroade, J. R. (2002). A method for modeling the intrinsic dynamics of intraindividual variability: Recovering the parameters of simulated oscillators in multi-wave panel data. *Multivariate Behavioral Research, 37*, 127–160.

Boker, S., Neale, M., & Rausch, J. (2004). Latent differential equation modeling with multivariate multi-occasion indicators. In K. van Montfort, J. Oud, & A. Satorra (Eds.), *Recent developments on structural equations models: Theory and applications* (pp. 151–174). Dordrecht, The Netherlands: Kluwer Academic Publishers.

Cummings, E. M., & Davies, P. T. (2002). Effects of marital conflict on children: Recent advances and emerging themes in process-oriented research. *Journal of Child Psychology and Psychiatry, 43*, 31–63.

Gard, T. C. (1988). *Introduction to stochastic differential equations.* New York: Marcel Dekker.

Gottschalk, A., Bauer, M. S., & Whybrow, P. C. (1995). Evidence of chaotic mood variation in bipolar disorder. *Archives of General Psychiatry, 52*, 947–959.

Hamerle, A., Nagl, W., & Singer, H. (1991). Problems with the estimation of stochastic differential equations using structural equations models. *Journal of Mathematical Sociology, 16*, 201–220.

Hamerle, A., Singer, H., & Nagl, W. (1993). Identification and estimation of continuous time dynamic systems with exogenous variables using panel data. *Econometric Theory, 9*, 283–295.

Itô, K. (1944). Stochastic integral. *Proceedings of Imperial Academy of Tokyo, 20*, 519–524.

Itô, K. (1951). *On stochastic differential equations* (American Mathematical Society Memoirs, No. 4). New York: American Mathematical Society.

Jazwinski, A.H. (1970). *Stochastic processes and filtering theory.* New York: Academic Press.

Jöreskog, K.G., & Sörbom, D. (1996). *LISREL 8: User's reference guide.* Chicago: Scientific Software International.

Marsh, H.W., & Hau, K. (1999). Confirmatory factor analysis: Strategies for small samples. In R. Hoyle (Ed.), *Statistical strategies for small sample research* (pp. 251-284). Thousand Oaks, CA: Sage.

Neale, M.C., Boker, S.M., Xie, G., & Maes, H.H. (1999). *Mx: Statistical Modeling* (4th ed.). Richmond, VA: Virginia Commonwealth University, Department of Psychiatry.

Oud, J. H. L. (2004). SEM state space modeling of panel data in discrete and continuous time and its relationship to traditional state space modeling. In K. van Montfort, J. Oud & A. Satorra (Eds.), *Recent developments on structural equations models: Theory and applications* (pp. 13–40). Dordrecht, The Netherlands: Kluwer Academic Publishers.

Oud, J. H. L. (2006). Continuous time modeling of reciprocal effects in the cross-lagged panel design. In S. M. Boker & M. J. Wenger (Eds.), *Data analytic techniques for dynamical systems in the social and behavioral sciences.* Mahwah, NJ: Lawrence Erlbaum Associates.

Oud, J. H. L., & Jansen, R. A. R. G. (2000). Continuous time state space modeling of panel data by means of SEM. *Psychometrika, 65,* 199–215.

Oud, J. H. L., Jansen, R. A. R. G., & Haughton, D. M. A. (1999). Small samples in structural equation state space modeling. In R. Hoyle (Ed.), *Statistical strategies for small sample research* (pp. 285–306). Thousand Oaks, CA: Sage.

Ruymgaart, P. A. & Soong, T. T. (1985). *Mathematics of Kalman-Bucy filtering.* Berlin: Springer.

Sarrias, M. J., Artigas, F., Martinez, E., & Gelpí, E. (1989). Seasonal changes of plasma serotonin and related parameters: Correlation with environmental measures. *Biological Psychiatry, 26,* 695–706.

Singer, H. (1990). *Parameterschätzung in zeitkontinuierlichen dynamischen Systemen* [Parameter estimation in continuous time dynamic systems]. Konstanz: Hartung-Gorre.

Singer, H. (1991). *LSDE - A program package for the simulation, graphical display, optimal filtering and maximum likelihood estimation of linear stochastic differential equations: User's guide.* Meersburg: Author.

Singer, H. (1992a). *Zeitkontinuierliche dynamische Systeme* [Continuous time dynamic systems]. Frankfurt: Campus.

Singer, H. (1992b). The aliasing-phenomenon in visual terms. *Journal of Mathematical Sociology, 17,* 39–49.

Singer, H. (1993). Continuous-time dynamical systems with sampled data, errors of measurement and unobserved components. *Journal of Time Series Analysis, 14*, 527–545.

Singer, H. (1995). Analytical score function for irregularly sampled continuous time stochastic processes with control variables and missing values. *Econometric Theory, 11*, 721–735.

Singer, H. (1998). Continuous panel models with time dependent parameters. *Journal of Mathematical Sociology, 23*, 77–98.

Singer, H. (1999). *Finanzmarktökonometrie* [Finance market econometrics]. Heidelberg: Physica.

Wiener, J. (1923). Differential space. *Journal of Mathematical Physics, 38*, 131–174.

Chapter 3

Modeling the Coevolution of Networks and Behavior

Tom Snijders, Christian Steglich, and Michael Schweinberger

University of Groningen, The Netherlands

3.1 INTRODUCTION: THE JOINT DYNAMICS OF NETWORKS AND BEHAVIOR

Social networks are representations of patterns of relations between actors (individuals, companies, countries, etc.; see Carrington, Scott, & Wasserman, 2005; Wasserman & Faust, 1994). Such networks are not static but evolve over time. Friendship ties form and dissolve again over the life course, trade relations between business partners typically cover only a limited time period – indeed, change over time occurs naturally for most social relations that are commonly studied, like trust, social support, communication, even web links and coauthorship ties. Such change can be due to purely structural, network-endogenous mechanisms like reciprocity (Sahlins, 1972), transitivity (friends of friends tend to be friends, Davis, 1970; Rapoport, 1953a, 1953b) or structural competition (Burt, 1987). However, also mechanisms related to individual characteristics of the network actors can be among the determinants of network change. Best known among these are patterns of homophily (i.e., preference for similarity) in friendship selection (McPherson, Smith-Lovin, & Cook, 2001), and a large variety of determinants of attractiveness as relational partner (e.g., the strong market position of a company as a determinant for strategic alliances, or the sociability of a classmate as a determinant for party invitations).

On the other side, actors' characteristics – indicators of performance and success, attitudes and other cognitions, behavioral tendencies – can depend on the social network in which the actor is situated. It is well-known that in many social situations, behavior and attitudes of individuals follow patterns of assimilation to others to whom they are tied. The examples are the diffusion of innovations in a professional community (Valente, 1995), pupils' copying of 'chic' behavior of their friends at school, or traders on a market copying the allegedly successful behavior of their competitors.

The change of network structure is often referred to as *selection* (Lazarsfeld & Merton, 1954), and the change of individual characteristics of social actors depending on the characteristics of others to whom they are tied is called *influence* (Friedkin, 1998). It is assumed here that the group of actors under study has been delineated in such a way that it is meaningful to investigate the selection and influence processes in this group without considering ties to others outside the group. The necessity of studying selection and influence processes in networks simultaneously was discussed both in detailed network investigations (e.g., Padgett & Ansell, 1993) and in theoretical discussion essays (Doreian & Stokman, 1997; Emirbayer & Goodwin, 1994). A concrete example is smoking initiation among adolescents, where it has been established in the literature that friends tend to have similar patterns of smoking behavior. What is unknown is to what extent this is a matter of selection of friends on the basis of common behavior, or adaptation of behavior toward that of one's friends (Bauman & Ennett, 1996).

This chapter proposes a statistical method for investigating network structure together with relevant actor attributes as joint dependent variables in a longitudinal framework, assuming that data have been collected according to a panel design. This is a more detailed exposition of the proposals sketched in Steglich, Snijders, and Pearson (2004). In the stochastic model, the network structure and the individual attributes evolve simultaneously in a dynamic process. The method is illustrated by an example on the dynamics of alcohol consumption among adolescent friends.

3.1.1 Overview

The principles of actor-driven, or actor-oriented, modeling were proposed in Snijders (1996). The model for dynamics of only networks, without behavior, was formulated in Snijders (2001, 2005). In Steglich et al. (2004), the sociological aspects of the model for dynamics of networks and behavior are discussed, with an extensive example about the interrelationship of the development of friendship networks and the dynamics in smoking and drinking behavior, on the basis of data from a Scottish high school. This chapter gives an overview of the specification of the stochastic model for dynamics of networks and behavior and then proceeds to parameter estimation and model selection.

The chapter is structured as follows. In Section 3.2, the data structure investigated is formalized. Section 3.3 formulates the family of stochastic models by which we propose to model and analyze network-behavioral coevolution. Section 3.4 is about parameter estimation. Goodness-of-fit issues and model selection are addressed in Section 3.5. These methods are illustrated by an example in Section 3.6. The final Section 3.7 gives a discussion of the main points raised in the article and some further developments.

3.2 NOTATION AND DATA STRUCTURE

A relation on a set $\mathcal{X}$ is defined mathematically as a subset $\mathcal{R}$ of the Cartesian product $\mathcal{X} \times \mathcal{X}$; if $(i, j) \in \mathcal{R}$, we say that there is a tie, or link, from i to j. When $\mathcal{X}$ is a set of social actors (e.g., individuals or companies), such a mathematical relation can represent a social relation like friendship, esteem, collaboration, and so forth. An introduction to the use of this type of model is given in Wasserman and Faust (1994), more recent developments in this area are presented in Carrington et al. (2005). This chapter is concerned with data structures consisting of one relation defined on a given set of n actors, changing over time, along with $H \geq 1$ changing actor attributes. The relation will be referred to as the *network*, the attributes as *behavior* or *actor characteristics*. The relation $\mathcal{R}$ is assumed to be nonreflexive, that is, for all i we have $(i, i) \notin \mathcal{R}$, and directed, that is, it is possible that $(i, j) \in \mathcal{R}$ but $(j, i) \notin \mathcal{R}$. The relation is represented by the $n \times n$ adjacency matrix $X = (X_{ij})$, where $X_{ij} = 0, 1$, respectively, represents that there is no tie [i.e., $(i, j) \notin \mathcal{R}$], or there is a tie [i.e., $(i, j) \in \mathcal{R}$], from actor i to actor j $(i, j = 1, ..., n)$. The relation can also be regarded as a directed graph, or digraph, and the existence of a tie from i to j is represented by the figure $i \rightarrow j$. The actor attributes are assumed to be ordered discrete, each having a finite interval of integer values as its range, and Z_{hi} denotes the value of actor i on the hth attribute. Time dependence is indicated by denoting $X = X(t)$ and $Z_h = Z_h(t)$, where t denotes time and Z_h is the column containing the Z_{hi} values.

This chapter presents models and methods for the dynamics of the stochastic process $(X(t), Z_1(t), \ldots, Z_H(t))$. In addition to the relation X and the attributes Z_h there can be other variables, called covariates, on which the distribution of this stochastic process depends; these can be individual (i.e., actor-dependent) covariates denoted by the letter v and dyadic covariates (depending on a pair of actors) denoted by w.

It is supposed that observations on $(X(t), Z_1(t), \ldots, Z_H(t))$ are available for discrete observation moments $t_1 < t_2 < \ldots < t_M$. The number M of time points is at least 2. In the discussion of the stochastic model, random variables are denoted by capital letters. For example, $X(t_m)$ denotes the random digraph of which $x(t_m)$ is the outcome.

The individual covariates $v_h = (v_{h1}, \ldots, v_{hn})$ and the dyadic covariates $w_h = (w_{hij})_{1 \leq i, j \leq n}$ may depend on the observation moments t_m or be constant. When covariates are time dependent, it is assumed that they are observed for all observation moments t_m, and their effect on the transition kernel of the stochastic process $\left(X(t), Z_1(t), \ldots, Z_H(t)\right)$ is determined by the most recently observed value, observed at time $\max\{t_m \mid t_m \leq t\}$. Because covariates are treated as deterministic, nonstochastic variables, they will often be treated implicitly and skipped in the notation.

To prevent an overload of notation, the stochastic process $\left(X(t), Z_1(t), \ldots, Z_H(t)\right)$ together with the covariate data (if any), will be represented by the symbol $Y(t)$. Thus, the totality of available data is represented by $y(t_1), \ldots, y(t_M)$.

3.3 MODEL DEFINITION

The process of network-behavioral coevolution is regarded here as an emergent group-level result of the network actors' individual decisions. These decisions are modeled as being the results of myopic optimization by each actor of an objective function that contains terms reflecting systematic tendencies and preferences, and also a random term representing nonsystematic (unexplained) change. This approach implies that the constituents of the actors' objective functions are the central model components; the myopic nature of the optimization implies that the objective functions represent the dynamic tendencies that actors have in the short term. Building on earlier work (Snijders, 1996, 2001, 2005), we denote this approach by the term *actor-driven modeling*. Each actor i is assumed to have, in principle, control over his/her outgoing ties X_{ij} ($j = 1, \ldots, n; j \neq i$) and over her/his characteristics Z_{hi} ($h = 1, \ldots, H$). These ties and characteristics have in this model, however, a great deal of inertia and it will be assumed that they change only by small steps.

To formulate a model containing separate causal processes of social influence (where an actor's characteristics are influenced by network structure and the properties of other network actors) and of social selection (where actor characteristics affect tie formation and tie dissolution), we make four reasonable simplifying assumptions. These simplifications provide a natural first choice for modeling the coevolution processes of networks and individual attributes in a host of applications.

The first of these assumptions is that the observations at the discrete time points $t_1 < t_2 < \ldots < t_M$ are the outcomes of an underlying process $Y(t) = \left(X(t), Z_1(t), \ldots, Z_H(t)\right)$ that is a Markov process with continuous time parameter t. Such an assumption was already proposed by Holland and Leinhardt (1977a, 1977b) and by Wasserman (1977) as a basis for longitudinal network modeling. Thus, changes in network ties and behavior happen in continuous time, at stochastically determined discrete moments, and the total difference between two consecutive observations $y(t_m)$ and $y(t_{m+1})$ is regarded as the result of usually many unobserved changes that occur between these observation moments. The Markov assumption means that given the current state $Y(t)$, the conditional distribution of the future $Y(t')$ for $t' > t$ is independent of the history before time t. In other words, the current state $Y(t)$ contains all information determining the future dynamics. The Markov assumption sets limits to the domain of applicability of these models: They are meaningful especially if the network $X(t)$ and the vector of behavioral variables $Z_h(t)$ together can be regarded as a *state*, which together with the covariates determines, in a reasonable approximation, the endogenous dynamics of these variables themselves. This excludes applications to ephemeral phenomena or brief events for which a dependence on latent variables would be plausible. Examples where such a Markov model could be applied are the dynamics of friendship and health-related or lifestyle-related behavior (Steglich et al., 2004) or strategic alliances and ownership ties between companies and their market performance (Pahor, 2003). Examples where such a model would be less suitable are ephemeral ties, or events, like going to a movie or email exchange.

The second assumption is that at any given moment t, all actors act conditionally independent of each other, given the current state $Y(t)$ of the process. This way, the possibility of simultaneous changes by two or more actors has probability zero. An example for such simultaneous changes would be binding contracts of the type "I'll start going out with you once you stop going out with that other person." Although such bargaining indeed may happen in real life, it would be modeled here as two subsequent decisions by the two actors involved, the connection of which cannot be enforced.

The third assumption is that the changes that an actor applies at time t to his/her network ties (thus, the changes in X_i) and the changes made about his/her behavioral characteristics (changes in Z_{hi}) all are conditionally independent of each other — again, given the current state of the process. This implies that simultaneous changes in network ties and actor behavior have probability zero. Thus the coevolution process is separated into a network change process (social selection) and a behavior change process (social influence), mutually linked because the transition distribution of each process is determined not only by its own current state but also by the current state of the other process; they are not linked by a joint choice process where an actor simultaneously determines a change in a network tie and a change in behavior.

The fourth assumption is that, when an actor makes a change in either the vector of outgoing tie variables X_{ij} ($j = 1, \ldots, n; j \neq i$) or in the behavior vector $(Z_{1i}, \ldots, Z_{Hi})$, not more than one variable X_{ij} or Z_{hi} can be changed at one instant, and in the value of Z_{hi}, only increases or decreases by one unit are permitted — recall that these variables are integer valued; larger changes are modeled as the result of several of these small steps. Thus, a change by actor i is either the creation of one new tie (X_{ij} changes from 0 to 1), the dissolution of one existing tie (X_{ij} goes from 1 to 0), or an increase or decrease in one behavior variable Z_{hi} by one unit.

The general principle of these assumptions is to specify the coevolution of the network and the behavior as a Markov process constructed from the smallest possible steps. This is proposed because it leads to a parsimonious and relatively simple model that in many applications seems a plausible first approximation to the coevolution process of network and behavior. Because only panel data are assumed to be available, perhaps collected at a quite limited number of moments like two or three, there is not much information available for a detailed check of this type of assumption, which underlines the requirement of parsimony. Depending on the application at hand, these assumptions may make more or less sense, which should be checked before applying these models as well as later, using the observed data.

The stochastic process is assumed to be a left-continuous function of time, that is,

$$\lim_{t' \uparrow t} Y(t') = Y(t) \, .$$

As is elaborated later, at randomly determined moments t, one of the actors i is assumed to have the opportunity to change either a tie variable X_{ij} or a behavioral variable Z_{hi}, and when the actor takes such a decision, this leads to a new value of this variable valid immediately after time t. When the actor has such an opportunity, it is also permitted not to change anything — that will happen if the actor is satisfied with the current situation, as is explained later. These small changes are referred to as *microsteps*. The often complex compound change between two consecutive observations $y(t_m)$ and $y(t_{m+1})$ is thus decomposed into many small, stochastically spaced microsteps that occur between observation moments. Altogether, this set of assumptions provides a simple way of expressing the feedback processes inherent in the dynamic process, where the currently reached state $Y(t)$ is always the initial state for further developments.

The first observation $y(t_1)$ is not modeled but conditioned upon, that is, the starting values of the network and the initial behaviors are taken for granted. This implies that the evolution process is modeled without contamination by the contingencies leading to the initial state, and that no assumption of a dynamic equilibrium needs to be invoked.

3.3.1 Rate Functions

The moments when any given actor i has the opportunity to make a decision to change the vector of outgoing tie variables $(X_{i1}, \ldots, X_{in})$ or a behavior variable Z_{hi} are randomly determined and follow Poisson processes, the waiting times being modeled by exponential distributions with parameters given by so-called *rate functions* λ. For each actor i, there is one rate function for the network (denoted $\lambda_i^{[X]}$) and one for each behavioral dimension (denoted $\lambda_i^{[Z_h]}$). The rate functions are allowed to depend not only on the time period m, but also on actor characteristics v_{hi} and Z_{hi} and on network characteristics (like indegree or outdegree of the actors). The latter two determinants can be expressed by calculating actor-dependent one-dimensional statistics $a_{ki}(Y(t))$. The rate functions during the time period $t_m < t < t_{m+1}$ then are given by

$$\lambda_i^{[X]}(Y, m) = \rho_m^{[X]} \exp\left(\sum_k \alpha_k^{[X]} a_{ki}^{[X]}(Y(t))\right) \tag{1}$$

for the timing of network decisions and

$$\lambda_i^{[Z_h]}(Y, m) = \rho_m^{[Z_h]} \exp\left(\sum_k \alpha_k^{[Z_h]} a_{ki}^{[Z_h]}(Y(t))\right) \tag{2}$$

for the timing of behavioral decisions. The rate functions depend on parameters ρ indicating period dependence and α indicating dependence on the statistics $a_{ki}(Y(t))$. The "forgetfulness property" of the exponential distribution used for modeling the rate function is a crucial condition for the Markov property of the stochastic process $Y(t)$. Multiplying the time scale by some amount will lead to an inversely proportional change in the multiplicative constants ρ_m. This implies that the numerical values of the durations $t_{m+1} - t_m$ are immaterial for modeling, and it is no restriction to assume that all time intervals have a unit duration, which will make the "real" durations be absorbed in the ρ_m parameters.

3.3.2 Objective Functions

Whereas the rate functions model the *timing* of the different actors' different types of decisions, the objective functions model *which* changes are made. It is assumed that actors i, once it is their turn to make a decision, myopically optimize an objective function over the set of possible microsteps they can make. This objective function is further assumed to be decomposable into three parts: the *evaluation function* f, the *endowment function* g, and a random term ϵ capturing residual noise, that is, unexplained influences. For network decisions taken by actor i, starting from the current state $Y(t)$ and optimizing the new state y under the constraints defined by the type of microstep, the objective function optimized is

$$f_i^{[X]}(\beta^{[X]}, y) + g_i^{[X]}(\gamma^{[X]}, y \mid Y(t)) + \epsilon_i^{[X]}(y), \tag{3}$$

while for behavioral decisions, it is the function

$$f_i^{[Z_h]}(\beta^{[Z_h]}, y) + g_i^{[Z_h]}(\gamma^{[Z_h]}, y \mid Y(t)) + \epsilon_i^{[Z_h]}(y). \tag{4}$$

The myopic optimization means that the actor chooses the change maximizing the value of the objective function that will be obtained by making the contemplated change, without taking into account the consequences later on.

The evaluation function f_i measures the satisfaction of actor i with a given network-behavioral configuration, independently of how this configuration is arrived at. The endowment function g_i, on the other hand, measures a component of the satisfaction with a given network-behavioral configuration that will be lost when the value of a variable X_{ij} or Z_{hi} is changed, but that was obtained without "cost" when this value was obtained. [Snijders' (2001) model used a so-called gratification function. This is mathematically equivalent to the model with the endowment function; the current formulation with the endowment function allows a more easily structured exposition.] The evaluation function depends only on the new state y whereas the endowment function depends both on the hypothetical new state y and the current state $Y(t)$ that is the immediate precursor of y.

By including network endowment effects into a model specification, it becomes possible to assess systematic differences between the creation and the dissolution of ties that cannot be captured by the evaluation function. An example is the phenomenon that the cost in loosing a reciprocal friendship tie is greater than the gain in establishing such a tie — one could say that the existence of a reciprocated tie gives a reward without cost; theoretical and empirical support for the endowment inherent in reciprocated friendships is given by Van de Bunt (1999) and Van de Bunt, Van Duijn, and Snijders (1999). By including behavioral endowment effects, it becomes possible to assess similar asymmetries between moving upward on a behavioral dimension and moving downward (e.g., the empirical phenomenon that some behaviors like smoking or drug consumption are started more easily than abandoned later on). The endowment effect is defined in microeconomics (Thaler, 1980) as the difference between "selling prices" and "buying prices": It is an empirical regularity that for most economic goods, the former are higher than the latter; related concepts of loss aversion and framing are discussed, for example, in Kahneman, Knetsch, and Thaler (1991) and Lindenberg (1993).

Both functions are modeled as weighted sums, the weights being statistical parameters in the model. The evaluation function is expressed as

$$f_i^{[X]}\big(\beta^{[X]}, y\big) = \sum_k \beta_k^{[X]} s_{ik}^{[X]}(y) \qquad (5)$$

for the evaluation of the network and

$$f_i^{[Z_h]}\big(\beta^{[Z_h]}, y\big) = \sum_k \beta_k^{[Z_h]} s_{ik}^{[Z_h]}(y) \qquad (6)$$

for the evaluation of behavior variable Z_h.

The endowment function gives the opportunity to entertain models where the gain in establishing a tie differs from the loss in breaking the same tie; and the gain in increasing a behavioral variable differs from the loss in decreasing it by the same amount. The parts of these gains and losses that perfectly compensate each other can be put into the evaluation function. Therefore it is assumed here that the satisfaction associated with *increasing* values of tie variables X_{ij} and behavior variables Z_{hi} is totally represented by the evaluation functions, whereas the endowment function represents only the extra satisfaction lost when *decreasing* these variables. Thus, for increases of the tie and behavior variables, only the evaluation function needs to be taken into account, whereas for decreases, both the evaluation and the endowment functions must be reckoned with.

The endowment function for network changes is written, for the change from y^0 to y, as

$$g_i^{[X]}\left(\gamma^{[X]}, y \mid y^{(0)}\right) = \sum_k \sum_{j \neq i} \gamma_k^{[X]} \, I\{x_{ij} < x_{ij}^{(0)}\} \, s_{ijk}^{[X]}(y^{(0)}) \qquad (7)$$

where $\gamma_k^{[X]} s_{ijk}^{[X]}(y^{(0)})$ is the endowment value of the tie $x_{ij}^{(0)} = 1$, which will be lost when this tie is withdrawn ($x_{ij} = 0$). $I\{A\}$ is the indicator function of the condition A, defined as 1 if the condition is satisfied, and 0 otherwise.

For the endowment function for the behavior variable Z_h, again for the change from y^0 to y, a slightly more complicated expression is used, because this variable may have an arbitrary number of integer values. The endowment function is

$$g_i^{[Z_h]}\left(\gamma^{[Z_h]}, y \mid y^{(0)}\right) = \sum_k \gamma_k^{[Z_h]} \, I\{z_{hi} < z_{hi}^{(0)}\} \left(s_{ik}^{[Z_h]}(y^{(0)}) - s_{ik}^{[Z_h]}(y)\right).$$
$$(8)$$

Here, $s_{ik}^{[Z_h]}(y^{(0)})$ is the satisfaction with the behavior variable Z_{hi} that is diminished to $s_{ik}^{[Z_h]}(y)$ when decreasing this variable, but that does not play a role for actor i when increasing it.

The third component of the objective function is defined by the random residuals ϵ, which are assumed to be independent and to follow a *type-I extreme value* distribution (also known as standard Gumbel distribution). This is a common and convenient choice in random utility modeling, which allows us to write the resulting choice probabilities for the possible microsteps in a *multinomial logit* form (Maddala, 1983; McFadden, 1974).

For network decisions, the resulting choice probabilities are

$$
\Pr\left(x(i \rightsquigarrow j) \mid x(t), z(t)\right) =
$$
$$
\frac{\exp\left([f + g]_i^{[X]}(\beta^{[X]}, \gamma^{[X]}, x(i \rightsquigarrow j)(t), z(t))\right)}{\sum_k \exp\left([f + g]_i^{[X]}(\beta^{[X]}, \gamma^{[X]}, x(i \rightsquigarrow k)(t), z(t))\right)} \quad (9)
$$

where $[f + g]_i^{[X]}$ is defined in a self-evident way, $x(i \rightsquigarrow j)$ denotes for $j \neq i$ the network resulting from a microstep in which actor i changes the tie variable to actor j (from 0 to 1, or vice versa), and $x(i \rightsquigarrow i)$ is defined to be equal to x. Thus, for $i \neq j$, $x(i \rightsquigarrow j)_{ij} = 1 - x_{ij}$ whereas all other elements of $x(i \rightsquigarrow j)$ are equal to those of x.

For behavioral decisions the formula is

$$
\Pr\left(z(i \updownarrow_h \delta) \mid x(t), z(t)\right) =
$$
$$
\frac{\exp\left([f + g]_i^{[Z_h]}(\beta^{[Z_h]}, \gamma^{[Z_h]}, x(t), z(i \updownarrow_h \delta)(t))\right)}{\sum_{\tau \in \{-1,0,1\}} \exp\left([f + g]_i^{[Z_h]}(\beta^{[Z_h]}, \gamma^{[Z_h]}, x(t), z(i \updownarrow_h \tau)(t))\right)} \quad (10)
$$

where $z(i \updownarrow_h \delta)$ denotes the behavioral configuration resulting from a microstep in which actor i changes the score on behavioral variable Z_h by δ. Thus, $z(i \updownarrow_h \delta)_{hi} = z_{hi} + \delta$, whereas all other elements of $z(i \updownarrow_h \delta)$ are equal to those of z.

3.3.3 Model Components

Possible components $s_{ik}^{[X]}$ in the network evaluation function (5) are presented and discussed in Snijders (2001, 2005). A limited number of such components include the following; more examples and interpretation can be found in the cited references.

1. Outdegree effect, the number of outgoing ties
   $s_{i1}(x) = x_{i+} = \sum_j x_{ij}$;

2. Reciprocity effect, the number of reciprocated ties
   $s_{i2}(x) = x_{i(r)} = \sum_j x_{ij} x_{ji}$;

3. Transitivity effect, the number of transitive patterns in i's ties. A transitive triplet for actor i is an ordered pairs of actors (j, h) for which $i \rightarrow j \rightarrow h$ and also $i \rightarrow h$, as indicated in Figure 3–1. The transitivity effect is defined by
   $s_{i3}(x) = \sum_{j,h} x_{ij} x_{ih} x_{jh}$;

4. Number of geodesic distances two effect, or indirect relations effect, defined by the number of actors to whom i is indirectly tied (through one

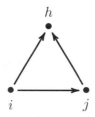

Figure 3–1. Transitive triplet

intermediary, i.e., at geodesic distance 2),
$$s_{i4}(x) = \sharp\{j \mid x_{ij} = 0,\ \max_h(x_{ih}\,x_{hj}) > 0\}\ ;$$

5. Attribute-related similarity, sum of similarities with respect to variable Z_h between i and those to whom i is tied
$$s_{i5}(x, z) = \textstyle\sum_j x_{ij}\left(1 - |z_{ih} - z_{jh}|/R_h\right), \tag{11}$$
where R_h is the range of variable Z_h ;

6. Main effect of a dyadic covariate w, defined by the sum of the values of w_{ij} for all others to whom i is tied,
$$s_{i6}(x) = \textstyle\sum_j x_{ij}\,w_{ij}\,.$$

Possibilities for components $s_{ijk}^{[X]}$ of the endowment function in Equation (7) for the network are given by the same formulae but skipping the summation over j.

Many possibilities for components $s_{ik}^{[Z_h]}$ in the behavior evaluation function in Equation 6 are discussed in Steglich et al. (2004). The foremost examples are listed here.

1. Tendency, indicating the preference for high values,
$$s_{i1}(x, z) = z_{ih}.$$

2. Attribute-related similarity, the sum of similarities with respect to variable Z_h between i and those to whom this actor is tied,
$$s_{i2}(x, z) = \textstyle\sum_j x_{ij}\left(1 - |z_{ih} - z_{jh}|/R_h\right), \tag{12}$$
where again Z_h has range R_h.

3. Dependence on other behaviors h' $(h \neq h')$,
$$s_{i3}(x, z) = z_{ih}\,z_{ih'}\,.$$

These formulae are also possibilities for components $s_{ik}^{[Z_h]}$ for the behavior endowment function (8).

Note that components $s_{i5}(x, z)$ for the network evaluation function and $s_{i2}(x, z)$ for the behavior evaluation function are the same formulae. This is basic to the difficulties in distinguishing these two effects: Positive values of the parameters for either component will contribute to positive correlations between the behavior values of actors with the behavior values of those to whom they are tied; network autocorrelation (Doreian, 1989).

3.3.4 Transition Intensities

The model described thus far amounts to a continuous-time Markov process $Y(t)$. Such a process is fully described by its starting value [here the first observation $y(t_1)$] and its matrix of transition intensities between the states at any moment t. This matrix of transition intensities has the following elements, where $y = (x, z)$ is the current and $\hat{y}$ the next outcome:

$$q(y; \hat{y}) = \begin{cases} \lambda_i^{[X]}(y) \Pr\left(x(i \rightsquigarrow j) \mid x, z\right) & \text{if } \hat{y} = \left(x(i \rightsquigarrow j), z\right), \\ \lambda_i^{[Z_h]}(y) \Pr\left(z(i \updownarrow_h \delta) \mid x, z\right) & \text{if } \hat{y} = \left(x, z(i \updownarrow_h \delta)\right), \\ -\sum_i \left\{ \sum_{j \neq i} q\left(y; (x(i \rightsquigarrow j), z)\right) + \right. \\ \qquad \left. \sum_{\delta \in \{-1,1\}} q\left(y; (x, z(i \updownarrow_h \delta))\right) \right\} & \text{if } \hat{y} = y, \\ 0 \text{ otherwise} \end{cases} \tag{13}$$

(dropping the dependence on parameters ρ, α, β, γ, as well as on time t). Integration over this infinitesimal generator gives transition probabilities for the process Y from one given time point to another, later moment.

3.4 METHODS OF MOMENTS ESTIMATION

The likelihood function for this model cannot be computed explicitly in the general case, which makes maximum likelihood or Bayesian estimation hard. Several other estimation methods, however, are possible within the general framework of Markov chain Monte Carlo (MCMC) estimation. Snijders (1995, 1996, 2001) proposed, for models with network evolution only, estimation procedures according to the method of moments (MoM). MoM estimators are specified here for the case of network-behavior coevolution. The elaboration of maximum likelihood estimators and the efficiency comparison between MoM and ML estimators is the topic of current work.

For a general statistical model with data Y and parameter θ, the MoM estimator based on the statistic $u(Y)$ is defined as the parameter value $\hat{\theta}$ for which the expected and observed values of $u(Y)$ are the same,

$$E_{\hat{\theta}}\left(u(Y)\right) = u(y), \tag{14}$$

$u(y)$ being the observed value. A review of the MoM is presented by Bowman and Shenton (1985). Equation 14 is called the *moment equation*. Usually θ and $u(Y)$ will be vectors with the same dimension, and the solution will be locally unique and often globally unique. Using the delta method (Lehmann, 1999) and the implicit function theorem, it can be proven under regularity conditions that if $\hat{\theta}$ is a consistent solution to the moment equation (where the dependence on the index n is left implicit), the asymptotic covariance matrix of the moment estimator is

$$\mathrm{cov}_\theta\left(\hat{\theta}\right) \approx D_\theta^{-1} \Sigma_\theta D_\theta'^{-1} , \tag{15}$$

where D_θ is the matrix of partial derivatives,

$$D_\theta = \left(\frac{\partial \mathrm{E}_\theta\big(u(Y)\big)}{\partial \theta} \right) , \tag{16}$$

and Σ_θ is the covariance matrix

$$\Sigma_\theta = \mathrm{cov}_\theta\big(u(Y)\big) .$$

This shows, at least in principle, how the efficiency of the MoM estimator depends on the statistic $u(Y)$.

3.4.1 Statistics for Moment Estimation

This section gives statistics $u(Y)$ for the network-behavior coevolution model that are intuitively plausible and have been shown to give useful estimates.

The intuition behind statistics that are useful for the construction of MoM estimators is that for each separate one-dimensional parameter θ_h in the total parameter vector θ, there must be a real-valued statistic included as a component in $u(Y)$ that tends to become larger as θ_h increases; its distribution should preferably be a stochastically increasing function of θ_h when the other components of the parameter θ are kept constant. The components of θ in this model are the parameters previously indicated by the letters ρ, α, β, γ. Suitable statistics are discussed separately for the constant factors ρ_m in the rate functions; for the other parameters α in the rate functions; the weights β in the evaluation functions; and the weights γ in the endowment functions. The proposed statistics for the network evolution were mentioned already in Snijders (2001).

The panel design, where observations on the stochastic process are available at several discrete time moments, together with the Markov property, leads to a slightly adapted version of the moment Equation 14. For parameters that influence only the stochastic process as it evolves in the period from t_{m-1} to t_m, that have no effect before t_{m-1} or after t_m, and that are estimated on the basis of some statistic $u_m\big(Y(t_{m-1}), Y(t_m)\big)$, the moment equation is

$$\mathrm{E}_\theta\big\{u_m\big(Y(t_{m-1}), Y(t_m)\big) \,|\, Y(t_{m-1}) = y(t_{m-1})\big\} = u_m\big(y(t_{m-1}), y(t_m)\big) . \tag{17}$$

On the other hand, for parameters that are constant across all time periods and thereby affect the distribution of the stochastic process from the first to the last observation, and for which statistics $u_m\big(Y(t_{m-1}), Y(t_m)\big)$ are relevant for all $m = 2 \ldots, M$, the moment equation is

$$\sum_{m=2}^{M} \mathrm{E}_\theta\big\{u_m\big(Y(t_{m-1}), Y(t_m)\big) \,|\, Y(t_{m-1}) = y(t_{m-1})\big\}$$

$$= \sum_{m=2}^{M} u_m\big(y(t_{m-1}), y(t_m)\big) . \quad (18)$$

Rate Function Parameters. The basic parameters in the rate functions are the constant factors $\rho_m^{[X]}$ for the rate of change of the network and $\rho_m^{[Z_h]}$ for the rate of change of behavior variable Z_h. Natural statistics for estimating these parameters are, respectively,

$$\sum_{i,j} \big|X_{ij}(t_m) - X_{ij}(t_{m-1})\big| \qquad \text{for estimating } \rho_m^{[X]} \qquad (19)$$

and

$$\sum_{i} \big|Z_{hi}(t_m) - Z_{hi}(t_{m-1})\big| \qquad \text{for estimating } \rho_m^{[Z_h]} . \qquad (20)$$

These are the only statistics for which the stochastic monotonicity property can be proved generally; for the statistics proposed below for other parameters, this property is plausible but has not yet been proven.

When the rates of change for actors i depend on one-dimensional statistics $a_{ki}^{[X]}\big(Y(t)\big)$ and $a_{ki}^{[Z_h]}\big(Y(t)\big)$, such as covariates or nodal degrees, relevant statistics are

$$\sum_{i,j} a_{ki}^{[X]}\big(Y(t_{m-1})\big) \big|X_{ij}(t_m) - X_{ij}(t_{m-1})\big| \qquad (21)$$

for parameters $\alpha_k^{[X]}$ influencing network change, and

$$\sum_{i} a_{ki}^{[Z_h]}\big(Y(t_{m-1})\big) \big|Z_{hi}(t_m) - Z_{hi}(t_{m-1})\big| \qquad (22)$$

for parameters $\alpha_k^{[Z_h]}$ determining the rate of change in behavior Z_h .

Evaluation Function Parameters. The evaluation functions f are specified in Equations 5 and 6, and operate uniformly through the period from t_1 to t_M. For both network and behavior, higher values of β_k will tend to lead to higher values of $s_{ik}(Y)$ — for all actors i and for all observation moments later than t_1. This reasoning leads to the statistics

$$u_m\big(Y(t_m)\big) = \sum_i s_{ik}^{[X]}\big(Y(t_m)\big) \qquad \text{for estimating } \beta_k^{[X]*}, \qquad (23)$$

and

$$u_m\big(Y(t_m)\big) = \sum_i s_{ik}^{[Z_h]}\big(Y(t_m)\big) \qquad \text{for estimating } \beta_k^{[Z_h]}, \qquad (24)$$

not depending explicitly on $Y(t_{m-1})$.

However, these equations do not distinguish between influence and selection. If the same statistic $s_{ik}(Y)$ is used in the models for the network dynamics and for the behavior dynamics of a variable Z_h, then these two equations would lead to identical moment equations and hence be inadequate for estimating two separate parameters.

The special property exploited to separate influence from selection is the time order that is basic to causality. Selection means that an earlier configuration of attributes leads later on to a change in ties; whereas influence means that an earlier configuration of ties leads later on to a change in attributes. Accordingly, writing the functions in Equations 5 and 6 as

$$s_{ik}^{[X]}(y) = s_{ik}^{[X]}(x, z), \quad s_{ik}^{[Z_h]}(y) = s_{ik}^{[Z_h]}(x, z), \qquad (25)$$

the statistics used in the moment equations are

$$u_m\big(Y(t_{m-1}), Y(t_m)\big) = \sum_i s_{ik}^{[X]}\big(X(t_m), Z(t_{m-1})\big) \qquad (26)$$

for estimating the parameters $\beta_k^{[X]}$ driving the network change, and

$$u_m\big(Y(t_{m-1}), Y(t_m)\big) = \sum_i s_{ik}^{[Z_h]}\big(X(t_{m-1}), Z(t_{m-1}), Z(t_m)\big) \qquad (27)$$

for estimating the parameters $\beta_k^{[Z_h]}$ driving the change in behavioral variable Z_h. Here the statistic $s_{ik}^{[Z_h]}\big(X(t_{m-1}), Z(t_{m-1}), Z(t_m)\big)$ is defined by employing for the behavioral variables the value at t_m for Z_h and the value at t_{m-1} for $Z_{h'}$ for all other h'. With some abuse of notation, this is expressed by

$$s_{ik}^{[Z_h]}\big(X(t_{m-1}), Z(t_{m-1}), Z(t_m)\big) = s_{ik}^{[Z_h]}\big(X(t_{m-1}), Z^*\big) \qquad (28)$$

with

$$Z_{h'}^* = \begin{cases} Z_{h'}(t_{m-1}) & \text{if } h' = h \\ Z_{h'}(t_m) & \text{if } h' \neq h . \end{cases} \qquad (29)$$

Also when the same components occur in the evaluation function for several different behavioral variables, the statistics in Equation 27 can be used to separate these effects from one another.

Endowment Function Parameters. The endowment functions g are specified in Equations 7 and 8. These functions are effective only for *downward* changes in the tie variables X_{ij} or the behavior variables Z_{hi}. This implies that similar statistics can be used for estimating the parameters in the endowment function, but these should sum only over those indices where X_{ij} or Z_{hi}, respectively, decreases when going from observation $Y(t_{m-1})$ to $Y(t_m)$. A larger endowment value will lead to a smaller tendency to decrease these variables, hence the minus signs in the following definitions of statistics.

For estimating $\gamma_k^{[X]}$, the statistic sums the loss $s_{ijk}^{[X]}$ only over those pairs (i, j) where the tie X_{ij} disappears when going from t_{m-1} to t_m,

$$u_m\big(Y(t_{m-1}), Y(t_m)\big) = \\ -\sum_i \sum_{j\neq i} I\{X_{ij}(t_m) < X_{ij}(t_{m-1})\}\, s_{ijk}^{[X]}\big(Y(t_{m-1})\big). \quad (30)$$

For estimating $\gamma_k^{[Z_h]}$ the statistic sums over the individuals for whom the value of the behavioral variable Z_{hi} decreases in the time period,

$$u_m\big(Y(t_{m-1}), Y(t_m)\big) = \\ -\sum_i I\{Z_{hi}(t_m) < Z_{hi}(t_{m-1})\} \left(s_{ik}^{[Z_h]}\big(Y(t_{m-1})\big) - s_{ik}^{[Z_h]}\big(Y(t_m)\big)\right). \\ (31)$$

3.4.2 Stochastic Approximation

The conditional expectations in the moment Equations 17 and 18 cannot be calculated explicitly except for some trivially simple models. However, the stochastic process can be easily simulated. Therefore, stochastic approximation methods, in particular, versions of the Robbins and Monro (1951) procedure (for recent treatments see, e.g., Pflug, 1996, or Kushner & Yin, 2003) can be used to solve the moment equations.

These methods are stochastic iterative algorithms using provisional values $\hat{\theta}_N$ as tentative approximate solutions of Equation 14. The basic iteration step in such algorithms is

$$\hat{\theta}_{N+1} = \hat{\theta}_N - a_N\, D_0^{-1}\left(U_N - u(y)\right), \quad (32)$$

where U_N is generated according to the probability distribution defined by the parameter value $\hat{\theta}_N$. For a_N, a sequence is used that converges slowly to 0. In principle, the optimal choice of D_0 might depend on the distribution of U_N and could be determined adaptively. However, Polyak (1990) and Ruppert (1988) showed (also see Pflug, 1996, Section 5.1.3, and Kushner & Yin, 2003) that if all eigenvalues of the matrix of partial derivatives in Equation 16 have positive real parts and certain regularity conditions are satisfied, then convergence at an optimal rate can be achieved when D_0 is fixed, for example, the identity matrix, with a_N a sequence of positive numbers converging to 0 at the rate N^{-c}, where $0.5 < c < 1$. To obtain this optimal convergence rate, the solution of Equation 14 must be estimated not by the last value $\hat{\theta}_N$ itself, but by the average of the consecutively generated $\hat{\theta}_N$ values. This algorithm is a Markov chain Monte Carlo algorithm because the iteration rule (Equation 32) indeed defines a Markov chain. The algorithm is further discussed and specified for network dynamics models in Snijders (2001, 2005).

The application to coordinates where the moment equation used is given by Equation 17 follows the general lines, because this equation has the form of Equation 14. For the parameter coordinates where Equation 18 is used, the corresponding coordinate of statistic U_N is defined as follows. For each $m = 2, \ldots, M$, the process $Y(t)$ is simulated starting at time t_{m-1} with the observed value $Y(t_{m-1}) = y(t_{m-1})$, letting time run from t_{m-1} to t_m, for parameter value $\hat{\theta}_N$. The simulated value obtained for time t_m is denoted $Y^{\text{sim}}(t_m)$. The coordinate of U_N then is defined as

$$\sum_{m=2}^{M} u_m\big(y(t_{m-1}), Y^{\text{sim}}(t_m)\big) \tag{33}$$

and its observed outcome $u(y)$ as

$$\sum_{m=2}^{M} u_m\big(y(t_{m-1}), y(t_m)\big). \tag{34}$$

This is precisely in accordance with Equation 18.

The MoM estimator presented in this section is what is called in Snijders (2001) the *unconditional estimator*. The *conditional* MoM estimator is similar except that it conditions on the outcome of exactly one of the sets of $M - 1$ statistics in Equation 19 or 20 ($h = 1, \ldots, H$); and the simulations of the process $Y(t)$ used to generate $Y^{\text{sim}}(t_m)$ start with the value $y(t_{m-1})$ and continue until the first time point where the observed outcome of Equation 19 or 20, respectively, is exactly reproduced. Expressed informally, either the network or one of the behaviors is chosen as the conditioning variable, and the condition consists of the requirement that the simulated "distance" on this variable — defined by Equation 19 for the network and 20 for behavior h — is equal to the observed distance. This is further explained (for network dynamics only) in Snijders (2001, 2005).

3.4.3 Standard Errors

The standard errors are obtained as the square roots of the diagonal elements of the asymptotic covariance matrix in Equation 15.

The two ingredients of Equation 15, the covariance matrix Σ_θ and the partial derivatives matrix D_θ, can be estimated by Monte Carlo methods. Snijders (1996) outlines Monte Carlo integration methods to estimate Σ_θ and Monte Carlo-based finite-difference methods to estimate D_θ.

Schweinberger and Snijders (2006) elaborated an alternative method to estimate D_θ, which is preferable on two grounds: (1) In contrast to the first method it produces unbiased estimates of the partial derivatives, and (2) the computational burden is reduced by the factor $L + 1$ compared to the first method, where L is the dimension of θ. The latter argument is important because in practice, computation time is an important issue, and L is in most applications larger than 5.

3.5 FORWARD MODEL SELECTION

It may be argued that in the present case forward model selection is preferable to backward model selection. One reason is that the time required to estimate these models is linear in L, the number of parameter coordinates. Because computation time is an important practical issue, it is preferable to start with simple models (as in forward model selection) and proceed to more complicated and, in terms of estimation time, more expensive models only when there is empirical evidence against the simple models. A second reason is that the data and model structures under consideration are complicated even in the simplest cases, and thus, starting model selection in high-dimensional parameter spaces (as in backward selection) may invalidate the selection procedure due to convergence problems.

To derive test statistics suitable for forward model selection, the "holy trinity" test statistics, being the Wald, the likelihood ratio, and the Lagrange multiplier / Rao efficient score (RS) tests, are of primary interest. The RS test is a good choice for forward model selection, because only the restricted model needs to be estimated, whereas the other two tests are computationally more expensive.

As the likelihood function is in general intractable (leaving aside some close-to-trivial cases), the RS test cannot readily be derived. Schweinberger (2005) proposed generalized Neyman-Rao score tests which can be based on estimators other than maximum likelihood estimators; in the present case, MoM estimators. Let the L-dimensional parameter vector θ be partitioned according to $(\theta_1', \theta_2')'$, where θ_1 represents nuisance parameters, and θ_2 the parameters of primary interest. Suppose that it is desired to test $H_0 : \theta_2 = 0$ against $H_1 : \theta_2 \neq 0$. (Hypotheses concerning more general functions of θ can be tested in the same way.) A test can be based on the quadratic form statistic

$$b'(\hat{\theta}_0)\,\hat{C}^{-1}\,(\hat{\theta}_0)\,b(\hat{\theta}_0)$$

where $b(\theta)$ is some function of the estimating function $E_\theta u(Y) - u(y)$ (cf. Equation 14), $\hat{\theta}_0$ is a suitable estimator for θ under H_0, and C is the asymptotic covariance matrix of $b(\theta)$. Given some regularity conditions, under H_0 the test statistic is asymptotically chi-square distributed with R degrees of freedom, where R is the dimension of θ_2.

The test statistic is associated with at least two appealing features. First, because θ_0 is estimated under H_0, θ_2 needs not be estimated, and thus only $L - R$ parameters are estimated compared to L under H_1. Second, it turns out (see Schweinberger, 2005) that $b(\hat{\theta}_0)$ is some function of $E_{\hat{\theta}_0} u_2(Y) - u_2(y)$, where the partition $u = (u'_1, u'_2)'$ conforms with the partition of θ. In other words, the test statistic is a function of the statistics corresponding to the tested parameter coordinates. Hence, when the restrictions on θ defining H_0 are valid, the observed values of the statistics corresponding to the restricted parameter coordinates should be close to their expected values; on the other hand, when these restrictions are not valid, the observed value of the statistics should depart from the expected value. Thus, the test statistic has an appealing interpretation in terms of goodness-of-fit.

Model selection may proceed in three main steps.

1. First the network dynamics are considered without taking the behavior into account. In network modelling, it is appealing to start simple and use the dyads $\big(X_{ij}(t), X_{ji}(t)\big)$ as the units of analysis, because many social relations, and in particular friendship and collaboration, have been shown to exhibit strong tendencies toward reciprocity; hence models postulating independent ties processes and thus ignoring reciprocity are hardly tenable. A classical continuous-time Markov model that postulates that the processes shaping the dyads are independent and governed by the same probability law, and at the same time captures reciprocity, is the so-called "reciprocity" model (Leenders, 1995a, 1995b; Snijders, 2005; Wasserman, 1980). The state space of the continuous-time Markov chain for each dyad is given by $\{(0,0), (1,0), (0,1), (1,1)\}$. The infinitesimal generator follows from the transition rates

$$\lambda_{0ij} = \zeta_0 + \mu_0 x_{ji}$$
$$\lambda_{1ij} = \zeta_1 + \mu_1 x_{ji}$$

where λ_{0ij} is the rate of changing $x_{ij} = 0$ into $x_{ij} = 1$, and λ_{1ij} is the rate of changing $x_{ij} = 1$ into $x_{ij} = 0$. The parameters $\zeta_0 > 0$ and $\zeta_1 > 0$ are basic rates governing transitions from 0 to 1 and from 1 to 0, respectively, and μ_0 and μ_1 represent the change in the rate that is due to the other tie being present in the dyad ($x_{ij} = 1$), subject to the constraints $\zeta_0 + \mu_0 > 0$ and $\zeta_1 + \mu_1 > 0$.

It is possible to incorporate covariates into the model that are constant between observation points (Leenders, 1995a).

Before proceeding with actor-driven models, it is meaningful to test the null hypothesis of independent dyad processes. Snijders and van Duijn (1997) showed that there exist parameterizations of the family of stochastic actor-driven models (with network dynamics but without action dynamics) that are equivalent to the reciprocity model. It is possible to extend such model specifications by including triadic dependencies, like the number of transitive triplets, in the evaluation function $f_i^{[X]}$. The resulting models are not equivalent to the reciprocity model any more, and violate the dyad independence (DI) assumption. Let the parameters corresponding to the triadic dependencies be collected in θ_2. Then the DI assumption can be tested by testing the null hypothesis of the reciprocity model extended by suitable covariate effects, and test this as the null hypothesis $H_0 : \theta_2 = 0$ against $H_1 : \theta_2 \neq 0$. Rejection of this null hypothesis would indicate that the DI assumption is indefensible in the light of the observed panel data, and it is an argument for continuing the analysis with actor-driven models.

2. If it is established that dyads do not follow independent processes, the main dependencies between dyad processes should be captured by actor-driven models for the network dynamics along with simple specifications of the behavior dynamics. It is sensible first to specify a model for the network and behavior dynamics that does not contain cross-references in the form of the statistics in Equations 11 and 12, implying independence of the network and behavior dynamics. Once a seemingly adequate specification of the network and behavior dynamics has been found, such a model then can be tested against an alternative that does contain such cross-references and therefore implies dependence between the network and behavior dynamics. For this purpose, again a generalized Neyman-Rao score test can be used.

3. Rejection of this independence hypothesis provides the empirical evidence for continuing the statistical modeling by actor-driven models for joint network and behavioral dynamics as proposed in the preceding sections.

It is often natural to start modeling with a focus on the evaluation functions. Given that seemingly adequate specifications of the evaluation functions have been found, more advanced specifications of the rate functions and endowment functions may be worthwhile to consider, as well as homogeneity tests with respect to nodes and periods (see Schweinberger, 2005).

3.6 EXAMPLE: THE DYNAMICS OF FRIENDSHIP AND ALCOHOL CONSUMPTION

Steglich et al. (2004) investigated the role played by tobacco and alcohol use for the formation of friendship networks, and vice versa — the role played by social network structure in propagating or inhibiting these risk-taking behaviors. In this section, a more restricted example is given of the methods described in the preceding sections using the same data set.

3.6.1 Some Background Theory

Starting with the study of *Elmtown's Youth* by de Belmont Hollingshead (1949), literature on adolescents' health consistently reports that friends tend to behave similarly with respect to health-endangering activities such as smoking, drug use, and alcohol consumption: smokers tend to be friends of smokers, whereas nonsmokers tend to be friends with nonsmokers, and so forth (Cohen, 1977; Kandel, 1978; Newcomb, 1962). In methodological terms, this pattern is known by the name of *network autocorrelation* (Doreian, 1989). These early cross-sectional studies have led to alternative strands of theory explaining the phenomenon. On the one hand, there is the literature on *social influence* processes (Friedkin, 1998, 2001; Homans, 1974; Oetting & Donnermeyer, 1998), arguing that peers condition (or "socialize") each other into compliance with group norms. By this line of reasoning, adolescents will seek to minimize deviance from their friends, and will adapt their own risk-taking behavior accordingly. On the other hand, there is the literature on *social selection* processes (Byrne, 1971; Lazarsfeld & Merton, 1954; McPherson & Smith-Lovin, 1987; McPherson et al., 2001), arguing that peers select each other based on similarity on a range of individual characteristics ("birds of a feather flock together"). By this line of reasoning, adolescents are likely to break their relationships with others who are not like them (e.g., do not drink as much as they do), and seek out new friends who are more similar.

For some time, researchers have been contemplating the question whether selection processes or processes of social influence play a stronger role in the explanation of particular network autocorrelation phenomena (Ennet & Bauman, 1994; Fisher & Bauman, 1988; Haynie, 2001; Kirke, 2004; Leenders, 1995b; Pearson & Michell, 2000; Steglich et al., 2004). This is an important question because its answer is crucial for success or failure of potential intervention strategies.

Research seems to indicate that the prevalence of either process type is domain-specific (cf. the cited references), with alcohol consumption being a domain where both processes occur. In the following exemplary analyses, it is shown how the actor-driven modeling approach previously introduced can be applied to assessing the strength of both selection and influence processes simultaneously, controlling the effects for each other. For a critique of the methods applied in the other studies mentioned, see Steglich et al. (2004).

3.6.2 Data

The data being analyzed were collected as part of the "Teenage Friends and Lifestyle Study." They contain three measurements of the friendship network among 160 students of a school cohort in Glasgow (Scotland), some demographic variables, and self-reported smoke and alcohol consumption (next to other health and lifestyle oriented data not considered here). The measurements were collected in three waves at intervals of one year, starting in 1995 when the pupils were 13 years old and ending in 1997 when they were aged 15. Alcohol consumption was measured by a self-report question on a scale ranging from 1 (never) to 5 (more than once a week). Previous results obtained through these data were reported by Michell and Amos (1997), Pearson and Michell (2000), Pearson and West (2003), and Steglich et al. (2004).

3.6.3 Statistical Analyses

The analyses reported here were run on the subset of 129 pupils that were present at all three measurement points. They follow the principle of forward model selection as outlined in Section 3.5 and use the score tests of Schweinberger (2005).

The first model fitted to the data is a model of dyadic independence ("reciprocity model") extended with some relevant actor characteristics and dyadic covariates. As actor characteristics, main effects of the gender of ego ("sender" of the tie), gender of alter ("receiver" of the tie), alcohol consumption of ego, and alcohol consumption of alter were included. Dyad characteristics included are the similarity effects of gender and alcohol consumption, representing homophily effects in network choices.

The focal interest of this first analysis is whether the fit of this model would benefit from the inclusion of triadic effects — whether a "true" network approach adds to the explanatory power of the analysis. Therefore, the score test was applied to two triadic parameters, each of which implies between-dyad dependence. The tested parameters are the transitivity effect and the number of geodesic distances two effect, described in Section 3.3.

The joint score test statistic for inclusion of the network closure effects was 1035 ($df = 2$), which is highly significant. Tested separately, the statistic for the number of transitive triplets was 29 ($df = 1$, $p < 0.0001$) while for the number of distance 2, the statistic was 1.9 ($df = 1$, $p = 0.17$). (Being based on simulated random samples, these test statistics are not exact, but independent repetitions give qualitatively similar results.) The comparatively high value of the joint test statistic illustrates that the bivariate test for these two effects jointly may have a higher power than the two univariate tests separately.

The significant result gives strong arguments for continuing with models that account for network interdependence. This is achieved by the following actor-driven models.

The second model fitted to the data assumes conditional independence of network dynamics and behavioral dynamics. This model was estimated for the purpose of investigating whether it is warranted to fit models where the dynamics of the friendship network and of alcohol consumption are interdependent.

In the submodel for network dynamics, the covariates included are the same as mentioned for the reciprocity model, except for the effects related to alcohol consumption. In the submodel for behavioral dynamics, only the main effect of gender on alcohol consumption was included, plus an intercept ("tendency") parameter. The effects tested for assessing interdependence of the network and behavior dynamics are effects of alcohol homophily in the network dynamics (a selection effect, corresponding to $s_{i5}^{[X]}$), and assimilation of alcohol consumption to one's friends in the behavioral dynamics (an influence effect, expressed by $s_{i2}^{[Z]}$). In Table 3–1, the estimation results are reported. The p-values given refer to tests based on the t-ratio defined as parameter estimate divided by standard error, testing whether the corresponding parameter differs from zero. Because such a test does not make sense for the rate parameters (the fact that any change has occurred indicates that the rate cannot be zero), these are only given for the parameters in the evaluation function.

TABLE 3–1

Estimates of the Conditional Independence Model

Parameter	Estimate	S.E.	p
X: Network dynamics			
X: outdegree	−2.11	0.08	<0.001
X: reciprocity	2.06	0.09	<0.001
X: transitive triplets	0.17	0.03	<0.001
X: distance-2	−0.80	0.11	<0.001
X: gender homophily	0.82	0.12	<0.001
X: gender ego (F)	0.18	0.09	0.05
X: gender alter (F)	−0.25	0.10	0.02
X: rate period 1	12.46	2.45	
X: rate period 2	9.33	2.66	
Z: Behavior (i.e., alcohol) dynamics			
Z: tendency	0.27	0.06	<0.001
Z: gender (F)	0.08	0.15	0.57
Z: rate period 1	1.36	0.21	
Z: rate period 2	2.18	0.12	

The parameter estimates demonstrate strong tendencies toward reciprocity of choice and toward transitivity (expressed both by a tendency toward transitive triplets and a tendency to have few other actors at a sociometric distance of 2; the latter result differs from that of the score test reported earlier, which is understandable because the tested null hypothesis is quite different). There is a preference for friends of the same sex, and girls tend to be slightly more active in having friends but less popular than boys. The rate parameters show that, whereas friendship dynamics slow down from the first to the second observation year (friendship stabilizes), the dynamics of alcohol consumption speed up. The score test statistic is $\chi^2 = 25.80$ ($df = 2$, $p < 0.001$). This means strong evidence for interdependence of the network and behavior dynamics. Separate score tests give values of $\chi^2 = 9.47$ for the alcohol homophily effect ($p = 0.002$) and $\chi^2 = 12.51$ for the alcohol assimilation effect ($p < 0.001$).

TABLE 3–2

Estimates of the Interdependence Model

Parameter	Estimate	S.E.	p
X: Network dynamics			
X: outdegree	−2.06	0.16	<0.001
X: reciprocity	2.03	0.11	<0.001
X: transitive triplets	0.17	0.04	<0.001
X: distance-2	−0.79	0.10	<0.001
X: gender homophily	0.84	0.11	<0.001
X: gender ego (F)	0.21	0.13	0.11
X: gender alter (F)	−0.24	0.13	0.06
X: alcohol homophily	0.89	0.30	0.003
X: alcohol ego	−0.04	0.05	0.48
X: alcohol alter	0.00	0.05	0.93
X: rate period 1	12.37	3.38	
X: rate period 2	9.22	3.50	
Z: Behavior (i.e., alcohol) dynamics			
Z: tendency	0.33	0.09	<0.001
Z: gender (F)	0.05	0.14	0.73
Z: assimilation	3.91	1.08	<0.001
Z: rate period 1	1.53	0.23	
Z: rate period 2	2.37	0.25	

In the next model, therefore, social selection and social influence effects with respect to alcohol consumption are included; an effect of alcohol homophily (along with main effects of alcohol consumption of ego and of alter) in the network dynamics part of the model, and an effect of assimilation to the network neighbors in the behavioral (alcohol) dynamics part of the model. This allows mutual dependence of the friendship dynamics and the alcohol consumption dynamics. To illustrate the possible use of endowment effects, score tests are used furthermore to test whether making new friends and dropping existing friends is influenced differently by the alcohol consumption of the other persons; and whether assimilation to the alcohol consumption of one's current friends is different when this assimilation means drinking more than when it means drinking less. The former distinction can be made by testing for an endowment effect in the network part of the model related to alcohol homophily. The latter distinction can be made by testing an endowment effect in the behavioral part of the model related to alcohol assimilation. Results of this model are reported in Table 3–2.

What can be seen from these results is that indeed, alcohol consumption influences network dynamics according to homophily patterns ($\hat{\beta}_k^{[X]} = 0.89$, $p = 0.003$). The nonsignificance of the alcohol-ego and alcohol-alter effects shows that there is no evidence for alcohol consumption-related differences in the tendency to have friends, or for a differential popularity depending on alcohol use. There is also evidence for a social influence effect: Alcohol consumption is affected by friends' alcohol consumption according to assimilation patterns ($\hat{\beta}_k^{[Z]} = 3.91$, $p < 0.001$). Tests for endowment effects in the behavior dynamics are currently not implemented in the software. Therefore, no results are given here of tests for the last mentioned endowment effects.

3.7 DISCUSSION

This chapter presents a statistical model for the simultaneous, mutually dependent, dynamics of a relation (or social network) on a given set of social actors, and the behavior of these actors as represented by one or more ordinal categorical variables. Longitudinal observations are assumed to be available at some discrete moments according to a panel design, but the dynamics of the network and behavior are assumed to take place in continuous time, unobserved between the panel waves. The mutual dependence is represented in a relatively simple way by a Markov model, where the state is defined by the network (X) together with the behavior (Z), and where the dynamics are composed of a sequence of microsteps, each microstep consisting of a change in at most one variable X_{ij} or Z_{hi} by one unit. These changes are represented as the consequence of choices by the actors: The model is actor-driven. The dependence between network and behavior is the result of the fact that network and behavior constitute each other's context, where both change endogenously and determine the transition probability distribution.

Statistical models for the dynamics of networks only were reviewed in Snijders (1995, 2005). Although models for simultaneous dynamics of a social network and actor behavior have been discussed in the literature according to various theoretical approaches (some examples are Bala & Goyal, 2000; Carley, 1991; Durlauf & Young, 2001; Ehrhardt, Marsili, & Vega-Redondo, 2005; Latané & Nowak, 1997; Macy, Kitts, Flache, & Benard, 2003; Mark, 1991) this is, to our knowledge, the first model of this kind that can be used for statistical inference. The model proposed here is more flexible than the models proposed in these references, and can represent a wider variety of dynamics, due to the flexibility in specifying the rate, evaluation, and endowment functions. This is required to obtain a good fit between the model and empirical data. The present model is limited by the assumption of an underlying continuous-time Markov process and the other assumptions in Section 3.3 that cut down the coevolution dynamics to the smallest possible microsteps. The proposal to use continuous-time Markov chains for the statistical modeling of network dynamics dates back to Holland and Leinhardt (1977a, 1977b) and Wasserman (1977). In situations where only a few panel observations on an evolving social network are available, a Markov chain model is natural and convenient. Because there is no information on the dynamics in between the panel waves, it seems unfruitful to go very far in specifying quite detailed models for these unobservables. The plausibility of a Markov model is increased by including covariates reflecting relevant characteristics of actors or pairs of actors. An extension is to include nonobserved variables into the state of the process, which can lead to various kinds of hidden Markov models. Extensions of this type, allowing unobserved actor heterogeneity, are currently being investigated by one of us (M.S.). It is also possible to extend the model by relaxing the second to fourth assumptions in Section 3.3, that is, by allowing simultaneous changes in network and behavior, or coordination between actors. Such extensions may be useful in specific applications, where it can be argued how such simultaneous changes or coordination should be modeled.

The results obtained by the application of this model depend on the plausibility and fit of the model. Further work on how to find good specifications of the model will be important; the generalized Neyman-Rao score tests of Schweinberger (2005) can be useful for this purpose. More practical applications and simulation studies of this model, and of its future extensions, are necessary to obtain a good understanding of the type of social situations where it can be fruitfully applied. For such applications, the SIENA program (Snijders, Steglich, Schweinberger, & Huisman, 2005) can be used, which implements the methods presented here.

Next to the method of moments elaborated in this chapter, it will be useful also to have likelihood-based estimation methods. For network dynamics, Bayesian estimation methods were proposed by Koskinen (2004), and further work is under way. The elaboration of maximum likelihood and Bayesian estimation methods for these models will not only increase efficiency in parameter estimation but also yield more insight in the performance of alternative models for this type of longitudinal data.

ACKNOWLEDGMENTS

We thank the Chief Scientist's Office of the Scottish Home and Health Department for permission to use the data of the "Teenage Friends and Lifestyle Study". Research by the second author is supported by the Netherlands Organization for Scientific Research (NWO), grant 401-01-550. Research by the third author is supported by the Netherlands Organization for Scientific Research (NWO), grant 401-01-551.

REFERENCES

Bala, V., & Goyal, S. (2000). A noncooperative model of network formation. *Econometrica, 68,* 1181–1229.

Bauman, K., & Ennett, S. (1996). On the importance of peer influence for adolescent drug use: Commonly neglected considerations. *Addiction, 91,* 185–198.

Bowman, K. O., & Shenton, L. R. (1985). Method of moments. In *Encyclopedia of statistical sciences, vol. 5* (pp. 467–473). New York: Wiley.

Burt, R. (1987). Social contagion and innovation: Cohesion versus structural equivalence. *American Journal of Sociology, 92,* 1287–1335.

Byrne, D. (1971). *The attraction paradigm.* New York: Academic Press.

Carley, K. (1991). A theory of group stability. *American Sociological Review, 56,* 331–354.

Carrington, P. J., Scott, J., & Wasserman, S. (2005). *Models and methods in social network analysis.* New York: Cambridge University Press.

Cohen, J. M. (1977). Sources of peer group homogeneity. *Sociology of Education, 50,* 227–241.

Davis, J. A. (1970). Clustering and hierarchy in interpersonal relations: Testing two theoretical models on 742 sociograms. *American Sociological Review, 35,* 843–852.

de Belmont Hollingshead, A. (1949). *Elmtown's youth: The impact of social classes on adolescents.* New York: Wiley.

Doreian, P. (1989). Two regimes of network autocorrelation. In M. Kochen (Ed.), *The small world* (pp. 280–295). Norwood, N.J.: Ablex.

Doreian, P., & Stokman, F. N. (1997). *Evolution of social networks.* Amsterdam: Gordon and Breach.

Durlauf, S. N., & Young, H. P. (Eds.). (2001). *Social dynamics.* Cambridge, MA: MIT Press.

Ehrhardt, G. C. M. A., Marsili, M., & Vega-Redondo, F. (2005). Emergence and resilience of social networks: A general theoretical framework. *Arxiv preprint physics/0504124.*

Emirbayer, M., & Goodwin, J. (1994). Network analysis, culture, and the problem of agency. *American Journal of Sociology, 99*, 1411–1454.

Ennett, S., & Bauman, K. (1994). The contribution of influence and selection to adolescent peer group homogeneity: The case of adolescent cigarette smoking. *Journal of Personality and Social Psychology, 67*, 653–663.

Fisher, L., & Bauman, K. (1988). Influence and selection in the friend-adolescent relationship: Findings from studies of adolescent smoking and drinking. *Journal of Applied Social Psychology, 18*, 289–314.

Friedkin, N. (1998). *A structural theory of social influence.* Cambridge, UK: Cambridge University Press.

Friedkin, N. (2001). Norm formation in social influence networks. *Social Networks, 23*, 167–189.

Haynie, D. L. (2001). Delinquent peers revisited: Does network structure matter? *American Journal of Sociology, 106*, 1013–1057.

Holland, P. W., & Leinhardt, S. (1977a). Social structure as a network process. *Zeitschrift für Soziologie, 6*, 386–402.

Holland, P. W., & Leinhardt, S. (1977b). A dynamic model for social networks. *Journal of Mathematical Sociology, 5*, 5–20.

Homans, G. C. (1974). *Elementary forms of social behavior.* New York: Harcourt, Brace, & Hollingshead.

Kahneman, D., Knetsch, J., & Thaler, R. (1991). Anomalies: The endowment effect, loss aversion and status quo bias. *Journal of Economic Perspectives, 5*, 193–206.

Kandel, D. B. (1978). Similarity in real-life adolescent friendship pairs. *Journal of Personality and Social Psychology, 36*, 306–312.

Kirke, D. M. (2004). Chain reactions in adolescents' cigarette, alcohol and drug use: Similarity through peer influence or the patterning of ties in peer networks? *Social Networks, 26*, 3–28.

Koskinen, J. (2004). *Essays on bayesian inference for social networks.* Unpublished doctoral dissertation, Department of Statistics, Stockholm University.

Kushner, H. J., & Yin, G. G. (2003). *Stochastic approximation and recursive algorithms and applications* (2nd ed.). New York: Springer.

Latané, B., & Nowak, A. (1997). Self-organizing social systems: Necessary and sufficient conditions for the emergence of clustering, consolidation and continuing diversity. *Progress in Communication Science, 13*, 43–74.

Lazarsfeld, P. F., & Merton, R. K. (1954). Friendship as social process. In M. Berger, T. Abel, & C. Page (Eds.), *Freedom and control in modern society.* New York: Octagon.

Leenders, R. T. A. J. (1995a). Models for network dynamics: A Markovian framework. *Journal of Mathematical Sociology, 20*, 1–21.

Leenders, R. T. A. J. (1995b). *Structure and influence: Statistical models for the dynamics of actor attributes, network structure and their interdependence.* Amsterdam: Thesis Publishers.

Lehmann, E. L. (1999). *Elements of large sample theory.* New York: Springer.

Lindenberg, S. (1993). Framing, empirical evidence and applications. In P. Herder-Dorneich, K.-E. Schenk, & D. Schmidtchen (Eds.), *Jahrbuch für Neue Politische Ökonomie* (pp. 11–38). Tübingen: Mohr (Siebeck).

Macy, M., Kitts, J., Flache, A., & Benard, S. (2003). A Hopfield model of emergent structure. In R. Breiger, K. Carley, & P. Pattison (Eds.), *Dynamic social network modeling and analysis: Workshop summary and papers* (pp. 162–173). Washington, DC: National Academies Press.

Maddala, G. S. (1983). *Limited-dependent and qualitative variables in econometrics* (3rd ed.). Cambridge, UK: Cambridge University Press.

Mark, N. (1991). Beyond individual differences: Social differentiation from first principles. *American Sociological Review, 63,* 309–330.

McFadden, D. (1974). Conditional logit analysis of qualitative choice behavior. In P. Zarembka (Ed.), *Frontiers in econometrics* (pp. 105–142). New York: Academic Press.

McPherson, J. M., & Smith-Lovin, L. (1987). Homophily in voluntary organizations: Status distance and the composition of face-to-face groups. *American Sociological Review, 52,* 370–379.

McPherson, J. M., Smith-Lovin, L., & Cook, J. (2001). Birds of a feather: Homophily in social networks. *Annual Review of Sociology, 27,* 415–444.

Michell, L., & Amos, A. (1997). Girls, pecking order and smoking. *Social Science and Medicine, 44,* 1861–1869.

Newcomb, T. M. (1962). Student peer-group influence. In N. Sanford (Ed.), *The american college: A psychological and social interpretation of the higher learning* (pp. 469–488). New York: Wiley.

Oetting, E. R., & Donnermeyer, J. F. (1998). Primary socialization theory: The etiology of drug use and deviance. I. *Substance Use and Misuse, 33,* 995–1026.

Padgett, J., & Ansell, C. (1993). Robust action and the rise of the Medici, 1400-1434. *American Journal of Sociology, 98,* 1259–1319.

Pahor, M. (2003). *Causes and consequences of companies' activity in ownership network.* Unpublished doctoral dissertation, Faculty of Economics, University of Ljubljana, Slovenia.

Pearson, M., & Michell, L. (2000). Smoke rings: Social network analysis of friendship groups, smoking, and drug-taking. *Drugs: Education, Prevention and Policy, 7,* 21–37.

Pearson, M., & West, P. (2003). Drifting smoke rings: Social network analysis and Markov processes in a longitudinal study of friendship groups and risk-taking. *Connections, 25,* 59–76.

Pflug, G. C. (1996). *Optimization of stochastic models. the interface between simulation and optimization.* Boston: Kluwer Academic.

Polyak, B. T. (1990). New method of stochastic approximation type. *Automation and Remote Control, 51*, 937–946.

Rapoport, A. (1953a). Spread of information through a population with socio-structural bias: II. Various models with partial transitivity. *Bulletin of Mathematical Biophysics, 15*, 535–546.

Rapoport, A. (1953b). Spread of information through a population with socio-structural bias: I. Assumption of transitivity. *Bulletin of Mathematical Biophysics, 15*, 523–533.

Robbins, H., & Monro, S. (1951). A stochastic approximation method. *Annals of Mathematical Statistics, 22*, 400–407.

Ruppert, D. (1988). *Efficient estimation from a slowly convergent Robbins-Monro process* (Tech. Rep.). Cornell University, School of Operations Research and Industrial Engineering, Ithaca, NY.

Sahlins, M. (1972). *Stone age economics.* New York: Aldine De Gruyter.

Schweinberger, M. (2005). *Statistical modeling of digraph panel data: Goodness-of-fit.* Manuscript submitted for publication.

Schweinberger, M., & Snijders, T. A. B. (2005). *Markov models for digraph panel data: Monte Carlo-based derivative estimation.* Manuscript submitted for publication.

Snijders, T. A. B. (1995). Methods for longitudinal social network data. In E. M. Tiit, T. Kollo, & H. Niemi (Eds.), *New trends in probability and statistics, vol. 3: Multivariate statistics and matrices in statistics* (pp. 211–227). Utrecht, The Netherlands: VSP.

Snijders, T. A. B. (1996). Stochastic actor-oriented dynamic network analysis. *Journal of Mathematical Sociology, 21*, 149–172.

Snijders, T. A. B. (2001). The statistical evaluation of social network dynamics. In M. Sobel & M. Becker (Eds.), *Sociological methodology* (pp. 361–395). Boston, MA: Blackwell.

Snijders, T. A. B. (2005). Models for longitudinal network data. In P. J. Carrington, J. Scott, & S. Wasserman (Eds.), *Models and Methods in Social Network Analysis* (pp. 215–247). New York: Cambridge University Press.

Snijders, T. A. B., Steglich, C. E. G., Schweinberger, M., & Huisman, M. (2005). *Manual for Siena version 2.* Groningen. (`http://stat.gamma.rug.nl/snijders/siena.html`)

Snijders, T. A. B., & van Duijn, M. A. J. (1997). Simulation for statistical inference in dynamic network models. In R. Conte, R. Hegselmann, & P. Terna (Eds.), *Simulating Social Phenomena* (pp. 493–512). Berlin: Springer.

Steglich, C. E. G., Snijders, T. A. B., & Pearson, M. (2004). *Dynamic networks and behavior: Separating selection from influence.* Manuscript submitted for publication.

Thaler, R. (1980). Toward a positive theory of consumer choice. *Journal of Economic Behavior and Organization, 1*, 39–60.

Valente, T. (1995). *Network models of the diffusion of innovations.* Cresskill, N.J.: Hampton Press.

Van de Bunt, G. G. (1999). *Friends by choice: An actor-oriented statistical network model for friendship networks through time.* Amsterdam: Thesis Publishers.

Van de Bunt, G. G., Van Duijn, M. A. J., & Snijders, T. A. B. (1999). Friendship networks through time: An actor-oriented statistical network model. *Computational and Mathematical Organization Theory, 5*, 167–192.

Wasserman, S. (1977). *Stochastic models for directed graphs.* Unpublished doctoral dissertation, Harvard University, Boston.

Wasserman, S. (1980). Analyzing social networks as stochastic processes. *Journal of the American Statistical Association, 75*, 280–294.

Wasserman, S., & Faust, K. (1994). *Social network analysis: Methods and applications.* Cambridge, UK: Cambridge University Press.

Chapter 4

Stochastic Differential Equation Models with Sampled Data

Hermann Singer

FernUniversität Hagen, Germany

4.1 INTRODUCTION

4.1.1 Continuous Time Models

Continuous time models coincide with the feeling that time is a continuously flowing quantity without steps. On the other hand, data are mostly available at certain time points, for example, daily, weekly, quarterly, and so forth, or at arbitrary times. Therefore, there has been a tendency to formulate dynamical models in discrete time (times series analysis). Thus, the causal relations are specified between the arbitrary measurement times. Bartlett (1946) argued as follows:

> It will have been apparent that the discrete nature of our obser-
> vations in many economic and other time series does not reflect
> any lack of continuity in the underlying series. Thus theoreti-
> cally it should often prove more fundamental to eliminate this
> imposed artificiality. *An unemployment index does not cease
> to exist between readings, nor does Yule's pendulum cease to
> swing.* [italics added]

Indeed there are many disadvantages of discrete time models. One of the most basic defects is that the dynamics are modeled between the (arbitrarily sampled) measurements and not between the system states. For example, a physical system like a pendulum fulfills a simple linear relation between the state and its velocity change (acceleration), whereas the relation between sampled measurements (e.g., daily) is very complicated and nonlinearly dependent on the parameters (mass, length of the pendulum, etc.) and the sampling interval.

Studies with different sampling intervals cannot be compared, because the causal parameters relate to the chosen interval. Moreover, if the same data set is analyzed with different intervals (select a weekly or monthly data set from daily measurements), one gets estimates corresponding to these intervals, which can be in contradiction. In the sequel, it is shown that the strength and even sign of causal relations depends on the chosen sampling interval, even if the underlying process is the same.

Nevertheless there is a theory that can combine both points of view:

1. A continuous time dynamical model,

2. Discrete time (sampled) measurements.

One attempts to estimate the parameters of the continuous time model from time series or panel measurements. This can be done by computing the conditional probability density between the measurement times. In the linear Gaussian case, only the time-dependent conditional mean and covariance is needed. More generally, in the presence of latent states and errors of measurement, a so-called measurement model can be defined, mapping the continuous time state to observable discrete time data. The corresponding hybrid model is called *continuous-discrete state space model*. It first appeared in engineering (Jazwinski, 1970), but is now well-known in econometrics, sociology, and psychology.

4.1.2 Differential Equations

Mathematically speaking, *differential equations* are the continuous time analog of time series models, that is, the state vector $Y(t)$ is a function of the real parameter t (time) and the desired time function is implicitly given in terms of time derivatives. For example, the simple *growth model*

$$dY(t)/dt = aY(t) \tag{1}$$

states that the time change of $Y(t)$ in the interval $[t, t + dt]$ is proportional to the state at this time point. Examples are the growth of populations or the attenuation of radioactive rays in media ($a < 0$). The solution of Equation 1 with initial condition $Y(t_0)$ is given by

$$Y(t) = \exp[a(t - t_0)]Y(t_0), \tag{2}$$

which can be verified by computing the derivative $dY(t)/dt$. In a social science context, the simple deterministic equation must be extended by a random initial condition $Y(t_0, \omega)$ and stochastic equation errors that model neglected variables and misspecifications in the functional form of the differential equation. A linear specification is given by the *stochastic differential equation* (SDE)

$$dY(t)/dt = aY(t) + g\zeta(t) \qquad (3)$$

where $\zeta(t)$ is a zero mean *Gaussian white noise* process with autocorrelation function $\gamma(t-s) = E[\zeta(t)\zeta(s)] = \delta(t-s)$ (Dirac delta function). This means that the noise process is only autocorrelated for very short time spans. The solution of Equation 3 is given by

$$Y(t) = \exp[a(t - t_0)]Y(t_0) + \int_{t_0}^{t} \exp(a(t-s))g\zeta(s)ds. \qquad (4)$$

Because the continuous time white noise process is a generalized random function (cf. Arnold, 1974, ch. 3), the solution is usually rewritten by the replacement $\zeta(s)ds = dW(s)$, where $W(s)$ is the Wiener process, a continuous, but not differentiable random walk process (cf. Arnold, ch. 4). Thus, in order to avoid derivatives of nondifferentiable processes, one writes symbolically

$$dY(t) \quad = \quad aY(t)dt + gdW(t) \qquad (5)$$

$$Y(t) \quad = \quad \exp[a(t - t_0)]Y(t_0) + \int_{t_0}^{t} \exp[a(t-s)]gdW(s). \qquad (6)$$

and interprets the first equation as an integral equation. This is the so-called *Itô calculus*, which is a well-defined method for the treatment of stochastic differential equations (cf. Arnold, 1974). From the explicit solution (Equation 6), it is seen that the solution process is Gaussian if the initial condition is Gaussian or constant as well.

In the context of parameter estimation, it is helpful to write the solution as a discrete time series (*exact discrete model, EDM*; Bergstrom, 1976, 1988)

$$Y_{i+1} \quad = \quad \exp[a(t_{i+1} - t_i)]Y_i + \int_{t_i}^{t_{i+1}} \exp[a(t_{i+1} - s)]gdW(s), \qquad (7)$$

$Y_i := Y(t_i)$, or more concisely as

$$Y_{i+1} \quad = \quad \Phi(t_{i+1}, t_i)Y_i + u_i, \qquad (8)$$

where Φ is the fundamental matrix (scalar case in Equation 8), but it should be noted that the parameters of the EDM are highly nonlinearly restricted (e.g., $\mathrm{Var}(u_i) = \int \Phi(t_{i+1}, s)^2 g^2 ds$).

This is the main problem for the task of parameter estimation. Software must be able to *implement the required nonlinear restrictions*, especially in the multivariate case where (time ordered) matrix exponentials are involved (some references are Hamerle, Nagl, & Singer, 1991; Hamerle, Singer, & Nagl, 1993; Jones, 1984; Phillips, 1976b; Singer, 1998). The term *time ordered* means, that the matrices $A(t)$ (see Equation 9), which contain the causal effects, do not commute in general, that is, $A(t)A(s) \neq A(s)A(t)$. This is a general property of matrices that must be considered in computing the fundamental matrix and the EDM (Equation 14).

Models with time-varying matrices are of empirical interest, because fluctuating exogenous variables may influence a time invariant system or the system itself changes its dynamics over time. For example, in the context of developmental psychology, the children get older in the course of a longitudinal study, so the causal effects are time dependent (cf. Singer, 1998). Similarly, the factor structure of a depression questionnaire may be time dependent due to the psychological state of the subjects.

4.1.3 Advantages of Differential Equation Models

Although the estimation of differential equations is more difficult than for discrete time models, there are many *advantages* of the approach (cf. Möbus & Nagl, 1983) :

1. The model specification of the system dynamics is independent of the measurement scheme and is given at the process level of the phenomenon (microcausality in the infinitesimal time interval dt).

2. The design of the study is specified by a measurement model, independently of the systems dynamics.

3. Changes of the variables can occur at any time, at and between the measurements. The state is defined for any time point, even if it can't be measured.

4. Extrapolation and interpolation of the data points can be obtained for arbitrary times and is not constrained to the sampling interval of the panel waves.

5. Studies with different or irregular sampling intervals can be compared, because the continuous time structural parameters of the system do not depend on the measurement intervals.

6. Data sets with different sampling intervals can be analyzed together as one vector series.

7. Irregular sampling and missing data are treated in a unified framework. The parameterization is parsimonious, because only the fundamental continuous time parameters must be estimated.

8. Cumulated or integrated data (flow data) can be represented explicitly.

9. Nonlinear transformations of data and variables can be handled by a differential calculus (Itô calculus).

4.2 LINEAR CONTINUOUS-DISCRETE STATE SPACE MODEL

4.2.1 Exact Discrete Model

In order to incorporate higher order derivatives (ARMA models), latent factors and errors of measurement, the *linear continuous/discrete state space model* (Jazwinski, 1970, ch. 7.2)

$$dY(t) = [A(t, \psi)Y(t) + b(t, \psi)]dt + G(t, \psi)dW(t) \qquad (9)$$
$$Z_i = H(t_i, \psi)Y(t_i) + d(t_i, \psi) + \epsilon_i \qquad (10)$$

with random initial condition $Y(t_0) \sim N(\mu, \Sigma)$ is introduced. In the state Equation 9, $W(t)$ denotes an r-dimensional *Wiener process* and the state is described by the p-dimensional state vector $Y(t)$. It fulfills a system of stochastic differential equations in the sense of Itô (cf. Arnold, 1974). The matrix $A : p \times p$ is called drift and $G : p \times r; \Omega = GG'$ is the square root of the diffusion matrix Ω. Furthermore, the vector b models deterministic control variables [stochastic control variables are already included in the model by extending the state vector $Y(t)$)].

In the measurement Equation 10, the measurement error $\epsilon_i \sim N(0, R(t_i, \psi)), R : k \times k$ is discrete time white noise and $H : k \times p$ contains factor loadings.

It should be noted that model Equations 9 and 10 are very general and include continuous time autoregressive integrated moving average (CARIMA) specifications, models with colored noise, regression models with CARMA errors and dynamic factor analysis.

Parametric estimation is based on the u-dimensional parameter vector ψ and the time dependence t also incorporates deterministic regressor variables $x(t)$. Moreover, panel data may be treated by joining a panel index $n, n = 1, \dots, N$ (cf. Singer, 1998). In this case, the system matrices may depend on deterministic regressors $x_n(t)$, that is, $A(t, \psi) \to A(t, x_n(t), \psi) := A_n(t)$, and so forth.

Random effects may be added by specifying $d\pi_n = 0$ in the state equation and by extending the state $Y_n \to \{Y_n, \pi_n\}$. In the panel case, the parameters of the random initial condition $Y_n(t_0) \sim N(\mu(x_n(t_0), \psi), \Sigma(x_n(t_0), \psi))$ can be estimated as well.

Example 1: CAR(2) Model. As mentioned earlier, the state space model is very general and allows the specification of models with higher order deriva-

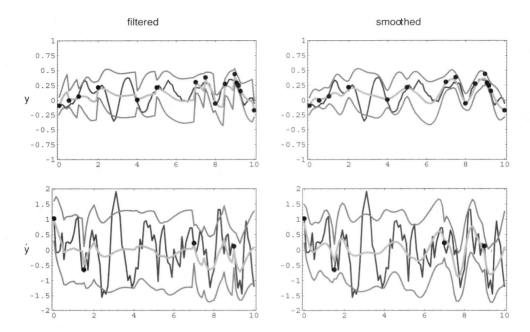

Figure 4–1.   Linear oscillator with irregularly measured states (dots):   Filtered state (left), smoothed state (right) with 95%-HPD confidence intervals.   Measurements at $\tau_1 = \{0, .5, 1, 2, 4, 5, 7, 7.5, 8, 8.5, 9, 9.1, 9.2, 9.3, 10\}$ (first component; 1 st line), $\tau_2 = \{0, 1.5, 7, 9\}$ (2 nd component, 2 nd line).   Discretization interval $\delta t = 0.1$.   The controls $x(t)$ were measured at $\tau_3 = \{0, 1.5, 5.5, 9, 10\}$ (see main text).

tives where only the first component is measured at the sampling times t_i. It should be noted that no approximation whatsoever is involved. For example, the CAR(2) process (pendulum, linear oscillator; γ = friction, $\omega_0 = 2\pi/T_o =$ angular frequency, T_o = period of oscillation)

$$\ddot{y} + \gamma\dot{y} + \omega_0^2 y = bx(t) + g\zeta(t) \qquad (11)$$

with exogenous controls $x(t)$ has state space representation

$$d\begin{bmatrix} y_1(t) \\ y_2(t) \end{bmatrix} := \begin{bmatrix} 0 & 1 \\ -\omega_0^2 & -\gamma \end{bmatrix}\begin{bmatrix} y_1(t) \\ y_2(t) \end{bmatrix}dt + \begin{bmatrix} 0 \\ b \end{bmatrix}x(t)dt + \begin{bmatrix} 0 & 0 \\ 0 & g \end{bmatrix}d\begin{bmatrix} W_1(t) \\ W_2(t) \end{bmatrix}$$

$$(12)$$

$$z_i \quad := \quad \begin{bmatrix} 1 & 0 \end{bmatrix} \begin{bmatrix} y_1(t_i) \\ y_2(t_i) \end{bmatrix} + \epsilon_i \tag{13}$$

and there is *no need to approximate differentials by finite differences*. The unobservable derivative $y_2 = \dot{y}$ is reconstructed by the filter as $E[y_2(t)|Z^T]$ (smoothed, filtered, or predicted state depending on time t; cf. Singer, 1993). Approximating the derivatives by finite differences introduces unnecessary specification error and biased estimates. Figure 4–1 shows the true, filtered and smoothed trajectories of a irregularly sampled oscillator with measurement error $R = \mathrm{diag}(.01, .01)$ (cf. Singer, 1995) and 95% highest probability density (HPD) confidence intervals. Here the second component is measured, but at other time points than the first one. The ML estimates were inserted in the filter. The EDM in this example was formulated on a grid with spacing $\delta t = 0.1$ and all time points are expressed as multiples of this (arbitrary) discretization interval (cf. Section 2.4). Figure 4–2 demonstrates, that the strength and even sign of the discrete time matrices of the EDM may change over time. *Thus, the interpretation of data should rely on the fundamental structural parameters of the SDE and not on the arbitrarily sampled discrete time models.*

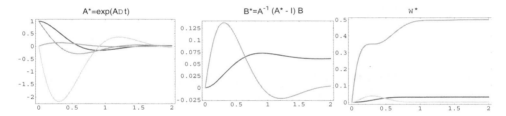

Figure 4–2. Linear oscillator: Exact discrete matrices $A^* = \exp(A\Delta t)$, $B^* = A^- (A^*-I)B$, $\Omega^* = \int_0^{\Delta t} \exp(As)\Omega \exp(A's)ds$ as a function of measurement interval Δt. Note that the discrete time coefficients change their strength and even sign.

The AR(2) model has been used for the sunspot activity (Bartlett, 1946; Singer, 1993), and more recently, for modeling the dynamics of married couples (Boker & Poponak, 2004). In this case, two oscillators (pendulums) are connected by a spring with coupling term $d(y_1 - y_2)$ representing the force.

The state Equation 9 can be solved for the times of measurement $t_i, i = 0, \dots, T$ (*exact discrete model; EDM*)

$$Y(t_{i+1}) \quad = \quad \Phi(t_{i+1}, t_i)Y(t_i) +$$
$$+ \quad \int_{t_i}^{t_{i+1}} \Phi(t_{i+1}, s)b(s)ds + \int_{t_i}^{t_{i+1}} \Phi(t_{i+1}, s)G(s)dW(s) \tag{14}$$

with the parameter functionals (for a proof, see Arnold, 1974)

$$A_i^* := \Phi(t_{i+1}, t_i) = \overleftarrow{T} \exp[\int_{t_i}^{t_{i+1}} A(s)ds] \tag{15}$$

$$b_i^* := \int_{t_i}^{t_{i+1}} \Phi(t_{i+1}, s)b(s)ds \tag{16}$$

where $\overleftarrow{T} A(t)A(s) = A(s)A(t); t < s$ is the Wick time ordering operator (cf. Abrikosov, Gorkov, & Dzyaloshinsky, 1963) and $\Phi(t_{i+1}, t_i)$ is the state transition matrix solving

$$\frac{d}{dt}\Phi(t, t_i) = A(t)\Phi(t, t_i) \tag{17}$$

$$\Phi(t_i, t_i) = I. \tag{18}$$

In shorthand, one obtains the vector autoregression VAR(1) scheme

$$Y_{i+1} = A_i^* Y_i + b_i^* + u_i \tag{19}$$

$$Z_i = H_i Y_i + d_i + \epsilon_i. \tag{20}$$

with covariance matrix

$$\text{Var}(u_i) := \Omega_i^* = \int_{t_i}^{t_{i+1}} \Phi(t_{i+1}, s)G(s)G'(s)\Phi'(t_{i+1}, s)ds. \tag{21}$$

Example 2: Growth Model With Time-Dependent Rates. The time-dependent model of growth rates with constant part

$$A_0 = \begin{bmatrix} \lambda_{11} & \lambda_{12} \\ \lambda_{21} & \lambda_{22} \end{bmatrix} \tag{22}$$

and a linearly changing part (due to development processes)

$$A_1(t) = \begin{bmatrix} \alpha t & 0 \\ 0 & \beta t \end{bmatrix} \tag{23}$$

yields a drift matrix $A(t) = A_0 + A_1(t)$. Because $A(t)$ does not commute with $A(s)$, that is, $A(t)A(s) - A(s)A(t) \neq 0$, the state transition matrix is not simply given by the matrix exponential

$$\Phi(t|t_i) = \exp[\int_{t_i}^{t} A(s)ds] \tag{24}$$

but by the time-ordered expression

$$\Phi(t|t_i) = \overleftarrow{T} \exp[\int_{t_i}^{t} A(s)ds] \tag{25}$$

Using the moment Equations 26 and 27 with a respective numerical approximation (Euler- or higher order Runge-Kutta scheme) automatically produces the time ordered expressions in the Kalman filter or the exact discrete model (Equation 14). This is the crucial step a software package must take in order to implement the correct parameter functionals (for details see Singer, 1998).

4.2.2 Filtering and Likelihood Function

The likelihood function can be computed recursively by means of the *Kalman filter algorithm* (Harvey & Stock, 1985; Jazwinski, 1970, Liptser & Shiryayev, 2001; Singer, 1998). The computation proceeds in steps of time updates and measurement updates involving the conditional moments $\mu(t|t_i) = E[Y(t)|Z^i]$ and $\Sigma(t|t_i) = \mathrm{Var}[Y(t)|Z^i]$, where $Z^i = \{Z_i, \ldots, Z_0\}$ are the measurements up to time t_i. The *time updates* fulfill ($t \in [t_i, t_{i+1}]$)

$$(d/dt)\mu(t|t_i) = A(t,\psi)\mu(t|t_i) + b(t,\psi) \tag{26}$$

$$(d/dt)\Sigma(t|t_i) = A(t,\psi)\Sigma(t|t_i) + \Sigma(t|t_i)A'(t,\psi) + \Omega(t,\psi) \tag{27}$$

where $\Omega(t,\psi) = GG'(t,\psi)$ is the diffusion matrix. Initial conditions are $\mu(t_i|t_i)$ and $\Sigma(t_i|t_i)$ (a posteriori moments at time t_i). The moment Equations 26 and 27 may be solved explicitly. Using the fundamental matrix, one obtains (dropping ψ)

$$
\begin{aligned}
\mu(t_{i+1}|t_i) &= \Phi(t_{i+1},t_i)\mu(t_i|t_i) + \\
&+ \int_{t_i}^{t_{i+1}} \Phi(t_{i+1},s)b(s)ds
\end{aligned}
\tag{28}
$$

$$
\begin{aligned}
\Sigma(t_{i+1}|t_i) &= \Phi(t_{i+1},t_i)\Sigma(t_i|t_i)\Phi'(t_{i+1},t_i) + \\
&+ \int_{t_i}^{t_{i+1}} \Phi(t_{i+1},s)\Omega(s)\Phi'(t_{i+1},s)ds.
\end{aligned}
\tag{29}
$$

These results may be obtained as well by taking the conditional (on Z^i) mean and variance of the EDM (Equation 14).

At the measurement times, the time update (optimal prediction) is corrected by the measurement Z_{i+1} using the Bayes formula leading to the *measurement update*

$$\mu(t_{i+1}|t_{i+1}) = \mu(t_{i+1}|t_i) + K(t_{i+1}|t_i)\nu(t_{i+1}|t_i) \tag{30}$$

$$\Sigma(t_{i+1}|t_{i+1}) = [I - K(t_{i+1}|t_i)H(t_{i+1})]\Sigma(t_{i+1}|t_i) \tag{31}$$

$$\nu(t_{i+1}|t_i) = Z_{i+1} - Z(t_{i+1}|t_i) \tag{32}$$

$$Z(t_{i+1}|t_i) = H(t_{i+1})\mu(t_{i+1}|t_i) + d(t_{i+1}) \tag{33}$$

$$\Gamma(t_{i+1}|t_i) = H(t_{i+1})\Sigma(t_{i+1}|t_i)H'(t_{i+1}) + R(t_{i+1}) \tag{34}$$

$$K(t_{i+1}|t_i) := \Sigma(t_{i+1}|t_i)H'(t_{i+1})\Gamma(t_{i+1}|t_i)^{-1} \tag{35}$$

where $K(t_{i+1}|t_i)$ is the *Kalman gain*, $Z(t_{i+1}|t_i)$ is the optimal predictor of the measurement Z_{i+1}, $\nu(t_{i+1}|t_i)$ is the *prediction error* and $\Gamma(t_{i+1}|t_i)$ is the *prediction error covariance matrix*. Fortunately, the updated state $Y(t_{i+1})|Z^{i+1}$ is again conditionally Gaussian and one can proceed with two conditional moments. After T steps one obtains the likelihood

$$l(\psi; Z) = \log p(Z_T, \ldots, Z_0; \psi) = \sum_{i=0}^{T-1} \log p(Z_{i+1}|Z^i; \psi) p(Z_0), \qquad (36)$$

where the transition densities are given in terms of the Gaussian distribution

$$p(Z_{i+1}|Z^i; \psi) = \phi[\nu(t_{i+1}|t_i); 0, \Gamma(t_{i+1}|t_i)]. \qquad (37)$$

Thus the Kalman filter computes the likelihood recursively in terms of predictions, prediction errors, and their conditional variance (cf. Jazwinski, 1970). The time update is the dynamical prediction starting from the information at time t_i, whereas the measurement update incorporates the new measurement information at t_{i+1}. It has the form of a linear regression model (Equation 30), where the Kalman gain is the regression parameter matrix and the time update is the intercept. This replicates the well-known fact that in a Gaussian system, information is optimally incorporated by a linear regression model. If there are deviations from normality, it is still the best linear estimate (cf. Liptser & Shiryayev, 2001, vol. 2, lemma 14.1).

It may be stated that the *parameter estimation task for the linear state space model can be carried out efficiently by the Kalman filter algorithm*. This works with only one trajectory and/or with panel data. One only has to sum up the N likelihood contributions. References are Jones (1993), Jones and Ackerson (1990), Jones and Boadi-Boateng (1991), Singer (1995, 1998).

4.2.3 Conditionally Gaussian Models

It should be noted that the system matrices may also depend on earlier measurements (i.e. $A(t) = A(t, Z^i), t_i \leq t, H(t_i) = H(t_i, Z^{i-1})$, but the distributions in the filter are still conditionally Gaussian if $Y(t_0)|Z(t_0)$ is such (cf. Liptser & Shiryayev, 2001, ch. 13). Thus, although the latent states $Y(t_i)$ may be non-Gaussian due to the Z-dependence, the conditionally Gaussian filtering scheme is still valid. For example, the diffusion matrix $\Omega(t)$ may contain delayed prediction errors $\Omega[t, \nu(t_i|t_{i-1}), \ldots]$ and thus autoregressive conditional heteroskedasticity (ARCH) effects in a continuous time model.

4.2.4 Computational Aspects and Simplifications

The moment Equations 28 and 29 and the EDM (Equation 14) contain integrals over the fundamental matrix that must be solved numerically. Because the solution

$$\Phi(t_{i+1}, t_i) \quad = \quad \overset{\leftarrow}{T} \exp[\int_{t_i}^{t_{i+1}} A(s)ds] \tag{38}$$

for the fundamental matrix is only formal, one seeks a numerical solution of

$$\frac{d}{dt}\Phi(t, t_i) \quad = \quad A(t)\Phi(t, t_i) \tag{39}$$

$$\Phi(t_i, t_i) \quad = \quad I, \tag{40}$$

for example, the Euler approximation

$$\Phi(\tau_{j+1}, t_i) \quad \approx \quad [I + A(\tau_j)\delta t]\Phi(\tau_j, t_i) \tag{41}$$

$$\tau_j \quad = \quad t_i + j\delta t; j = 0, \dots, J - 1; J = \Delta t_i/\delta t \tag{42}$$

on a fine grid with (arbitrary) spacing $\delta t \to 0$. This expression is analogous to the formula $e^x = \lim_{n\to\infty}(1 + x/n)^n$ and automatically incorporates the time ordering of $A(s)$. More generally, one solves the moment equations (Equations 26–27) by appropriate discrete schemes in the intervals $[t_i, t_{i+1}]$, for example,

$$\mu(\tau_{j+1}|t_i) \quad \approx \quad [I + A(\tau_j)\delta t]\mu(\tau_j|t_i) + b(\tau_j)\delta t \tag{43}$$

or higher order Runge-Kutta schemes. The EDM may be treated analogously.

In many cases, simplified models are sufficient, for example the panel model with constant coefficients (Singer, 1991, 1993)

$$dY_n(t) \quad = \quad [A(\psi)Y_n(t) + B(\psi)x_n(t)]dt + G(\psi)dW_n(t) \tag{44}$$

$$Z_{ni} \quad = \quad H(\psi)Y_n(t_i) + D(\psi)x_n(t_i) + \epsilon_{ni}. \tag{45}$$

Here, the influence of exogenous (control) variables is parameterized by setting $b(t) = Bx_n(t)$. Because $x_n(t)$ is in general only known at times t_i, the parameter functional (Equation 16) can be computed only approximately if $x_n(t_i)$ is interpolated. For example, the EDM is given by the explicit matrices

$$A_i^* \quad = \quad \exp(A\Delta t_i) \tag{46}$$

$$B_i^* \quad = \quad A^{-1}(A_i^* - I)B \tag{47}$$

$$\Omega_i^* \quad = \quad \int_0^{\Delta t_i} \exp(As)\Omega \exp(A's)ds \tag{48}$$

if the control variables are (approximated by) piecewise constant regressors (step functions). Similar, but more complicated formulas may be obtained if the controls are polygonal lines or other approximations between measurements (cf. Hamerle et al., 1993; Phillips, 1976a).

The numerical solution of the moment equations (Equations 26–27) is more convenient, however, because arbitrary interpolations of $x_n(t_i)$ can be used without explicit computation of the EDM (cf. Singer, 1995, 1998). The exogenous variables may even be measured at other times than the endogenous state.

A variant of the EDM is formulated on a fine uniform grid with spacing $\delta t, \tau_j = t_0 + j\delta t; t_i = t_0 + j_i \delta t, i = 0, \ldots, T$, such that all sampling times can be expressed as multiples of this unit. Then, one obtains the EDM scheme

$$Y_{j+1} = A_j^* Y_j + b_j^* + u_j \tag{49}$$

$$Z_j = H_j Y_j + d_j + \epsilon_j. \tag{50}$$

$j = 0, \ldots, j_T - 1; j_T = (t_T - t_0)/\delta t$, with matrices

$$A_j^* := \Phi(\tau_{j+1}, \tau_j) = \overleftarrow{T} \exp\left[\int_{\tau_j}^{\tau_{j+1}} A(s)ds \right] \approx \exp(A_j \delta t) \tag{51}$$

$$b_j^* := \int_{\tau_j}^{\tau_{j+1}} \Phi(\tau_{j+1}, s)b(s)ds \approx b_j \delta t \tag{52}$$

$$\text{Var}(u_j) := \Omega_j^* = \int_{\tau_j}^{\tau_{j+1}} \Phi(\tau_{j+1}, s)\Omega(s)\Phi'(\tau_{j+1}, s)ds \approx \Omega_j \delta t. \tag{53}$$

If the discretization interval δt is short, one can approximate (piecewise constant) $A_j^* \approx \exp(A_j \delta t); A_j = A(\tau_j), b_j^* \approx A_j^{-1}(A_j^* - I)b_j \approx b_j \delta t, \text{row}(\Omega_j^*) \approx L_j^{-1}(A_j^* \otimes A_j^* - I)\text{row}(\Omega_j) \approx \text{row}(\Omega_j)\delta t, L_j = A_j \otimes I + I \otimes A_j$ (cf. Singer, 1995, 1998).[1] Then, the irregular sampling intervals $\Delta t_i = (j_{i+1} - j_i)\delta t$ can be bridged by a missing data treatment if Z_j is not observed (cf. Figure 4–1). In the limit $\delta t \to 0$, one obtains an alternative numerical scheme for the parameter functionals of the irregular EDM (Equations 15 and 16) and/or the conditional moments (Equations 28 and 29). In the case of constant parameter matrices, only one set of EDM matrices must be computed and the exogenous variables $x(t)$ can vary arbitrarily between sampling times.

4.2.5 Estimation with Structural Equations Models (SEM)

The EDM

$$Y_{i+1} = A_i^* Y_i + b_i^* + u_i \tag{54}$$

$$Z_i = H_i Y_i + d_i + \epsilon_i. \tag{55}$$

---

[1]"row" is the rowwise vector operator and $\otimes$ is the Kronecker product.

$i = 0, \ldots, T - 1$ may be represented by the matrix equation (cf. Oud & Jansen, 2000; Oud, van Leeuwe, & Jansen, 1993)

$$\eta = B\eta + \Gamma + \zeta \tag{56}$$

$$Y = \Lambda\eta + \tau + \epsilon \tag{57}$$

where $\eta' = [Y_0', \ldots, Y_T']$ is the sampled trajectory, Γ is a *deterministic* intercept term, $\zeta' = [\zeta_0', u_0', \ldots, u_{T-1}']$ is the vector of process errors,

$$B = \begin{bmatrix} 0 & 0 & 0 & \ldots & 0 \\ A_0^* & 0 & 0 & \ldots & 0 \\ 0 & A_1^* & 0 & \ldots & 0 \\ \vdots & 0 & \ddots & 0 & 0 \\ 0 & 0 & \ldots & A_{T-1}^* & 0 \end{bmatrix} \tag{58}$$

$$\Gamma = \begin{bmatrix} \mu \\ b_0^* \\ b_1^* \\ \vdots \\ b_{T-1}^* \end{bmatrix} \tag{59}$$

$$\mathrm{Var}(\zeta) = \begin{bmatrix} \Sigma & 0 & 0 & \ldots & 0 \\ 0 & \Omega_0^* & 0 & \ldots & 0 \\ 0 & 0 & \Omega_1^* & \ldots & 0 \\ \vdots & 0 & 0 & \ddots & 0 \\ 0 & 0 & \ldots & 0 & \Omega_{T-1}^* \end{bmatrix} \tag{60}$$

are the structural matrices, and

$$\Lambda = \begin{bmatrix} H_0 & 0 & 0 & \ldots & 0 \\ 0 & H_1 & 0 & \ldots & 0 \\ 0 & 0 & H_2 & \ldots & 0 \\ \vdots & 0 & 0 & \ddots & 0 \\ 0 & 0 & \ldots & 0 & H_T \end{bmatrix} \tag{61}$$

$$\tau = \begin{bmatrix} d_0 \\ d_1 \\ d_2 \\ \vdots \\ d_T \end{bmatrix} \tag{62}$$

$$\mathrm{Var}(\epsilon) = \begin{bmatrix} R_0 & 0 & 0 & \ldots & 0 \\ 0 & R_1 & 0 & \ldots & 0 \\ 0 & 0 & R_2 & \ldots & 0 \\ \vdots & \vdots & 0 & \ddots & 0 \\ 0 & 0 & \ldots & 0 & R_T \end{bmatrix} \tag{63}$$

are the factor loading, *deterministic* intercept and error matrices of the measurement model. Solving for η one obtains the solution of the SDE for the time points t_i

$$\eta = (I - B)^{-1}(\Gamma + \zeta). \tag{64}$$

In this equation, the initial condition is represented by $\eta_0 = y(t_0) = \mu + \zeta_0 \sim N(\mu, \Sigma)$. If the matrices do not depend on measurements Z_t, the system is multivariate Gaussian[2] and the log likelihood function is given by (omitting constants)

$$l = -\tfrac{1}{2}(\log |\Sigma_y| + \text{tr}[\Sigma_y^{-1}(Y - \mu_y)(Y - \mu_y)']), \tag{65}$$

where

$$\mu_y = E[Y] = \Lambda(I - B)^{-1}\Gamma + \tau \tag{66}$$

$$\Sigma_y = \text{Var}(Y) = \Lambda(I - B)^{-1}\Sigma_\zeta(I - B)^{-T}\Lambda' + \Sigma_\epsilon. \tag{67}$$

In the panel case, one has N trajectories $Y_n, n = 1, \dots, N$ and the likelihood is given by (assuming $b(t) = b_n(t), d(t) = d_n(t)$)

$$l = -\tfrac{N}{2}(\log |\Sigma_y| + \text{tr}[\Sigma_y^{-1}\tfrac{1}{N}\sum(Y_n - \mu_{yn})(Y_n - \mu_{yn})']). \tag{68}$$

where $\mu_{yn} = E[Y_n] = \Lambda(I - B)^{-1}\Gamma_n + \tau_n$, and $\Gamma_n' = [\mu_n', (b_{0n}^*)', \dots, (b_{T-1,n}^*)'], \tau_n' = [d_{0n}', \dots, d_{T-1,n}'].$[3]

These expressions may again be simplified by

$$b_n(t) = B(t, \psi)x_n(t) \tag{69}$$

$$d_n(t) = D(t, \psi)x_n(t) \tag{70}$$

and stepwise constant controls yielding

$$b_{ni}^* = [\int_{t_i}^{t_{i+1}} \Phi(t_{i+1}, s)B(s, \psi)ds]x_{ni} \tag{71}$$

$$:= B_i^* x_{ni}. \tag{72}$$

In this case, one can factorize $\Gamma_n = \Gamma X_n, \tau_n = \tau X_n$, where

$$X_n = \begin{bmatrix} 1 \\ x_{n0} \\ x_{n1} \\ \vdots \\ x_{nT} \end{bmatrix} : (T+2)q \times 1 \tag{73}$$

---

[2] But cf. Section 4.2.3.
[3] Assuming that the matrices A, G, etc. do not depend on n, but see Section 2.1.

$$\Gamma = \begin{bmatrix} \mu & 0 & 0 & \dots & 0 & 0 \\ 0 & B_0^* & 0 & \dots & 0 & 0 \\ 0 & 0 & B_1^* & \dots & 0 & 0 \\ \vdots & 0 & \ddots & 0 & 0 & 0 \\ 0 & 0 & \dots & 0 & B_{T-1}^* & 0 \end{bmatrix} : (T+1)p \times (T+2)q \quad (74)$$

$$\tau = \begin{bmatrix} 0 & D_0 & 0 & \dots & 0 & 0 \\ 0 & 0 & D_1 & 0 & \dots & 0 \\ 0 & 0 & 0 & D_2 & \dots & 0 \\ 0 & \vdots & 0 & \ddots & 0 & 0 \\ 0 & 0 & 0 & \dots & 0 & D_T \end{bmatrix} : (T+1)k \times (T+2)q. \quad (75)$$

The SEM now reads (X_n are *deterministic* controls) [4]

$$\eta_n = B\eta_n + \Gamma X_n + \zeta_n \quad (76)$$
$$Y_n = \Lambda\eta_n + \tau X_n + \epsilon_n \quad (77)$$

and one can rewrite the likelihood for the N independent panel units in terms of data matrices $Y' = [Y_1, \dots, Y_N] : (T+1)p \times N$, $X' = [X_1, \dots, X_N] : (T+1)k \times N$ as

$$l = -\frac{N}{2}(\log|\Sigma_y| + \text{tr}[\Sigma_y^{-1}(M_y + CM_xC' - M_{yx}C' - CM_{xy})]), \quad (78)$$

where

$$E[Y_n] = [\Lambda(I-B)^{-1}\Gamma + \tau]X_n := CX_n \quad (79)$$

and the moment matrices are $M_y = Y'Y : (T+1)p \times (T+1)p$, $M_x = X'X : (T+2)k \times (T+2)k$, $M_{yx} = Y'X : (T+1)p \times (T+2)k$.

In the case of constant parameter matrices, further simplifications are possible.

Discussion. SEM software must be able to incorporate the nonlinear restrictions as created by the EDM or by the moment Equations 26 and 27. It is very easy to implement the likelihood function (Equation 78) in a matrix language (e.g., Mathematica or SAS/IML) and to write all matrices as nonlinear functions of a parameter vector ψ.

The Kalman filter (KF) and the SEM approach are different in some respects:

1. The KF computes the likelihood recursively for the data $Z = \{Z_0, \dots, Z_T\}$, that is, the conditional distributions $p(Z_{t+1}|Z^t)$ are up-

---

[4]This model was implemented as a Mathematica program, called SEM (Singer, 2004b), and is available from the author.

dated step by step, whereas the SEM representation utilizes the joint distribution of the vector $\{Z_0, \ldots, Z_T\}$.

2. Therefore, the KF can work online, because new data update the conditional moments and the likelihood, whereas the SEM uses the batch of data $Z = \{Z_0, \ldots, Z_T\}$ with dimension $(T+1)k$. The KF only involves the data point $Z_t : k \times 1$ and one has to invert matrices of order $k \times k$ (prediction error covariance). The SEM must invert the matrices $\Sigma_y : (T+1)k \times (T+1)k$ and $B : (T+1)p \times (T+1)p$ in each likelihood computation. This will be a serious problem if long data sets $T > 100$ are analyzed, but not for short panels.

3. The KF also works in the conditionally Gaussian case, because $p(Z_{t+1}|Z^t)$ is still Gaussian, whereas the joint distribution of $Z = \{Z_0, \ldots, Z_T\}$ is not.

4. As a consequence, the KF approach can be easily generalized to nonlinear systems (extended Kalman filter EKF etc.), since the transition probabilites are still approximately conditionally Gaussian (see ch. 3).

5. The SEM approach is more familiar to many scientists used to work with LISREL and other programs. In the early days of SEM modeling, only linear restrictions could be implemented, but now the system (Equations 76–77) and its likelihood (Equation 78) can be easily programmed and maximized using matrix software like Mathematica, SAS/IML.

6. Filtered estimates of the latent states are computed recursively by the KF (the conditional moments), and smoothed trajectories can be computed by a (fixed interval) smoother algorithm. On the other hand, in the SEM approach, one can compute the conditional expectations $E[\eta|Y]$ and $\text{Var}[\eta|Y]$ yielding the smoothed estimates, but again matrices of order $(T+1)k \times (T+1)k$ are involved.

7. Missing data may be treated in both cases by modifying the measurement model. The Kalman filter processes the data $z_n(t_i) : k \times 1$ for each time point and panel unit. Thus, the missing data treatment can be automatically included in the measurement update by dropping missing entries in the matrices. In the SEM approach, the so-called individual likelihood approach may be utilized.

In my opinion, software with a direct implementation of the Kalman filter (KF) is preferable. The KF is the recursive, most direct and efficient implementation of the continuous/discrete state space model.

4.2.6 Other Issues

Flow Data. In economics, many variables (such as gross national product) are cumulated or averaged over a certain period of time. These so-called *flow data* can be naturally modelled by differential equations if additional derivatives are included in the state space model that generate integrated measurements (cf. Bergstrom, 1984; Singer, 1995). Then, the dynamics are between stocks and latent differentiated flows, but only integrated measurements are needed.

Missing Data. Often, *missing data* occur in panel designs or data are measured at *arbitrary frequencies.* Sometimes, one may want combine different time series collected at different frequencies (daily, quarterly, etc.). The continuous-discrete state space model can handle all these cases easily, because the system model proceeds in continuous time but is only measured at certain irregular times t_i. Even different sampling intervals of the panel units and/or exogenous variables are possible. Thus, in principle, one could collect data at arbitrary times (no panel waves; see clinical example Section 4.2.7). Missing data can be treated easily by the Kalman filter measurement update, if missing components are canceled in the respective matrices. In fact, the discrete time measurement of a continuous time model may be viewed as a missing data problem and all nonmeasured states are reconstructed by the filter.

Random Effects. Individual specific random effects π_n can be treated in the state space model by writing ($n = 1, \ldots, N$)

$$d\begin{bmatrix} y_n \\ \pi_n \end{bmatrix} = \begin{bmatrix} A & I \\ 0 & 0 \end{bmatrix}\begin{bmatrix} y_n \\ \pi_n \end{bmatrix} dt + \begin{bmatrix} G \\ 0 \end{bmatrix} dW_n(t) \tag{80}$$

$$z_{ni} = \begin{bmatrix} H & 0 \end{bmatrix}\begin{bmatrix} y_{ni} \\ \pi_{ni} \end{bmatrix} + \epsilon_{ni},$$

From this, one gets estimates of the covariance matrix $\text{Var}(\pi_n)$ of the several unobserved components and is able to specify correlations between initial states and the random effects $\text{Cov}(y_n(t_0), \pi_n)$.

4.2.7 Clinical Application

The differential equation method was applied to clinical data that were collected in a psychiatric hospital at arbitrary time points. [5] The data set contains many behavioral, socioeconomic, and medical variables. Here we choose the three variables $y(t) = \{weight, neuroleptica\ dose, clinical\ impression\}$,

[5] I would like to thank Dr. Matthias Dobmeier, Arbeitsgruppe Psychopharmakologie, Harald Binder, Dipl. Psych., Arbeitsgruppe Versorgungsforschung, Klinik und Poliklinik für Psychiatrie und Psychotherapie der Universitat Regensburg am Bezirksklinikum, Direktor: Prof. Dr. H.E. Klein, for the sampling, preparation, and permission to analyze the data set.

where "clinical impression": 2, ... ,8, is a rating scale with lower values corresponding to a better health state.

The data set is highly irregular, because the number $T + 1$ of measurement times ranges between persons from 2 to 21 time points, and the sampling intervals Δt_i vary from 1 to 1574 days corresponding to 4.31 years (cf. Figures 4–4, 4–5, and 4–6). Moreover, missing values are present in some components of the state vector. Nevertheless, the proposed methodology is able to model and estimate the dynamical connection between the state components $y = \{y_1, y_2, y_3\}$. In a first step, I used a linear SDE of the form of a vector CAR(1) model (the panel index n is dropped)

$$dy(t) = A[y(t) - m]dt + G dW(t) \qquad (81)$$

or explicitly

$$dy_1 = [a_{11}(y_1 - m_1) + a_{12}(y_2 - m_2) + a_{13}(y_3 - m_3)]dt + g_{11}dW_1(t) \quad (82)$$
$$dy_2 = [a_{21}(y_1 - m_1) + a_{22}(y_2 - m_2) + a_{23}(y_3 - m_3)]dt + g_{22}dW_2(t) \quad (83)$$
$$dy_3 = [a_{31}(y_1 - m_1) + a_{32}(y_2 - m_2) + a_{33}(y_3 - m_3)]dt + g_{33}dW_3(t) \quad (84)$$

where $y_1 = $ weight (kg), $y_2 = $ neuroleptica dose (mg), $y_3 = $ clinical impression [2 (better), ... ,8 (worse)]. The parameter vector m can be interpreted as the asymptotic mean value $(t \to \infty)$ of $y(t)$. Using only subjects with at least 2 measurement times a number of $N = 384$ persons was selected and the parameters in $A, m, G, \mu = E[y_{n0}], \Sigma = \mathrm{Var}(y_{n0})$ were estimated with the EDM $[A^* = \exp(A\delta t)$, etc.] and a linearized EDM $(A^* \approx I + A\delta t$, etc.) by using the Kalman filter. Because all sampling times can be expressed as multiples of $\delta t = 1$ day, the exact discrete model is formulated for this discretization interval (cf. Section 2.4).

The model specification is motivated by the fact that the panel is nonstationary, because neuroleptica are known to increase the weight of the subjects. Thus we have an initial level expressed by the parameters μ and Σ and a mean level expressed by m. Indeed, comparing the estimates $\hat{\mu}_1$ and $\hat{m}_1$ we see a mean increase of about 5 kg (over all persons and times). The coefficients a_{ij} are rate constants of the action of variables $i \leftarrow j$, that is, the relative change of variable $dy_i / [(y_j - m_j)dt]$ in a small time interval dt, by keeping the other variables at their mean level m. The action over the interval Δt is given by the regression parameter $A^*(\Delta t) := \exp(A\Delta t)$. Thus, the results of the SDE estimation are independent of any sampling intervals and different persons can be analyzed jointly in a panel. The parameter matrices relate to the fundamental infinitesimal change in the interval dt. In contrast, a discrete time model would have to use many autoregressive and error parameter matrices, each one for the different sampling intervals within and between subjects. Thus, a SDE model is parsimonious, because all measured quantities are expressed in terms of only one set of matrices A, B, Ω.

TABLE 4–1

ML Estimates of the Continuous Time Panel Model Based on the EDM with Variables *Weight*,
Neuroleptica Dose and *Clinical Impression*.

θ	$\hat{\theta}$	Std	t-value	Interpretation
a_{11}	-0.00529433	0.000598578	-8.84483	weight← weight
a_{12}	0.00299021	0.00301962	0.990259	weight← neuroleptica
a_{13}	0.0234382	0.0437436	0.535809	weight← clinical impression
a_{21}	0.00198898	0.00143129	1.38964	neuroleptica← weight
a_{22}	-0.0505835	0.00470394	-10.7534	neuroleptica← neuroleptica
a_{23}	-0.0090749	0.0614409	-0.147701	neuroleptica← clinical imp.
a_{31}	0.00008002	0.000453001	0.176651	clinical impression← weight
a_{32}	0.00167256	0.000670036	2.49623	clinical imp.← neuroleptica
a_{33}	-0.0933535	0.0127247	-7.33641	clinical imp.← clinical imp.
m_1	80.0107	1.50742	53.0779	mean weight
m_2	16.0973	0.36628	43.9481	mean dose
m_3	4.50905	0.0439121	102.684	mean impression
g_{11}	1.72074	0.0497599	34.5808	error weight
g_{22}	2.54972	0.0979298	26.0362	error dose
g_{33}	0.38952	0.0237472	16.4028	error impression
μ_1	75.4199	0.922667	81.7412	initial weight
μ_2	14.8932	0.43461	34.2681	initial dose
μ_3	4.39445	0.0472563	92.9919	initial impression
σ_{11}	283.029	21.9171	12.9136	initial weight variance
σ_{12}	-3.16446	13.6215	-0.2323	initial weight-dose covar.
σ_{13}	0.5679	0.872826	0.6506	initial weight-imp. covar.
σ_{22}	72.533	5.23379	13.8586	initial dose variance
σ_{23}	0.66783	0.452169	1.4769	initial dose-imp. covar.
σ_{33}	0.79420	0.0601353	13.2068	initial dose variance

Results. Table 4–1 shows the ML estimates, asymptotic standard deviations, and t values. Comparing the initial level μ and the asymptotic saturation mean level m, the weight changes from 75.42 to 80.01 kilograms. A Wald test

$$H_0 \quad : \quad R\theta = b \tag{85}$$
$$W \quad = \quad (R\hat{\theta} - b)'(RCR)^{-1}(R\hat{\theta} - b) \sim \chi^2(\text{rank} R), \tag{86}$$

$C = F^{-1}$ (asymptotic covariance of $\hat{\theta}$; F= Fisher information matrix), shows that this difference is significant [$W = 6.62881$, $\chi^2(0.95, 1)$-quantile = 3.84].

Here, the hypothesis matrix is $R = [0, 0, \ldots, 1, 0, \ldots, -1, 0, \ldots, 0]$, where the 1 entries are at columns 10 and 16 (cf. the parameter list in Table 4–1) and $b = 0$.

The neuroleptica dose slightly increases [14.89 to 16.01; $W = 4.49$, $\chi^2(0.95, 1) = 3.84$] and the clinical impression is about the same [4.39 to 4.51; $W = 3.13$, $\chi^2(0.95, 1) = 3.84$]. There is a nonsignificant negative initial covariance $\hat{\sigma}_{12} = -3.16$ between weight and dose, but the action weight← neuroleptica is positive ($\hat{a}_{12} = 0.003$ with t-value of 0.99). The only significant ($\alpha = 5\%$) interaction parameter is $\hat{a}_{32} = 0.0017$ (clinical impression← neuroleptica), which means that higher dose leads to a higher clinical impression score (worse) later. The reverse effect is negative, but nonsignificant (this effect would mean an influence of clinical impression on the medication). The model shows that an initial level μ changes asymptotically to a saturation mean level m with higher weight and slightly higher dose (Figure 4–3), but this effect cannot be significantly explained by the causal action of dose on weight. Figures 4–4 to 4–8 display the filtered and smoothed trajectories of 3 selected persons. At the points of measurement, the extrapolated state $E[y(t)|Z^i], t > t_i$ is corrected by newly incoming information. Between measurements, it tends to the asymptotic mean level m. Figure 4–7 shows the case, when a nonmeasured state component (weight at time $t = 63$ days) is corrected by the other measured states. Finally, the smoothed trajectory $E[y(t)|Z^T]$ uses information from the past and future and yields a smooth interpolation of the data points.

Further analysis of the data would impose restrictions on the parameter matrices followed by a comparision of the models with information criteria like AIC (Akaike's information criterion). Also, higher order derivatives could be added, such as a CAR(2) vector autoregression. Furthermore, using the EKF (cf. Section 3.1), nonlinear specifications could be estimated. However, in contrast to the linear case, an infinity of possible drift and diffusion specifications is conceivable.

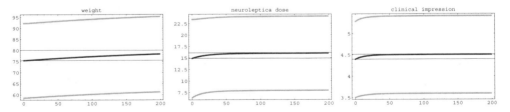

Figure 4–3. Mean level change from initial condition $\hat{\mu}(t_0) = \hat{\mu}$ to $\hat{\mu}(t \to \infty) = \hat{m}$ (interval $t = 0, \ldots, 200$ days). Also shown is the standard deviation std $= \sqrt{\widehat{\text{Var}}(y(t))}$.

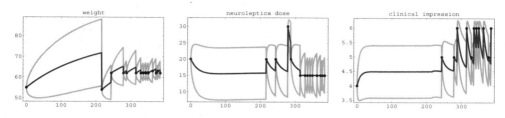

Figure 4–4. Filtered estimates with data points and 67%-HPD confidence intervals. Female with age 49 and ICD 10 diagnosis F20.

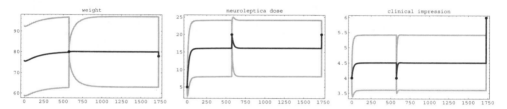

Figure 4–5. Filtered estimates with data points and 67%-HPD confidence intervals. Male, age 28, ICD diagnosis F20.

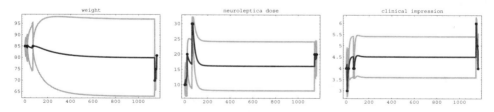

Figure 4–6. Filtered estimates with data points and 67%-HPD confidence intervals. Female, age 48, diagnosis F20.

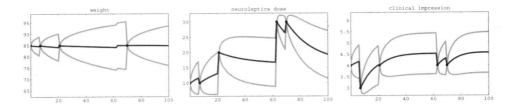

Figure 4–7. Same person, enlarged graph in the interval [0,100]. The weight is missing at time point $t = 63$, but corrected due to the measurements of dose and impression at the same time.

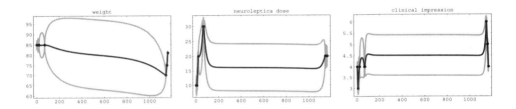

Figure 4–8. Same person. Smoothed estimates with data points and 67%-HPD confidence intervals.

Computational Aspects. The data set was analyzed by using a Mathematica/C-implementation of the SAS/IML package LSDE (Singer, 1991) [6], where each panel unit n can have different sample size T_n. The Mathematica code for the linear drift function $f(y, x, \psi) = Ay + b = A(y - m)$ is similar to Equations 82–84.

```
f[{y1_,y2_,y3_},x_,
   {a11_,a12_,a13_,a21_,a22_,a23_,a31_,a32_,a33_,
     m1_,m2_,m3_,g11_,g22_,g33_,
     mu1_,mu2_,mu3_,s11_,s12_,s13_,s22_,s23_,s33_}]:=

   {a11 (y1-m1) + a12 (y2-m2) + a13 (y3-m3),
```

[6]A new version called SDE (Stochastic Differential Equations) running on Mathematica/C will appear soon. It covers the linear models as well as nonlinear algorithms such as EKF, SNF etc.

```
a21 (y1-m1) + a22 (y2-m2) + a23 (y3-m3),
a31 (y1-m1) + a32 (y2-m2) + a33 (y3-m3)}
```

In the above code, x is the q-vector $x(t)$ of exogenous variables (not used here). One only has to specify the drift $f(y, x, \psi)$, diffusion function $G(x, \psi)$ and the measurement model given by $h(y, x, \psi) = Hy + d$ and $R(x, \psi)$. Also nonlinear specifications are possible (extended Kalman filter EKF; see Section 3.1). The software implements the EDM (Equations 49 and 50). The likelihood for unit n is obtained by the command

```
cEKFEDM[{Z, X}, psi, {{f, A, G, h, H, R, mue, sigma},
        {dt=1, k=3, p=3, q=1, r=3, u=24, T}},
        {miss, option, nonlin, constant}]
```

where $\mathrm{dt} = \delta t$ and $\mathrm{mue} = \mu(x, \psi)$, $\mathrm{sigma} = \Sigma(x, \psi)$ is the initial condition of the Kalman filter. Maximization of the likelihood is obtained by using a quasi-Newton algorithm with numerical derivatives and BFGS secant updates. The asymptotic Fisher information matrix is computed from a numerical Hessian with double sided differences.

4.3 NONLINEAR DIFFERENTIAL EQUATIONS AND STATE SPACE MODELS

Whereas the linear case can be treated completely and efficiently, there are many issues and competing approaches in the nonlinear field. It is presently an area of very active research due to the growing interest in finance models. The option price model of Black and Scholes relies on a SDE model for the underlying stock variable and Merton's (1990) monograph on continuous finance has been given the field a strong "continuous" flavor. This is in contrast to econometrics where still time-series methods dominate and also sociology, despite the old tradition of Coleman (1968) and others.

Here we have the *nonlinear continuous-discrete state space model* (Jazwinski, 1970, ch. 6.2)

$$dY(t) = f(Y(t), t, \psi)dt + g(Y(t), t, \psi)dW(t) \tag{87}$$
$$Z_i = h(Y(t_i), t_i, \psi) + \epsilon_i. \tag{88}$$

with nonlinear drift and diffusion functions f and g. In the nonlinear case, it is especially important to interpret the SDE correctly. We use the Itô interpretation yielding simple moment equations (for a thorough discussion of the system theoretical aspects see Arnold, 1974, ch. 10; Singer, 1999, ch. 3; van Kampen, 1981). A strong simplification occurs when the state is completely measured at times t_i, that is, $Z_i = Y_i = Y(t_i)$. Then, only the transition density $p(y_{i+1}, t_{i+1}|y_i, t_i)$ must be computed in order to obtain the likelihood function. Unfortunately, the transition probability can be computed analytically only in some special cases (including the linear), but in general approximation methods must be employed. Because the transition density fulfills a partial differential equation (PDE), the so-called *Fokker-Planck equation* (cf. Equation 96), approximation methods for the PDE such as *finite difference methods* can be used (cf. Jensen & Poulsen, 2002).

A large class of approximations rests on linearization methods that can be applied to the exact moment equations (*extended Kalman filter* EKF; *second order nonlinear filter* SNF; cf. Jazwinski, 1970 and Section 4.3.1) or directly to the nonlinear differential equation using Itô's lemma (*local linearization* LL; Shoji & Ozaki, 1997, 1998). Because the linearity is only approximate in the vicinity of a measurement or reference trajectory, the conditional Gaussian schemes are valid only for short measurement intervals $t_{i+1} - t_i$. Other linearization methods relate to the diffusion term, but are interpretable in terms of the EKF (Nowman, 1997).

Another class of approximations relates to the filter density. Generally, the filter density may be represented by Gaussian sums (Alspach & Sorensen, 1972). In the *unscented Kalman filter* (UKF; cf. Julier, Uhlmann, & Durrant-White, 2000), the true density is replaced by a singular density with correct first and second moment, whereas the *Gaussian filter* (GF) assumes a normal density. Integrals in the update equations are obtained using Gauss-Hermite quadrature (Ito & Xiong, 2000).

Alternatively, the *Monte Carlo method* can be employed to obtain approximate transition densities (Andersen and Lund, 1997; Elerian, Chib, & Shephard, 2001; Pedersen, 1995; Singer, 2002, 2003).

More recently, *Hermite expansions* of the transition density have been utilized by Ait-Sahalia (2002). In this approach, the expansion coefficients are expressed in terms of conditional moments and computed analytically by using computer algebra programs. The computations comprise the multiple action of the backward operator $L = F^\dagger$ on polynomials [7]. Alternatively, one can use systems of moment differential equations (Section 4.3.2, or Singer, 2004a). It seems that this approach is most efficient both in accuracy and computing time (cf. Ait-Sahalia, 2002, Figure 1; Jensen and Poulsen, 2002).

Nonparametric approaches attempt to estimate the drift function f and the diffusion function Ω without assumptions about a certain functional form. They typically involve kernel density estimates of conditional densities (cf. Bandi & Phillips, 2001). Other approaches utilize Taylor series expansions of the drift function and estimate the derivatives (expansion coefficients) as latent states using the LL method (similarly to the SNF; Shoji, 2002).

---

[7] $L = F^\dagger$ is the adjoint of the Fokker-Planck operator (Equation 99).

4.3.1 Extended Kalman Filter EKF

The continuous-discrete state space model (Equations 87 and 88) may be treated approximately by linearized moment equations, if one computes the exact evolution equations (the dependence on ψ is dropped; $Z^i = \{Z_i, \ldots, Z_0\}$)

$$(d/dt)\mu(t|t_i) \;=\; E[f(Y,t)|Z^i] \tag{89}$$

$$(d/dt)\Sigma(t|t_i) \;=\; E[f(Y,t)(Y(t) - \mu(t|t_i))'|Z^i] +$$
$$E[(Y(t) - \mu(t|t_i))f(Y,t)'|Z^i] + E[\Omega(Y,t)|Z^i]. \tag{90}$$

These are not differential equations, however, because they contain the conditional density $p(y,t|Z^i)$ that is already the complete solution of the filtering problem. Taylor expansion of f up to first order around the conditional mean $\mu(t|t_i) = E[Y(t)|Z^i]$ yields the *continuous-discrete extended Kalman filter* EKF

$$(d/dt)\mu(t|t_i) \;=\; f(\mu(t|t_i), t) \tag{91}$$

$$(d/dt)\Sigma(t|t_i) \;=\; A(t)\Sigma(t|t_i) + \Sigma(t|t_i)A'(t) + \Omega(\mu(t|t_i), t). \tag{92}$$

with Jacobian $A(t) = (\partial f/\partial y)(\mu(t|t_i), t) : p \times p$. In contrast to Equations 89 and 90, the EKF equations are a closed system of differential equations to be solved with standard numerical techniques (Runge-Kutta etc). Second order derivatives lead to the second order nonlinear filter (SNF).

At measurement time t_{i+1}, the output vector h may be expanded around the approximate conditional mean $\mu(t_{i+1}|t_i)$ to yield a locally linear measurement equation

$$Z_{i+1} \;=\; h(\mu(t_{i+1}|t_i), t_{i+1}) + H(t_{i+1}) * (Y_{i+1} - \mu(t_{i+1}|t_i)) + \epsilon_{i+1} \tag{93}$$

$$:= \; H(t_{i+1})Y_{i+1} + d(t_{i+1}) + \epsilon_{i+1} \tag{94}$$

with Jacobian $H(t_{i+1}) = (\partial h/\partial y)(\mu(t_{i+1}|t_i), t_{i+1}) : k \times p$. This permits the usage of the linear *measurement update* Equations 30 to 35. Because we approximate the probability density $p(Z_{i+1}|Z^i; \psi)$ by a Gaussian, we obtain the approximate likelihood function of observation Z_{i+1}

$$p(Z_{i+1}|Z^i; \psi) = \phi(Z_{i+1}; Z(t_{i+1}|t_i), \Gamma(t_{i+1}|t_i)). \tag{95}$$

In the linear case $f(Y, t) = A(t)Y + b(t)$, $g(Y, t) = G(t)$, $h(Y, t) = H(t)Y + d(t)$, the formulas of the KF are recovered. Panel data can be treated by summing the N likelihood contributions and filtered estimates may be computed for each panel unit.

4.3.2 General Nonlinear Filtering Scheme

For large measurement intervals Δt_i or strongly nonlinear systems, the conditionally Gaussian approach (EKF, SNF, or LL) is not sufficient and other approximation methods must be applied. The computation of the a priori density $p(y_{i+1}, t_{i+1}|Z^i)$ requires the solution of the Fokker-Planck equation and the measurement update is the Bayes formula leading to the *general nonlinear filtering scheme* (Jazwinski, 1970, ch. 6.3).

Time Update.

$$\frac{\partial p(y, t|Z^i)}{\partial t} = F(y, t)p(y, t|Z^i) \; ; t \in [t_i, t_{i+1}] \tag{96}$$

$$p(y, t_i|Z^i) := p(y_i|Z^i)$$

$$p(y, t_{i+1}|Z^i) := p(y_{i+1}|Z^i)$$

Measurement Update.

$$p(y_{i+1}|Z^{i+1}) = \frac{p(z_{i+1}|y_{i+1}, Z^i)p(y_{i+1}|Z^i)}{p(z_{i+1}|Z^i)} \tag{97}$$

$$:= p_{i+1|i+1}$$

$$p(z_{i+1}|Z^i) = \int p(z_{i+1}|y_{i+1}, Z^i)p(y_{i+1}|Z^i)dy_{i+1}, \tag{98}$$

$i = 0, \ldots, T - 1$, where F is the Fokker-Planck operator

$$F(y, t)p(y, t|x, s) = -\sum_i \frac{\partial}{\partial y_i}[f_i(y, t)p(y, t|x, s)]$$

$$+ \frac{1}{2}\sum_{ij} \frac{\partial^2}{\partial y_i \partial y_j}[\Omega_{ij}(y, t)p(y, t|x, s)]. \tag{99}$$

The filtering scheme yields a recursive computation of the likelihood function

$$l(\psi; Z) = \sum_{i=0}^{T-1} \log p(Z_{i+1}|Z^i; \psi) + \log p(Z_0; \psi). \tag{100}$$

Although the problem is completely described by the filtering scheme, the computation of the updates is difficult. Some numerical approximations use Monte Carlo integration (Pedersen, 1995; Singer, 2003). Other *simulation-based filtering methods* in discrete time have been used such as Markov chain Monte Carlo (MCMC; Carlin, Polson & Stoffer, 1992; Kim, Shephard, & Chib, 1998), rejection sampling using density estimators (Hürzeler & Künsch, 1998; Tanizaki, 1996; Tanizaki & Mariano, 1995), importance sampling and anti-thetic variables (Durbin & Koopman, 1997, 2000) and recursive bootstrap re-sampling (Gordon, Salmond, & Smith, 1993; Kitagawa, 1996). Moreover, *numerical integration* procedures have been utilized (Kitagawa, 1987).

4.3.3 Filtering Using Hermite Expansions

In the EKF approach, the non-Gaussian transition density $p(y, t|Z^i)$ was approximated by a Gaussian $p(y, t|Z^i) \approx \phi(y; \mu(t|t_i), \Sigma(t|t_i))$ and the conditional moments were obtained as solutions of approximate moment equations. Higher order approximations can be derived if the density is expanded into a Hermite orthogonal series with leading Gaussian term. The first terms in the series read (scalar case)

$$p(y, t|Z^i) \quad := \quad (1/\sigma)\phi(z)[1 + (1/6)\nu_3 H_3(z) + (1/24)(\nu_4 - 3)H_4(z) + ...] \tag{101}$$

where $z = (y - \mu)/\sigma$, and the standardized moments $\nu_k = E[(Y - \mu)^k]/\sigma^k := m_k/\sigma^k$ can be expressed in terms of the *centered moments*

$$m_k := E[M_k] := E[(Y - \mu)^k]; \quad \sigma^2 := m_2; \quad \mu := E[Y]. \tag{102}$$

In the previous expressions, the condition on the measurements Z^i was dropped and $H_n(x)$ are the Hermite polynomials, an orthogonal function system w.r.t the standard normal distribution $\phi(x)$

$$\int_{-\infty}^{\infty} H_n(x)H_m(x)w(x)dx \quad = \quad \delta_{nm}n! \tag{103}$$

The Hermite polynomials $H_n(x)$ are defined by (cf. Courant & Hilbert, 1968, ch. II, 9; Abramowitz & Stegun, 1965, ch. 22)

$$\phi^{(n)}(x) \quad := \quad (d/dx)^n \phi(x) = (-1)^n \phi(x) H_n(x). \tag{104}$$

and are given explicitly by $H_0 = 1, H_1 = x, H_2 = x^2 - 1, H_3 = x^3 - 3x, H_4 = x^4 - 6x^2 + 3$ etc.

Time Update. Between measurements $t_i \leq t < t_{i+1}$, the centered moments fulfill

$$\dot{\mu}(t|t_i) \quad = \quad E[f(Y(t), t)|Z^i] \tag{105}$$

$$\dot{m}_2(t|t_i) \quad = \quad 2E[f(Y(t), t) * (Y(t) - \mu(t|t_i))|Z^i] + \\ + \quad E[\Omega(Y(t), t)|Z^i] \tag{106}$$

$$\dot{m}_k = kE[f(Y, t) * (M_{k-1} - m_{k-1})|Z^i] + \tfrac{1}{2}k(k-1)E[\Omega(Y, t) * M_{k-2}|Z^i] \tag{107}$$

with initial condition $m_k(t_i|t_i) = E[(Y(t_i) - \mu(t_i|t_i))^k|Z^i]$. These moment equations may be obtained by inserting the Fokker-Planck Equation 96 in the time derivatives of the moments m_k. These are not differential equations, however, and Taylor expansion of f and Ω around μ yields

$$\dot{\mu} := \sum_{l=0}^{\infty} f^{(l)}(\mu, t) \frac{m_l}{l!} \tag{108}$$

$$= f(\mu, t) + \tfrac{1}{2} f''(\mu, t) m_2 + \tfrac{1}{6} f'''(\mu, t) m_3 + \dots$$

and $(k \geq 2)$

$$\dot{m}_k = k \sum_{l=1}^{\infty} \frac{f^{(l)}(\mu, t)}{l!} (m_{l+k-1} - m_l m_{k-1}) +$$

$$+ \tfrac{1}{2} k(k-1) \sum_{l=0}^{\infty} \frac{\Omega^{(l)}(\mu, t)}{l!} m_{l+k-2}. \tag{109}$$

Measurement Update. At the next measurement Z_{i+1}, the a priori density $p(y, t_{i+1}|Z^i)$ must be updated according to Equation 97. Because the density is represented in terms of the Hermite series, the likelihood and the a posteriori moments were computed using numerical integration. After the determination of $m_k(t_{i+1}|t_{i+1})$, the next time update is performed.

Example 3: CEV Model with Ordinal Measurements.   The algorithm was implemented in Mathematica (Wolfram, 1999) and tested with a heteroskedastic stock price model. The system model reads

$$dY(t) = rY(t)dt + \sigma Y(t)^{\alpha/2} dW(t), \tag{110}$$

the constant elasticity of variance (CEV) process. It is a generalization of the geometric Brownian motion (GBB) that models random rates of change, that is,

$$dY(t)/dt = [r + \sigma dW(t)/dt]Y(t). \tag{111}$$

This equation can be interpreted as Equation 1 with a stochastic rate $a(t) = r + \sigma dW(t)/dt$. The CEV model yields this as a special case ($\alpha = 2$). The measurement model

$$Z_i = h(Y(t_i)) + \epsilon_i \tag{112}$$

$$h(y) = \theta(y - c_1) + \theta(y - c_2) \tag{113}$$

$$\mathrm{Var}(\epsilon_i) = R \tag{114}$$

gives ordinal measurements ($Z \in \{0, 1, 2\}$) at sampling times t_i ($\theta =$ unit step function). Examples are rating classes for firms or dynamic threshold models in psychometrics. The true parameter values were $\psi = \{r = .1, \alpha =$

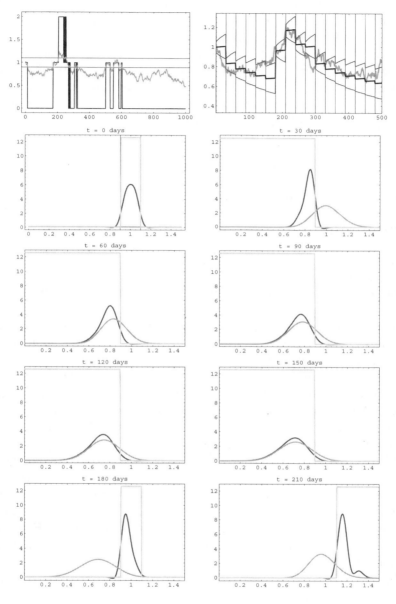

Figure 4–9. CEV model: trajectory $Y(t)$ and ordinal measurements $h(Y(t))$ with threshold values (left above). Filtered estimates with data points and 67%-HPD confidence intervals (right above). Film of a priori (light grey) and a posteriori densities (dark grey) at measurement points. Also shown is the measurement density ($\propto$ indicator function).

$1, \sigma = .2, R = .001, c_1 = .9, c_2 = 1.1\}$ (square root model). Note that the measurement density $p(z|y) = \phi(z; h(y), R)$ is proportional to the indicator function of the interval $h^{-1}(z)$, that is, $\chi_{\{y|z=h(y)\}}(y)$.

Figure 4–9 illustrates the sequence of measurement updates of a non-Gaussian density using the Hermite expansion (Equation 100). The moment equations were solved with $K = 4$ moments and the Taylor expansion was up to order $L = 3$. The unknown moments on the right hand side of Equations 108 and 109 were factorized by the Gaussian assumption

$$m_k = \begin{cases} (k-1)!!m_2^{k/2}; & k > K \quad \text{is even} \\ 0; & k > K \quad \text{is odd} \end{cases} \qquad (115)$$

(for a discussion see Singer, 2004a).

4.4 CONCLUSION

We have shown that the continuous/discrete state space model is a very flexible dynamical specification with many theoretical as well as practical advantages. Completely irregularly sampled data can be analyzed in a parsimonious way by separating the dynamical model from the measurement process. Moreover, the system state is defined for any continuous time point. Models with higher order derivatives, CAR(p), can be estimated efficiently without approximating the derivatives by finite differences.

Clinical survey data with irregular sampling intervals and different sample size for each person including missing values could be easily specified and estimated within the proposed framework. Kalman filter software like LSDE or SEM software with nonlinear parameter restrictions (Mx, SEM etc.) can be used to estimate the exact discrete model.

Whereas the linear continuous/discrete state space model (including conditionally Gaussian models) can be efficiently estimated by the Kalman filter algorithm, the nonlinear case (with and without measurement model) is presently an active field of research with competing methods (both analytical and numerical). The methods of extended Kalman filtering (EKF) and Hermite expansions were shortly discussed. Research is needed especially in the multivariate case.

ACKNOWLEDGMENT

I would like to thank two anonymous referees for their detailed and useful comments that helped to improve the presentation of the chapter.

REFERENCES

Abramowitz, M., & Stegun, I. (1965). *Handbook of mathematical functions.* New York: Dover.

Abrikosov, A. A., Gorkov, L. P., & Dzyaloshinsky, I. E. (1963). *Methods of quantum field theory in statistical physics.* New York: Dover.

Ait-Sahalia, Y. (2002). Maximum likelihood estimation of discretely sampled diffusions: A closed-form approximation approach. *Econometrica, 70,* 223–262.

Alspach, D. L., & Sorenson, H. W. (1972). Nonlinear Bayesian estimation using Gaussian sum approximations. *IEEE Transactions on Automatic Control, 17,* 439–448.

Andersen, T. G., & Lund, J. (1997). Estimating continuous-time stochastic volatility models of the short-term interest rate. *Journal of Econometrics, 77,* 343–377.

Arnold, L. (1974). *Stochastic differential equations.* New York: Wiley.

Bandi, F. M., & Phillips, P. C. B. (2001). *Fully nonparametric estimation of scalar diffusion models.* [Discussion paper 1332]. Cowles Foundation, Yale University.

Bartlett, M. (1946). On the theoretical specification and sampling properties of autocorrelated time-series. *Supplement to the Journal of the Royal Statistical Society, 8,* 27–41.

Bergstrom, A. R. (Ed.). (1976). *Statistical inference in continuous time models.* Amsterdam: North Holland.

Bergstrom, A. R. (1984). Continuous time stochastic models and issues of aggregation over time. In Z. Griliches & M. D. Intriligator (Eds.), *Handbook of Econometrics* (pp. 1145-1212). Amsterdam: North Holland.

Bergstrom. A. R. (1988). The history of continuous-time econometric models. *Econometric Theory, 4,* 365–383.

Boker, S. M., & Poponak, S., (2004). Multivariate multilevel models of dynamical systems using latent differential equations. In C. van Dijkum, J. Blasius, H. Kleijer & B. van Hilten (Eds.), *Recent developments and applications in social research methodology.* Amsterdam: SISWO (CD-ROM, ISBN 90-6706-176-x).

Carlin, B. P., Polson, N. G., & Stoffer, D. S. (1992). A Monte Carlo approach to nonnormal and nonlinear state-space modeling. *Journal of the American Statistical Association, 87,* 493–500.

Coleman, J. S. (1968). The mathematical study of change. In H.M. Blalock & A. B. Blalock (Eds.), *Methodology in social research* (pp. 428–478). New York: McGraw-Hill.

Courant, R., & Hilbert, D. (1968). *Methoden der mathematischen Physik.* Berlin: Springer.

Durbin, J., & Koopman, S. J. (1997). Monte Carlo maximum likelihood estimation for non-Gaussian state space models. *Biometrika, 84,* 669–684.

Durbin, J., & Koopman, S. J. (2000). Time series analysis of non-Gaussian observations based on state space models from both classical and Bayesian perspectives. *Journal of the Royal Statistical Association B, 62,* 3–56.

Elerian, O., Chib, S., & Shephard, N. (2001). Likelihood inference for discretely observed nonlinear diffusions. *Econometrica, 69,* 959–993.

Gordon, N. J., Salmond, D. J., & Smith, A. F. M. (1993). Novel approach to nonlinear/non-Gaussian Bayesian state estimation. *IEEE Transactions on Radar and Signal Processing, 140,* 107–113.

Hamerle, A., Nagl, W., & Singer, H. (1991). Problems with the estimation of stochastic differential equations using structural equations models. *Journal of Mathematical Sociology, 16,* 201–220.

Hamerle, A., Singer, H., & Nagl, W. (1993). Identification and estimation of continuous time dynamic systems with exogenous variables using panel data. *Econometric Theory, 9,* 283–295.

Harvey, A. C. & Stock, J. (1985). The estimation of higher order continuous time autoregressive models. *Econometric Theory, 1,* 97–112.

Hürzeler, M., & Künsch, H. (1998). Monte Carlo approximations for general state-space models. *Journal of Computational and Graphical Statistics, 7,* 175–193.

Ito, K., & Xiong, K. (2000). Gaussian filters for nonlinear filtering problems. *IEEE Transactions on Automatic Control, 45,* 910–927.

Jazwinski, A. H. (1970). *Stochastic processes and filtering theory.* New York: Academic Press.

Jensen, B. & Poulsen, R. (2002). Transition densities of diffusion processes: Numerical comparision of approximation techniques. *Institutional Investor, Summer 2002,* 18–32.

Jones, R. H. (1984). Fitting multivariate models to unequally spaced data. In E. Parzen (Ed.), *Time series analysis of irregularly observed data* (pp. 158–188). New York: Springer.

Jones, R. H. (1993). *Longitudinal data with serial correlation: A state space approach.* New York: Chapman and Hall.

Jones, R. H., & Ackerson, L. M. (1990). Serial correlation in unequally spaced longitudinal data. *Biometrika, 77,* 721–731.

Jones, R. H., & Boadi-Boateng, F. (1991). Unequally spaced longitudinal data with AR(1) serial correlation. *Biometrics, 47,* 161–175.

Julier, S., Uhlmann, J., & Durrant-White, H. F. (2000). A new method for the nonlinear transformation of means and covariances in filters and estimators. *IEEE Transactions on Automatic Control, 45,* 477–482.

Kim, S., Shephard, N., & Chib, S. (1998). Stochastic volatility: Likelihood inference and comparision with ARCH models. *Review of Economic Studies, 45,* 361–393.

Kitagawa, G. (1987). Non-Gaussian state space modeling of nonstationary time series. *Journal of the American Statistical Association, 82,* 1032–1063.

Kitagawa, G. (1996). Monte Carlo filter and smoother for non-Gaussian non-linear state space models. *Journal of Computational and Graphical Statistics, 5,* 1–25.

Liptser, R. S., & Shiryayev, A. N. (2001). *Statistics of random processes* (Vols. 1–2, 2nd ed.). New York: Springer.

Merton, R. C. (1990). *Continuous-time finance.* Cambridge, MA: Blackwell.

Möbus, C., & Nagl, W. (1983). Messung, Analyse und Prognose von Veränderungen [Measurement, analysis, and prediction of change]. In *Hypothesenprüfung, Band 5 der Serie Forschungsmethoden der Psychologie der Enzyklopädie der Psychologie.* Göttingen, Germany: Hogrefe.

Nowman, K. B. (1997). Gaussian estimation of single-factor continuous time models of the term structure of interest rates. *Journal of Finance, 52,* 695–703.

Oud, J. H. L., & Jansen, R. A. R. G. (2000). Continuous time state modeling of panel data by means of SEM. *Psychometrika, 65,* 199-215.

Oud, J. H. L., van Leeuwe, J. F. J., & Jansen, R. A. R. G. (1993). Kalman filtering in discrete and continuous time based on longitudinal LISREL models. In J. H. L. Oud & R. A. W. van Blokland-Vogelesang (Eds.), *Advances in longitudinal and multivariate analysis in the behavioral sciences* (pp. 3–26). Nijmegen, The Netherlands: ITS.

Pedersen, A. R. (1995). A new approach to maximum likelihood estimation for stochastic differential equations based on discrete observations. *Scandinavian Journal of Statistics, 22,* 55–71.

Phillips, P. C. B. (1976a). The estimation of linear stochastic differential equations with exogenous variables. In A. R. Bergstrom (Ed.), *Statistical inference in continuous time models* (pp. 135–173). Amsterdam: North Holland.

Phillips, P. C. B. (1976b). The structural estimation of a stochastic differential equation system. In A. R. Bergstrom (Ed.), *Statistical inference in continuous time models* (pp. 97–122). Amsterdam: North Holland.

Shoji, I. (2002). Nonparametric state estimation of diffusion processes. *Biometrika, 89,* 451–456.

Shoji, I. & Ozaki, T. (1997). Comparative study of estimation methods for continuous time stochastic processes. *Journal of Time Series Analysis, 18,* 485–506.

Shoji, I., & Ozaki, T. (1998). A statistical method of estimation and simulation for systems of stochastic differential equations. *Biometrika, 85,* 240–243.

Singer, H. (1991) *LSDE - A program package for the simulation, graphical display, optimal filtering and maximum likelihood estimation of linear stochastic differential equations, User's guide.* Meersburg: Author.

Singer, H. (1993). Continuous-time dynamical systems with sampled data, errors of measurement and unobserved components. *Journal of Time Series Analysis, 14,* 527–545.

Singer, H. (1995). Analytical score function for irregularly sampled continuous time stochastic processes with control variables and missing values. *Econometric Theory, 11,* 721–735.

Singer, H. (1996). Continuous panel models with time dependent parameters. *Journal of Mathematical Sociology, 23,* 77–98.

Singer, H. (1999). *Finanzmarktökonometrie: Zeitstetige Systeme und ihre Anwendung in Ökonometrie und empirischer Kapitalmarktforschung.* Heidelberg: Physica.

Singer, H. (2002). Parameter estimation of nonlinear stochastic differential equations: Simulated maximum likelihood vs. extended Kalman filter and Itô-Taylor expansion. *Journal of Computational and Graphical Statistics, 11,* 972–995.

Singer, H. (2003). Simulated maximum likelihood in nonlinear continuous-discrete state space models: Importance sampling by approximate smoothing. *Computational Statistics, 18,* 79–106.

Singer, H. (2004a). Moment equations and Hermite expansion for nonlinear stochastic differential equations with application to stock price models. In C. van Dijkum, J. Blasius, H. Kleijer & B. van Hilten (Eds.), *Recent developments and applications in social research methodology.* Amsterdam: SISWO (CD-ROM, ISBN 90-6706-176-x).

Singer, H. (2004b). SEM – Linear structural equations models with arbitrary nonlinear parameter restrictions (Version 0.1). [Mathematica program]. Hagen, Germany: Fernuniversität in Hagen.

Tanizaki, H. (1996). *Nonlinear filters: Estimation and applications* (2nd ed.). Berlin: Springer.

Tanizaki, H. & Mariano, R. S. (1995). Prediction, filtering and smoothing in nonlinear and non-normal cases using Monte-Carlo integration. In H. K. van Dijk, A. Monfort, & B. W. Brown (Eds.), *Econometric inference using simulation techniques* (pp. 245–261). New York: Wiley.

van Kampen, N. G. (1981). Itô vs. Stratonovich. *Journal of Statistical Physics, 24,* 175–187.

Wolfram S. (1999). *The Mathematica Book* (4th ed.). Cambridge, UK: Cambridge University Press.

Chapter 5

Factor Score and Parameter Estimation in Nonlinear Dynamical Systems Models

Sy-Miin Chow

University of Notre Dame

5.1 INTRODUCTION

Dynamical systems models are models used to represent a system's patterns of change over time, more often through a set of differential equations, difference equations, or neural network models (Alligood, Sauer, & Yorke, 1996; Martelli, 1999). In contrast to the widely known growth curve models, which are typically used to represent the levels of a system of variables as a linear, quadratic, or other nonlinear function of time (McArdle & Epstein, 1987; Meredith & Tisak, 1990), dynamical systems models are used to represent *changes* in the variables as functions of previous values of the variables—as opposed to the *levels* of such variables as functions of time as in conventional growth curve models—and how such changes are interrelated. Specifically, in growth curve models, the level of a variable at time t is represented as a function of an intercept and a latent slope times t, but typically not as a function of other possibly time-varying endogenous and/or exogenous variables. In certain special cases, dynamical systems models can be formulated as alternative versions of growth curve models (McArdle & Hamagami, 2001). However, in most other cases, the specific forms of many dynamical systems models deviate substantially from conventional growth curve modeling framework. Thus, by depicting change as a process, dynamical systems models offer a renewed way of conceptualizing intraindividual variability within a process-oriented framework.

Indeed, dynamical systems-related concepts have inspired a myriad of studies in the social and behavioral sciences in the last few decades (e.g., Newell & Molenaar, 1998; Vallacher & Nowak, 1994). Within the methodological realm, for instance, several researchers have continued to develop and further refine methodologies suited for fitting dynamical systems models. More often, such techniques are developed within the more familiar context of structural equation modelling (SEM; e.g., McArdle & Hamagami, 2001; Boker, Neale, & Rausch, 2004; Oud & Jansen, 2000). Yet, with few exceptions (e.g., Molenaar & Raijmakers, 1998; Singer, 2002), most methodologists are still somewhat reluctant to step out of the "comfort zone" grounded on the assumptions of normality and linearity. From polynomial regression to more complex nonlinear models (e.g., Browne & du Toit, 1991; Cobb, 1981), linear models are still the "gold standard" against which the appropriateness of nonlinear models is judged.

In the present context, nonlinear dynamical systems (or dynamic) models are defined specifically as differential/difference equation models that are nonlinear in the variables (e.g., involving multiplicative terms of a system of variables). Other models characterized by linear differential/difference equations are referred to as linear dynamic models, even though their integral solutions can be nonlinear functions (e.g., involving exponential terms), or other nonlinear parameterizations have to be imposed in the model-fitting process (e.g., models considered by McArdle & Hamagami, 2001; Nesselroade & Boker, 1994; Oud & Jansen, 2000). Taken together, the assumptions underlying linear models are well documented and more clearly understood. However, as evidenced in the work of many others, nonlinear dynamic models provide promising theoretical alternatives for conceptualizing more complex changes (e.g., Frederickson & Losada, 2005; Haken, Kelso, & Bunz, 1985; Van Geert, 1998). Unfortunately, such models are rarely evaluated empirically through direct model fitting.

5.1.1 Issues in Fitting Linear and Nonlinear Dynamic Models

Since Coleman (1968), the promises and methodological difficulties involved in fitting linear differential/difference equation models have become relatively well-known issues. In some of the early modelling approaches, reparameterized versions of the integral solutions of a set of differential equations were fitted as linear regression or structural equations models without the appropriate nonlinear constraints (e.g., Arminger, 1986; Hamblin, Hout, Miller, & Pitcher, 1977). As a result, the original differential/difference equations were not uniquely identified by the reparameterized models (Hamerle, Nagl, & Singer, 1990). More recently, Oud and Jansen (2000) illustrated how such nonlinear constraints can be imposed within the SEM context to fit the solution of a continuous-time linear stochastic (i.e., with process noise) differential equation as a discrete-time panel model (see also the related work of Singer, 1993). Still, the primary focus of many researchers is restricted to the special case of linear dynamic modeling techniques.

Much of the work in fitting nonlinear models in psychology was instigated by the work of Kenny and Judd (1984), who highlighted some issues in fitting a specific cross-sectional model with interaction between two latent variables. When such models are fitted in an SEM framework, the latent interaction term has to be identified using product terms derived from multiplying indicators of the individual components. Thus, the dependencies between the linear and nonlinear terms have to be specified analytically as part of the SEM models (see Jöreskog & Yang, 1996). In addition, the usual assumption of normality central to maximum likelihood estimation no longer holds in this case. Even though more practical ways of fitting these models have been proposed in recent years (Klein & Moosbrugger, 2000; McArdle & Ghisletta, 2000; Schumacker & Marcoulides, 1998), psychometricians' widespread interest in nonlinear cross-sectional models such as the Kenny-Judd model has not really generalized to the related case of nonlinear dynamic models. At most, nonlinearity in the form of interactions was examined within the more familiar context of growth curve modeling (e.g., interaction between the latent slopes of two variables; Li, Duncan, & Acock, 2000; Wen, Marsh, & Hau, 2002).

The advent of Markov chain Monte Carlo (MCMC) methods helps resolve much of the aforementioned issues (e.g., Bremer & Kaplan, 2001). This approach was also used by Arminger and Muthén (1998) to fit the Kenny-Judd model. However, MCMC methods require the evaluation of complex numerical integrals in cases involving nonlinear dynamic models, thus rendering them less conducive for handling time series data with a large number of measurement occasions, especially when online estimation is required (Gilks & Berzuini, 2001). Because all Kalman filter techniques—linear and nonlinear alike—are utilized primarily to handle time series data, [1] Kalman filter techniques and other related state-space modeling and particle filter methods have important features that have been adapted to supplement current MCMC methods (e.g., Gilks & Berzuini, 2001).

To add to the repertoire of modelling tools currently available to a broader social/behavioral sciences audience, the purpose of the present chapter is to present and summarize the key aspects of a nonlinear Kalman filter technique known as the unscented Kalman filter (UKF; Julier, Uhlmann, & Durrant-Whyte, 1995). This technique is suited for fitting nonlinear dynamical systems models as well as for estimating longitudinal factor scores. In particular, a chaotic dynamical systems model, the Lorenz system (Lorenz, 1963), is used

---

[1] Note however that a few exceptions do exist in social and behavioral sciences wherein Kalman filter techniques have been adapted for use with panel data (e.g., Oud & Jansen, 2000).

as the basis of several model-fitting examples. In addition, the algorithms presented in the present context are specifically developed for fitting discrete-time nonlinear dynamical systems models (e.g., difference equation models). Thus, I show how a fourth-order numerical integration procedure can be used to approximate a continuous differential equation model as a discrete difference equation model.

In the next sections, the mathematical basis of the linear Kalman filter is first reviewed, followed by a summary of concepts and algorithm underlying the UKF. I then highlight by means of a Monte Carlo simulation the aspects in which the UKF outperforms the extended Kalman filter (Anderson & Moore, 1979; Gelb, 1974), a benchmark nonlinear filter, as a longitudinal factor score estimator. I further explicate the ways in which the UKF can be combined with a maximum likelihood procedure known as prediction error decomposition function (Harvey, 1989; Schweppe, 1965) to yield quasi-maximum likelihood parameter estimates for a subclass of nonlinear dynamic models, and generalization of such procedures from single-subject, time series settings to multiple-subject settings. To conclude, I discuss how such techniques can and have been used as the basis of several modified Gaussian sum filters (Sorensen & Stubberud, 1968) and other related particle filter methods.

5.2 THE LINEAR KALMAN FILTER (KF)

The Kalman filter (KF; Kalman, 1960) is an estimation technique often used to track ongoing (i.e., online) changes in a system of variables (e.g., to track the current position of a vehicle; Gelb, 1974). When no prior information is available, the KF can be conceived as a sequential least-squares approach for estimating longitudinal factor scores (Dolan & Molenaar, 1991; Oud, van den Bercken, & Essers, 1990; Zarchan & Musoff, 2000). In social and behavioral sciences wherein factor score and parameter estimations are often performed after all the data have been collected (i.e., for off-line estimation), the KF is routinely used in conjunction with a maximum likelihood procedure termed prediction error decomposition to estimate parameters for dynamic and time series models (Durbin & Koopman, 2001; Kim & Nelson, 1999; Shumway & Stoffer, 2004). Central to the prediction algorithm of the KF is a state-space model that expresses the dynamic and measurement relations among a system of latent and manifest variables. Formulation of linear state-space models is highlighted next.

5.2.1 Linear State-Space Models

Different researchers diverge slightly on the exact formulation of—or even, what constitutes—state-space models. Here, I refer to state-space models more broadly as a general way of representing the measurement and dynamic relations of a set of latent and manifest variables. My rationale in doing so will become clear as I proceed to the case of nonlinear state-space models. Note that factor scores in the engineering and physical sciences literature are often referred to as latent states. In general, the term states is used to describe the "true scores" or status of a system regardless of the number of indicators used whereas a factor is typically associated with multiple indicators. Here, I use the terms states and factor scores interchangeably regardless of the number of indicators under consideration.

In a linear state-space model, the dynamics of a set of latent variables at time t are represented as

$$\eta_{it} = \alpha_t + B_t\eta_{i,t-1} + \zeta_{it}, \tag{1}$$

and the corresponding measurement model is expressed as

$$y_{it} = \tau_t + \Lambda_t\eta_{it} + \epsilon_{it}, \tag{2}$$

where η_{it} is a vector of length w that represents person i's latent states at time t, apprehended through a $p \times 1$ vector of manifest variables y_t; α_t is $w \times 1$ vector of constants at time t, B_t is a $w \times w$ transition matrix depicting the transition of the system from time t-1 to t, ζ_{it} is a $w \times 1$ vector of residuals or process noise representing uncertainties not accounted for by the assumed model. Λ_t is a $p \times w$ matrix of factor loadings at time t, τ_t is a $p \times 1$ vector of intercepts at time t, and ϵ_{it} is a p-variate vector of measurement errors for person i at time t.

The process and measurement noises (ζ_t and ϵ_t) are assumed to be Gaussian processes that are normally distributed over time and subjects with a mean of zero and covariance matrices Ψ and Θ respectively, represented as

$$\zeta_{it} \sim N(0, \Psi) \text{ and} \tag{3}$$
$$\epsilon_{it} \sim N(0, \Theta). \tag{4}$$

In short, η_t and y_t represent latent variables and noisy observations at time t, respectively. B_t, Λ_t, α_t, τ_t, Ψ, and Θ are either time-varying or time-invariant parameters to be estimated in conjunction with η_t. Equation 1 is thus a very general representation of a one-step-ahead prediction equation for linear processes with auto- and cross-regressions up to an arbitrary order s. A variety of time series, difference and even differential equation models (with appropriate discretization procedures) can thus be formulated and fitted as state-space models in the form of Equations 1–2 (Hamilton, 1994; Harvey, 1989). In some applications, additional exogenous input vectors are incorporated into Equations 1–2 to represent the effects of other external variables on η_t and y_t (Gelb, 1974) but this alternative representation form is not considered here.

5.2.2 Implementation of the KF

After a state-space model has been formulated, the Kalman filter (KF) can then be used to to estimate the current states of a system given information *up to the current time point*. This is known as *filtering*. Estimation of future states with information up to time t is known as *prediction*; estimation of current states given data beyond the current time point (e.g., given data from all time points) is known as *smoothing* (for implementation of the Kalman smoothers see Dolan & Molenaar, 1991; Harvey, 1989; Shumway & Stoffer, 2004). In probabilistic terms, filtering, prediction and smoothing are procedures used to derive the probability density of $p(\eta_t|y_u)$, where $t = u$ in the case of filtering, $t < u$ in smoothing, and $t > u$ in prediction. More details pertaining to various smoothing and prediction procedures can be found elsewhere (Anderson & Moore, 1979; Harvey, 1989; Oud, Jansen, van Leeuwe, Aarnoutse, & Voeten, 1999; Shumway & Stoffer, 2004).

For filtering purposes, the KF is first initiated by setting the states and their associated covariance matrix at time $t = 0$ (i.e., $a_{0|0}$ and $P_{0|0}$, respectively for all persons) to some user-specified (often uninformative) initial conditions (Harvey, 1989). Initial guesses on the parameters are then used to estimate person i's factor scores from time $t = 1$ to T. Specifically, person i's state estimates at time t and the associated covariance matrix are computed as

$$\eta_{i,t|t-1} = \alpha_t + B_t\eta_{i,t-1|t-1} \text{ and} \tag{5}$$
$$P_{t|t-1} = B_tP_{t-1|t-1}B_t' + \Psi, \tag{6}$$

where $\eta_{i,t|t-1}$ is person i's states estimates "projected" forward from time $t-1$ to time t, and $P_{t|t-1}$ is the associated covariance matrix for all persons. Ψ and Θ are process and measurement noise covariance matrices, respectively, as defined in Equations 3–4.

The estimates for η_{it} and P_t at time t are then updated based on manifest information available at time t using a gain function. These updates are defined as

$$K_{t|t} = P_{t|t-1}\Lambda_t'[\Lambda_tP_{t|t-1}\Lambda_t' + \Theta]^{-1}, \tag{7}$$
$$\eta_{i,t|t} = \eta_{i,t|t-1} + K_{t|t}[y_{it} - (\Lambda_t\eta_{i,t|t-1} + \tau_t)], \tag{8}$$
$$P_{t|t} = [I - K_{t|t}\Lambda_t]P_{t|t-1}, \tag{9}$$

where the difference $[y_{it} - (\Lambda\eta_{i,t|t-1} + \tau)]$ shown in Equation 8 is the one-step-ahead prediction error that reflects the discrepancy between predicted and actual measurements at time t. It is sometimes referred to as innovation because it represents the new information available at time t. $K_{t|t}$ is a gain function that determines how heavily the prediction error is weighted in updating the current estimate of η_i for person i. The same projection and update phases are then performed for person $i = 1$ to N. As mentioned earlier, in the absence of prior information, the linear KF is simply a recursive least squares approach. Thus, as demonstrated by several researchers (Dolan & Molenaar, 1991; Otter, 1986; Oud et al., 1990), the KF yields identical factor scores as the regression estimator in the special case of cross-sectional models (i.e., $T = 1$).

5.2.3 Prediction Error Decomposition

Several by-products of the KF from each time point can be used in conjunction with a maximum likelihood (ML) procedure termed *prediction error decomposition* to yield raw data ML estimates of the parameters. More specifically, letting

$$e_{i,t|t-1} = y_{it} - (\Lambda_t\eta_{i,t|t-1} + \tau_t) \text{ and} \tag{10}$$

$$E[(e_{i,t|t-1})(e_{i,t|t-1})'] = Py_t \tag{11}$$
$$= \Lambda_t P_{t|t-1}\Lambda_t' + \Theta \text{ for all persons,} \tag{12}$$

the loglikelihood function can be written as a function of the prediction error, $e_{i,t|t-1}$, and its associated covariance matrix, yielding

$$LL_{KF}(\theta) = \frac{1}{2}\sum_{i=1}^{N}\sum_{t=1}^{T}[-p_{it}log(2\pi) - log(|Py_t|) - (e_{i,t|t-1}')Py_t^{-1}(e_{i,t|t-1})],$$
$$\tag{13}$$

where p_{it} is the number of complete manifest variables at time t for person i. Maximizing Equation 13 with respect to the parameters in Λ, τ, B, α, Ψ, and Θ (collectively represented hereby as a vector θ) results in ML estimates of these parameters. Originally proposed by Schweppe (1965), the specific form of loglikelihood function shown in Equation 13 has come to be known as the prediction error decomposition function (by e.g., Caines & Rissanen, 1974; Harvey, 1989). It is based on the premise that the one-step-ahead prediction errors are normally and independently distributed after all the dynamic and measurement relationships in a system have been accounted for and it is referred to as the innovation form of the likelihood function by Shumway and Stoffer (2004). When all data are available for parameter estimation purposes, the prediction error decomposition procedure outlined earlier is routinely used. When online estimation has to be performed as new data arrive, two KF chains can be executed in parallel to estimate the states and the parameters successively. Alternatively, a joint KF approach wherein the $w \times 1$ vector of latent states is augmented to include unknown parameters to be estimated jointly with the unknown states can be implemented instead.

5.3 NONLINEAR STATE-SPACE MODELS AND FILTERING TECHNIQUES

5.3.1 Extended Kalman Filter (EKF)

Defined more broadly, state-space models can be represented as

$$\eta_{it|t-1} = f(\eta_{i,t-1}, \zeta_{it}) \text{ and} \tag{14}$$
$$y_{it} = h(\eta_{i,t}, \epsilon_{it}), \tag{15}$$

where $f(\eta_{i,t-1}, \zeta_{it})$ and $h(\eta_{it}, \epsilon_{it})$ can be used to depict any linear or nonlinear regression functions for the dynamic and structural models. Distributions of process and measurement noises across time and persons can be non-Gaussian, and the noise terms do not have to manifest additive relationships with the latent states η. Put in a probabilistic framework, Equations 14 and 15 can be expressed even more generally as the conditional prior and posterior density functions [namely, $p(\eta_t|\eta_{t-1}, \theta_t)$ and $p(y_t|\eta_t, \theta_t$, respectively]. The probabilistic representation form is useful when Monte Carlo methods are used e.g., to derive the posterior distributions of latent states and parameters (Kitagawa, 1998).

Because of the nonlinearity in Equations 14–15, the linear KF procedures have to be modified accordingly. For instance, the conditional densities $p(\eta_t|\eta_{t-1}, \theta_t)$ and $p(y_t|\eta_t, \theta_t)$ are only Gaussian distributed in certain special cases. One possible nonlinear extension to the linear KF is the extended Kalman filter (EKF) (Anderson & Moore, 1979; Gelb, 1974). Using this approach, the nonlinear dynamic and measurement functions are linearized locally around the current state estimates, $\eta_{t|t-1}$, by means of a Taylor series expansion. Keeping only the first-order terms gives rise to projection and update equations similar to those used for the linear KF. Specifically, the state estimates from time $t-1$ are first projected forward to time t as

$$\eta_{it|t-1} = f(\eta_{i,t-1}). \tag{16}$$

Predicted observations are obtained as

$$y_{it|t-1} = h(\eta_{it|t-1}). \tag{17}$$

The projected and updated state covariance matrices are then obtained by replacing B_t and Λ in Equations 6, 7, and 9 with the Jacobian matrices F_{it} and H_{it} written as

$$F_{it} = \frac{\partial f(\eta_{it})}{\partial \eta_{it}}\Big|_{\eta_{i,t-1|t-1}} \text{ and} \tag{18}$$

$$H_{it} = \frac{\partial h(\eta_{it})}{\partial \eta_{it}}\Big|_{\eta_{i,t|t-1}}, \tag{19}$$

where the jth row and kth column of F_{it} carries the partial derivative of the jth dynamic function with respect to the kth latent variable, evaluated at subject i's posterior state estimates from time $t - 1$, $\eta_{i,t-1|t-1}$. By the same token, the jth colum and kth row of H_{it} carries the partial derivative of the jth measurement function with respect to the kth latent variable, evaluated at subject i's prior state estimates at time t, $\eta_{i,t|t-1}$.[2] If process and measurement noises are also functions of the latent states, then Jacobian matrices composed of partial derivatives of these functions with respect to the latent states have to be provided as well.

Stated differently, the EKF approximates the possibly non-Gaussian $p(\eta_t|\eta_{t-1}, \theta_t)$ and $p(y_t|\eta_t, \theta_t)$ by means of single Gaussian distributions that are only accurate up to the first order. Thus, in cases involving high nonlinearity or if the sampling interval between two successive measurements is large, this approximation is no longer adequate and the resultant mean and in particular, the covariance estimates are biased. In such cases, higher order EKF will have to be used at the expense of substantially higher computational time (Gelb, 1974; Julier & Uhlmann, 2002). The need to provide the first- and possibly higher order Jacobian matrices also limits the class of state-space models to which the EKF can be applied (i.e., functions that are differentiable up to the appropriate orders with respect to the states). However, the intuitive appeal of the EKF and its straightforward relatedness to the linear KF remain important strengths from an implementation standpoint. Thus, it often forms the basis of other add-on algorithms to collectively constitute newer, more robust filtering or smoother techniques. For instance, the now-classic Gaussian sum filter is formulated based on executing multiple chains of EKF in parallel, the output

---

[2]The subject index in F_{it} and H_{it} is used to indicate that the associated Jacobian matrices have different numerical values because they are evaluated at each subject's respective current state estimates, not that the dynamic or measurement functions are subject dependent.

of which is used to form mixtures of Gaussian distributions to approximate $p(\eta_t|\eta_{t-1}, \theta_t)$ and $p(y_t|\eta_t, \theta_t)$ (Anderson & Moore, 1979).

5.3.2 Unscented Kalman Filter (UKF)

The unscented Kalman filter proposed by Julier et al. (1995) capitalizes on repeated applications of a transformation technique known as unscented transformation to generate expected means and variances for nonlinear state-space models. For each measurement occasion t, a set of deterministically selected points, termed *sigma points*, is used to approximate $p(\eta_t|\eta_{t-1}, \theta_t)$ and $p(y_t|\eta_t, \theta_t)$. Then, the means and variances of $p(\eta_t|\eta_{t-1}, \theta_t)$ and $p(y_t|\eta_t, \theta_t)$ (i.e., $\eta_{t|t-1}, P_{t|t-1}, \eta_{t|t}$ and $P_{t|t}$) are computed as weighted regression functions of these sigma points (Lefebvre, Bruyninckx, & Schutter, 2002). The UKF differs from Monte-Carlo based particle filter techniques in that the sigma points used for approximation purposes are constructed using the minimum possible set of points selected using a deterministic scheme. Unlike the EKF, however, the UKF does not require the derivation of analytical derivatives and it was specifically designed to capture the means as well as variances of the prior and posterior densities. In other words, the UKF is comparable to a second-order EKF with regard to computational accuracy, but at a much reduced computational cost (Julier & Uhlmann, 2002; Wan & Nelson, 2001). The additional scaling constants proposed later by Julier and Uhlmann (2002) can also be used to accommodate slight deviations from normality—namely, to reconstruct symmetric densities with higher or smaller kurtosis (i.e., with fatter or longer tails) than a Gaussian distribution. For ease of presentation, subject index i is omitted from the following presentation but note that the focus is still on the general case wherein parameters are allowed to be time-varying but invariant across subjects, and states are allowed to vary over time as well as over subjects.

Here, the UKF algorithm is outlined in relation to a computationally simpler subclass of state-space models with additive process and measurement noises also assumed in the case of the EKF. In cases with nonadditive noises (e.g., if the noise terms actually appear as part of $f[.]$ or $h[.]$), additional sigma points will have to be used to approximate the distributions around the current noise estimates.[3] The model under consideration is expressed as

$$\eta_{t|t-1} = f(\eta_{t-1}) + \zeta_t \text{ and} \qquad (20)$$
$$y_t = h(\eta_t) + \epsilon_t. \qquad (21)$$

---

[3]In models with additive noises, the number (and thus computational costs) of the sigma points is reduced substantially. Algorithms associated with the more general case of non-additive noises can be found in Julier and Uhlmann (2002) and Wan and Van der Merwe (2001).

State prediction and update are accomplished in five major steps as follows (Julier & Uhlmann, 2002; Wan & Van der Merwe, 2001).

● *Step 1. Selecting Sigma Points.* Given a $w \times 1$ vector of latent states, a set of $2w + 1$ sigma points is selected as

$$\chi_{0,t-1} = \eta_{t-1|t-1}, \tag{22}$$

$$\chi_{k,t-1} = \eta_{t-1|t-1} + [\sqrt{(w+\lambda)P_{t-1|t-1}}], k = 1, \ldots, w \tag{23}$$

$$\chi_{k,t-1} = \eta_{t-1|t-1} - [\sqrt{(w+\lambda)P_{t-1|t-1}}], k = w+1, \ldots, 2w, \tag{24}$$

where w is again the dimension of η.[4] The term λ is a scaling constant composed of two user-specified constants, written as

$$\lambda = \alpha^2(w + \kappa) - w. \tag{25}$$

The constant α is a value between 0 and 1 that determines the spread of the sigma points away from $\eta_{t-1|t-1}$. Typically, α is set to a small positive value. κ is a positive constant used to scale the kurtosis of the sigma point distribution when desired. In practice, the value of κ is not critical and it is usually set to 0, or to 3 - w to ensure that the kurtosis of the sigma point distribution agrees with the kurtosis of a Gaussian distribution (Julier & Uhlmann, 2002; Wan & Van der Merwe, 2001).

● *Step 2. Nonlinear Transformation of Sigma Points through Dynamic Function.* After these sigma points have been selected, each of them is propagated forward in time through the dynamic equation as

$$\chi*_{k,t|t-1} = f(\chi_{k,t-1}). \tag{26}$$

● *Step 3. Compute Prior State and Covariance Estimates for Latent States.* Prior state estimates (i.e., $\eta_{t|t-1}$) and covariance estimates (i.e., $P_{t|t-1}$) at time t are approximated by the weighted mean and variance of the transformed sigma points. Defining a set of weights for the sigma points as

---

[4]Note that the sigma-point index k goes from $1 \ldots w$, and $w+1 \ldots 2w$ to emphasize that half of the sigma points are placed to the left of the previous estimate $\eta_{t-1|t-1}$, and the other half to its right.

$$W_0^{(c)} = \frac{\lambda}{w + \lambda} + 1 - \alpha^2 + \beta \text{ for } k = 0, \tag{27}$$

$$W_0^{(m)} = \frac{\lambda}{w + \lambda}, \text{ for } k = 0 \text{ and} \tag{28}$$

$$W_k^{(c)} = W_k^{(m)} = \frac{1}{2(w + \lambda)} \text{ for } k > 0. \tag{29}$$

The prior state and covariance estimates are then computed using the sigma points and their associated weights as

$$\eta_{t|t-1} = \sum_{k=0}^{2w} W_k^{(m)} \chi *_{k,t|t-1} \text{ and} \tag{30}$$

$$P_{t|t-1} = W_k^{(c)} [(\chi_{k,t|t-1} - \eta_{t|t-1})(\chi *_{k,t|t-1} - \eta_{t|t-1})' + \Psi], \tag{31}$$

where β is another scaling constant used to incorporate prior knowledge of the distribution of η in the state prediction and update. For Gaussian distributions, $\beta = 2$ is optimal (c.f., Van der Merwe, Doucet, Freitas, & Wan, 2000). In short, the prior state estimates $\eta_{t|t-1}$ are derived from a weighted mean of the sigma points from step 2, and the prior covariance matrix $P_{t|t-1}$ is estimated as the weighted sum of the squared distances of all the sigma points from $\eta_{t|t-1}$.

• *Step 4. Transformation of Sigma Points through Measurement Function.* In a similar way, the manifest observations are predicted by subjecting the sigma points to the transformation dictated by the measurement function. More specifically, the predicted measurements and their estimated covariance matrix are generated by first augmenting the prior state sigma-point set (i.e., $\chi *_{k,t|t-1}$) to include the uncertainty constituted by the process noise as

$$\chi_{k,t|t-1} = [\chi *_{k,t|t-1} ; \chi *_{k,t|t-1} + \lambda\sqrt{\Psi}; \chi *_{k,t|t-1} - \lambda\sqrt{\Psi}], \tag{32}$$

and subsequently projecting the new sigma-point set, $\chi_{k,t|t-1}$, through the measurement function as

$$Y_{k,t|t-1} = h(\chi_{k,t|t-1}). \tag{33}$$

Because of the additive process noise, the uncertainty constituted by the process noise (i.e., Ψ) can be temporarily "dissociated" from the dynamic process and added *after* the transformation $f[.]$ in Equation 32. Otherwise, sigma points constructed around the current process noise estimates will have to be propagated through $f[.]$ with the state sigma points (i.e., $\chi_{k,t-1}$ in Equation

26) in step 2 as well. Next, predicted observations and the associated variance and covariance matrices are computed as

$$y_{t|t-1} = \sum_{k=0}^{2w} W_k^{(m)} Y_{k,t|t-1}, \tag{34}$$

$$Py_t = \sum_{k=0}^{2w} W_k^{(c)} [(Y_{k,t|t-1} - y_{t|t-1})(Y_{k,t|t-1} - y_{t|t-1})'] + \Theta \tag{35}$$

$$P\eta_t, y_t = \sum_{k=0}^{2w} W_k^{(c)} [(\chi_{k,t|t-1} - \eta_{t|t-1})(Y_{k,t|t-1} - y_{t|t-1})']. \tag{36}$$

By the same rationale, the additive measurement noise can also be temporarily dissociated from the measurement function and Θ is then added independently of the transformation $h[.]$ in Equation 35.

• *Step 5. Defining and Executing the Kalman Filter Function.* With output from step 4, actual observations are finally brought in and the discrepancy between model prediction and actual observations (i.e., the one-step ahead prediction error) is weighted by a Kalman gain function to yield posterior state and covariance estimates as

$$K_{t|t} = P\eta_t, y_t Py_t^{-1}, \tag{37}$$

$$\eta_{t|t} = \eta_{t|t-1} + K_{t|t}(y_t - y_{t|t-1}), \tag{38}$$

$$P_{t|t} = P_{t|t-1} - K_{t|t} Py_t K'_{t|t}, \tag{39}$$

where the element $P\eta_t, y_t$ in Equation 37 is also present in the linear case as $P_{t|t-1} \Lambda'_t$ (see Equation 7) but was omitted earlier for the sake of clarity. The covariance update function in Equation 39 is formulated in a different but equivalent form from that in Equation 9 to indicate more clearly how the state covariance matrix is updated using output from the sigma-point transformations (Wan & Van der Merwe, 2001). Step 1 to step 5 are then repeated until all the observations have been incorporated.

5.3.3 Combining the UKF with Prediction Error Decomposition.

As mentioned earlier, the prediction error decomposition function can be used to derive $L(\theta)$ based on one-step-ahead prediction errors in the context of the linear KF. In situations in which the one-step-ahead prediction errors are independently and normally distributed after all the nonlinear dynamic and measurement relations have been accounted for, my colleagues and I (Chow, Ferrer, & Nesselroade, in press) showed that the UKF provides the one-step-ahead prediction errors and Py_t (see Equation 35) that can be used in conjunction with the prediction error decomposition function to yield approximate ML parameter estimates. A similar approach was used by Young, McKenna, and Bruun (2001) to estimate parameters for nonlinear stochastic systems. This approach is used in one of the forthcoming illustrative examples to estimate part of the parameters of the Lorenz system. Generalization of this procedure to multiple-subject settings is also demonstrated.

5.4 SIMULATION EXAMPLES

5.4.1 The Lorenz System

Simulation examples based on the Lorenz system (Lorenz, 1963) are now presented to highlight several features of the UKF. The Lorenz system is a well-know nonlinear dynamical system that exhibits chaotic dynamics and properties such as sensitive dependence on initial conditions. In other words, slight differences in initial conditions could lead to cascading divergence in later dynamics of the system. I illustrate the use of a joint estimation approach wherein the state vector η is augmented to include unknown parameters to be estimated as states by means of the UKF. Furthermore, I used a fourth-order Runge-Kutta integration scheme to fit the associated differential equations of the Lorenz system as a discrete state-space model.

Originally used to represent the weather system, the Lorenz system is composed of three latent-state variables (denoted below as x_{1t}, x_{2t} and x_{3t}), the dynamics of which are expressed as

$$\dot{x}_{1t} = \sigma(x_{2t} - x_{1t}), \tag{40}$$
$$\dot{x}_{2t} = \rho x_{1t} - x_{2t} - x_{1t}x_{3t} \text{ and} \tag{41}$$
$$\dot{x}_{3t} = x_{1t}x_{2t} - \gamma x_{3t}, \tag{42}$$

where the system as a whole is a simple portrayal of the weather system. The atmosphere is described as a layer of air being heated from below by the earth and cooled at the top by the void of outer space. Here, x_{1t} represents the convective flow of the air at time t, x_{2t} the horizontal temperature distribution at time t and x_{3t} the vertical temperature distribution at time t, σ the ratio of viscosity to thermal conductivity, ρ is the temperature difference between the two ends of the layer, and γ is the width-to-height ratio of the layer (Martelli, 1999).

Many researchers have found the theoretical concept underlying the Lorenz system intriguing. For instance, Frederickson and Losada (2005) used the Lorenz equations to represent the ongoing "tension" between an individual's positive emotion and negative emotion (Frederickson & Losada, 2005).

Furthermore, at the specific parameters of $\sigma = 10$, $\rho = 46$, and $\gamma = 8/3$, the convection flow exhibits chaotic patterns that seem to be repeating themselves (i.e., self-similar) over time (see Figure 5–1); yet, the exact numerical values of the states can be very different with just slight differences in initial conditions. Such a "chaotic" emotional profile is thought to reflect higher emotional complexity and psychological resilience.

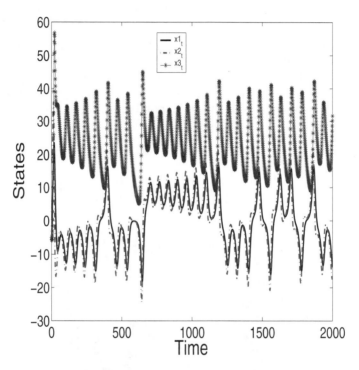

Figure 5–1. A plot of the clean dynamics of the Lorenz system. The three latent variables show seemingly random but self-similar long-term behaviors.

To highlight the key dynamics of the Lorenz system, a single time series ($T = 2000$, $N = 1$) was generated with $\sigma = 10$, $\rho = 46$ and $\gamma = 8/3$ (see clean time series in Figure 5–1). Each latent variable was identified by one indicator that was corrupted with measurement noise at approximately 70% signal-to-noise ratio. The process noise covariance matrix, Ψ, was set to a null matrix.[5] Although single-subject, intensive time series data are rarely encountered in the social sciences, such data sets are in fact the "norm," for instance,

---

[5]Chaotic systems are known to be nonlinear dynamical systems that are deterministic (i.e., no process noise) and yet manifest seemingly random behaviors.

in physiological, Electro-Encephalography (EEG) and perceptual-motor studies. Pairwise plots of the clean state variables are shown in Figure 5–2. The famous butterfly-shaped attractor associated with the Lorenz system is evident in the pairwise plots—the three state variables manifest very complex time-based dynamics, but they maintain lawful relationships with respect to one another.

Slight variations in simulation design were implemented in the three sets of forthcoming simulation examples but some common features concerning the use of a joint estimation approach, and a fourth-order Runge-Kutta procedure to fit the continuous-time differential equations (see Equation 42) as a discrete-time state-space model are first described here. Specifically, using a joint estimation approach, the parameters σ, ρ, and γ were represented as part of the state vector $\eta_t = [x_{1t}, x_{2t}, x_{3t}, \sigma_t, \rho_t, \gamma_t]'$ and the augmented state vector was estimated using the UKF. The corresponding dynamic model is written as

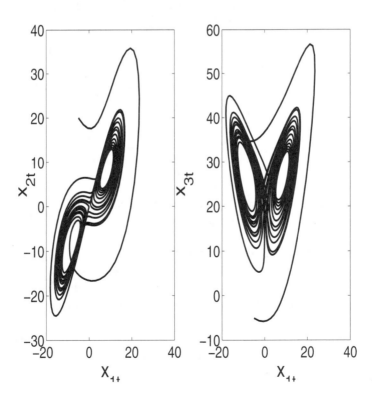

Figure 5–2. Pairwise plots of the clean time series against each other.

$$\begin{bmatrix} x_{1t} \\ x_{2t} \\ x_{3t} \\ \sigma_t \\ \rho_t \\ \gamma_t \end{bmatrix} = \begin{bmatrix} f_1(x_{t-1}) \\ f_2(x_{t-1}) \\ f_3(x_{t-1}) \\ \sigma_{t-1} \\ \rho_{t-1} \\ \gamma_{t-1} \end{bmatrix}, \tag{43}$$

where the terms $f_q(x_t), (q = 1, 2, 3)$ represent discrete approximations to the differential Equations 41–42 by means of a fourth-order Runge-Kutta approach. A fourth-order Runge-Kutta is a way to obtain a numerical integral solution to a set of differential equations. This is done by first deducing changes at four arbitrarily small intervals between two successive measurement occasions based on the dynamic functions, and subsequently computing the value of x_q at time t by smoothing over these changes. As the computation intervals become very small, a smooth, continuous trajectory is obtained (for implementation details see Press, Teukolsky, Vetterling, & Flannery, 2002). In this way, a fourth-order Runge-Kutta procedure allows a researcher to represent a continuous-time differential equation model as a discrete state-space model by first "filling in" and subsequently smoothing over the "missing observations" that exist between two measurement occasions. Alternatively, other lower order integration methods (i.e., involving the computation of changes over fewer intervals) such as the Euler method can be used (e.g., Martelli, 1999; Singer, 2002).

The corresponding measurement model is written as

$$\begin{bmatrix} y_{1t} \\ y_{2t} \\ y_{3t} \end{bmatrix} = \begin{bmatrix} 1 & 0 & 0 & 0 & 0 & 0 \\ 0 & 1 & 0 & 0 & 0 & 0 \\ 0 & 0 & 1 & 0 & 0 & 0 \\ 0 & 0 & 0 & 0 & 0 & 0 \\ 0 & 0 & 0 & 0 & 0 & 0 \\ 0 & 0 & 0 & 0 & 0 & 0 \end{bmatrix} \begin{bmatrix} x_{1t} \\ x_{2t} \\ x_{3t} \\ \sigma_t \\ \rho_t \\ \gamma_t \end{bmatrix} + \begin{bmatrix} \epsilon_{1t} \\ \epsilon_{2t} \\ \epsilon_{3t} \end{bmatrix}. \tag{44}$$

Although the parameters do not vary over time, they were incorporated into the time-varying state vector and were constrained to be invariant over time. Alternatively, a separate UKF chain can be run to estimate the parameters, again by treating them as state variables, or a quasi-maximum likelihood approach based on prediction error decomposition can be used to estimate the parameters. One advantage of the joint estimation approach utilized here is that it provides researchers with a more flexible way of representing the dynamics of time-varying parameters in conjunction with the dynamics of the state variables (for other conventional approaches see e.g., Harvey, 1989; Kim & Nelson, 1999). For instance, the parameters in a model can be hypothesized to follow a first-order autoregressive process (e.g., a random walk model) instead of being constant over the entire span of a study. Within-person deviations in parameters, especially in manner of discontinuous jumps can also be handled very easily using this approach.

I. Comparing the UKF and the EKF as Longitudinal Factor Score Estimators. Simulation results were organized into three major sections to highlight important features of the UKF. The current example is used to demonstrate the utility of the UKF as a factor score estimator in comparison with the EKF. A single time series generated using the Lorenz system with intensive repeated measures ($T = 2000$) was used. The measurement noise variances were set to yield a 55% signal-to-noise ratio. Using this example, the performance of the UKF as a longitudinal factor score estimator was compared to that of the EKF using very noisy time-series data. For illustration purposes, I used the special case wherein the measurement noise covariance matrix and all other parameters were not estimated and thus set to their true values. This special case is a typical modelling scenario in engineering and the physical sciences.

Results reported in this section were based on estimates averaged over 200 Monte Carlo simulations. On average, the two approaches took less than 2 minutes of CPU time to complete a single run on a 2 GHz IBM laptop with 1 GB RAM. As shown in Figure 5–3, both the UKF and the EKF were able to reconstruct and track the dynamics of x_{1t}, x_{2t}, and x_{3t} very accurately. The UKF was observed to outperform the EKF slightly in terms of its estimation accuracy. Across the 2000 time points, the UKF's estimates yielded root mean squared errors in magnitudes of 2.18, 2.76, and 2.49 for the three state variables, whereas the corresponding root mean squared errors of the EKF estimates were 4.45, 5.53, and 4.94. However, both techniques' margins of errors were quite low considering the complex patterns of change under consideration. In addition, in lower noise conditions (e.g., 70% signal-to-noise ratio), the two filters' performances were largely comparable to each other. More detailed analytic proofs and simulation results comparing the performances of the two approaches can be found elsewhere (Julier & Uhlmann, 1996; Van der Merwe et al., 2000; Wan & Van der Merwe, 2001).

II. Quasi-Maximum Likelihood Approach to Parameter Estimation. In the current example, a quasi-maximum likelihood approach that capitalizes on the prediction error decomposition method was used to estimate the process and measurement noise covariance matrices. Other parameters (σ, ρ and γ) were estimated using the UKF by means of joint estimation. This approach was used by my colleagues and I (Chow et al., in press) to estimate all the parameters of the classical predator-prey system in combination with a fourth-order Runge-Kutta procedure and was able to recover all the parameters very accurately. In

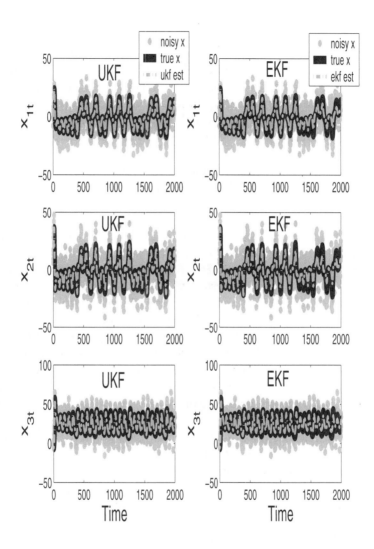

Figure 5–3. Estimates of x_{1t}. x_{2t} and x_{3t} obtained from the UKF and the EKF, plotted together with the noisy observations and the clean time series.

practice, the accuracy of the parameter estimates is rather robust toward slight overestimation of the magnitudes of noise variances, but the state and parameter variances are typically overestimated in such cases. In general, to increase numerical stability, it is advisable to dissociate the variance estimation procedure from the parameter estimation process—just as the approach used here, because estimation biases in any parameter can increase the chance of false convergence to local minima.

Parameter estimates obtained using this approach averaged over 50 Monte Carlo runs are summarized in Table Table 5–1. To speed convergence, I used a trick detailed in Wan and Van der Merwe (2001) to add a a small amount of process noise variances to the parameters. This approach helps prevent the parameter estimates from lingering in local minima for too long. A similar approach was adopted by Molenaar and Raijmakers (1998), for example. Parameter estimates recovered using the combined joint estimation and quasi-ML approach were very accurate.

Standard errors associated with the measurement noise variances were obtained by computing the finite difference Hessian matrix evaluated at the final parameter estimates. Square-root of the qth diagonal elements of $P_{t|t}$ ($q = 4, 5, 6$) associated with σ, ρ, and γ were taken as these parameters' standard error estimates (e.g., Sitz, Kurths, & Voss, 2002). The parallels between the standard error estimate given by the two approaches and their corresponding Monte Carlo standard error estimates[6] confirmed the utility of the former as an estimate of the variability or "uncertainty" in the resultant parameter estimates. Due the relatively few replications in the current Monte Carlo simulation, more extensive simulations are needed to further determine the accuracy of the parameter and standard error estimates, especially when certain modelling assumptions are violated. Note that if the number of measurement occasions available for estimation purposes is insufficient (e.g., if information from all measurement occasions is exhausted before the state variance estimates stabilize), biases in standard error as well as parameter estimates are typically observed.

As a whole, because maximum likelihood estimation requires multiple iterations of the aforementioned UKF algorithm until convergence criteria are met, the increase in computational time was substantial. For instance, over the 50 Monte Carlo runs, the quasi-maximum likelihood approach took an average of 24 minutes of CPU time to reach convergence for one single run. If maximum likelihood is used to estimate all the parameters, the increase in computational time is even more pronounced, and it typically takes days to complete one single run.

III. Extension to a Multiple-Subject Modeling Scenario. To extend the quasi-maximum likelihood approach to a multiple-subject setting, the loglikelihood function in Equation 13 can be readily used in conjunction with a joint UKF es-

---

[6]These are empirical standard deviations of the parameter estimates across Monte Carlo runs used to quantify the variability in parameter estimates. This specific index of empirical standard errors was also used in Monte Carlo simulations by Boomsma and Hoogland (2001).

TABLE 5–1

True Parameters and Parameter Estimates Recovered by the Quasi-Maximum Likelihood
Approach Together with a Joint UKF Estimation Approach Averaged over 50 Monte Carlo
Simulations

Parameters	*True values*	*Estimates*	*MC SE*
σ	10	9.998 (.69)	.58
ρ	28	28.069 (.43)	.33
γ	2.667	2.663 (.24)	.13
$\epsilon_{11}{}^{a}$	26	25.408 (.83)	1.08
ϵ_{22}	34	32.989 (1.06)	1.77
ϵ_{33}	32	32.467 (1.09)	1.02

Notes. Standard error estimates are included in parentheses.

    $^{a}\epsilon_{11}$ = measurement error variance for x_1 across all time points, ϵ_{22} = measurement error variance
    for x_2 across all time points and ϵ_{33} = measurement error variance for x_3 across all time points.

timation approach to estimate the subject-invariant parameters. Loglikelihood
values are computed by summing over the individual loglikelihood values from
$t = 1$ to T, and from $i = 1$ to N. One property of chaotic systems such as the
Lorenz system—namely, sensitive dependence on initial conditions—is worth
further elaboration here. An illustrative case in which data from 100 subjects
with different initial conditions over 300 time points were generated using the
same set of parameters. The property of sensitive dependence on initial conditions is clearly portrayed in Figure 5–4. Although all subjects were known
to conform to the same set of parameters, the slight differences in initial conditions [$M(x_{10}) = -5$, $SD(x_{10}) = 25$; $M(x_{20}) = 20$, $SD(x_{20}) = 25$;
$M(x_{30}) = -5$, $SD(x_{30}) = 25$] evolved into rather different behavioral trajectories over time. In particular, dynamics of the true states were completely
masked in the noisy data. Piecing together shorter segments of data from multiple subjects gave a similar but slightly distorted representation of the relationships among the state variables (e.g., see Figures 5–5A and 5–5B).

In this particular scenario, the trajectory of a "prototypical" individual
with the same parameters as all others and of average x_{10}, x_{20}, and x_{30} did
not have sufficient measurement occasions to reconstruct the butterfly-shaped
trajectories—or "attractor," thus creating the impression that the aggregate
curve did not in any way resemble the overall group dynamics. In addition,
the true dynamics among the state variables are completely obscured by the
measurement errors in the noisy data (see Figures 5–5C and 5–5D). A second
multiple–subject illustrative case was simulated with $T = 1000$ and $N = 10$.
The property of sensitive dependence on initial conditions still holds in this
case, but the more intensive repeated measurements at the individual level

gives an accurate portrayal of the butterfly-shaped attractor dynamics characteristic of the Lorenz system for each individual.

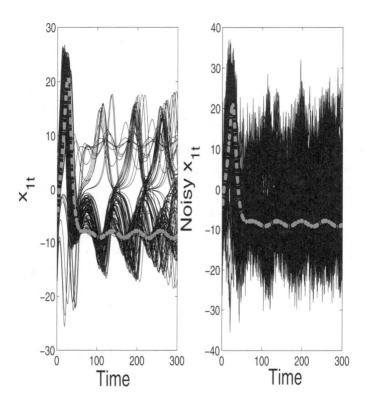

Figure 5–4. True states of x_{1t} over time (left panel) and the corresponding noisy observations (right panel) generated using $N = 100$ and $T = 300$ with the same set of parameters but different initial conditions (i.e., x_{10}, x_{20}, and x_{30}). Dashed lines indicate the trajectories of a "prototypical" subject with initial conditions that were right at the sample's averages. Because of the property of sensitive dependence on initial conditions, different "subjects" appear to conform to different behavioral dynamics even though all subjects were characterized by the same set of parameters.

Parameter estimates obtained using the quasi-maximum likelihood approach combined with the UKF are shown in Table 5–2. Each subject's noisy observations at time $t = 1$ were set as their respective initial conditions for the three state variables. Estimates presented in Table 5–2 were obtained by averaging estimates over 50 Monte Carlo simulations. With appropriate tuning, the two cases took approximately 1 hour and 17 minutes of CPU time,

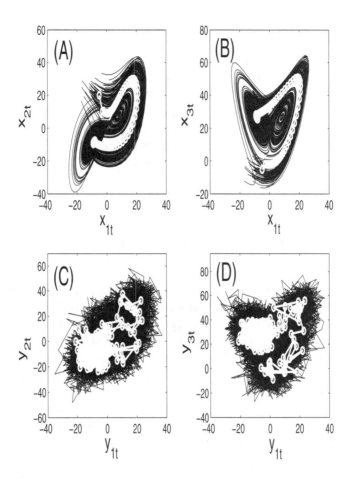

Figure 5–5. (A) Plot of the relationship between clean x_{1t} and x_{2t} among all subjects with $T = 300$ and $N = 100$, (B) plot of clean x_{1t} against x_{3t}, (C) plot of noisy observations of x_{1t} (i.e., y_{1t}) against noisy observations of x_{2t} (i.e., y_{2t}), and (D) plot of noisy observations of x_{1t} (i.e., y_{1t}) against noisy observations of x_{3t} (i.e., y_{3t}). In all plots, solid lines indicate trajectories at the individual level and dash lines with circles indicate the trajectories of a "prototypical" subject of average x_{10}, x_{20}, and x_{30}.

respectively, to complete one single run. The former was harder to "tune" and it required the addition of larger magnitudes of process noise for the ML estimation to converge. Some of the earlier simulations with smaller process noise variances took days to run and had not reached convergence.

TABLE 5–2

True Parameters and Parameter Estimates Recovered by Using Shorter Segments of Data from Multiple Subjects Averaged over 50 Monte Carlo Simulations.

Parameters	True values	Est (N=100, T=300)	Est (N=10, T=1000)
σ	10	9.787 (2.92^a/1.95^b)	9.674 (1.35/1.07)
ρ	28	27.790 (1.81/.97)	27.946 (.88/.51)
γ	2.667	2.659 (1.19/.69)	2.751 (.54/.31)
ϵ_{11}	26	26.513 ($.24^c$/.22)	26.325 (.39/.70)
ϵ_{22}	34	36.405 (.32/.60)	35.723 (.53/1.71)
ϵ_{33}	32	32.649 (.29/.33)	34.071 (.52/1.61)

Notes. Standard error estimates are included in parentheses.

[a] SE estimates by the UKF.

[b] Monte Carlo SE.

[c] SE estimates based on finite difference Hessian evaluated at the final parameter estimates.

The parameter estimates obtained in both cases were reasonably accurate (see Table 5–2). However, the SE estimates given by the UKF for the $T = 300$ and $N = 100$ case were relatively high. This is due to the fact that the individual trajectories generated using the Lorenz system can differ quite substantially from one another, thus making it difficult to track such dynamics without sufficient observations at the individual level. Thus, as mentioned earlier, larger magnitudes of process noise had to be added in this case to the state variables to yield final parameter estimates of comparable accuracy to the $T = 1000, N = 10$ case. In general, with less than 100 measurement occasions, it is extremely difficult to recover individual factor scores accurately and consequently, the overall parameter estimates as well. Even with $T = 300$, higher uncertainty in the UKF state and parameter estimates (i.e., higher state and parameter variances, $P_{t|t}$) was still observed in comparison with the $T = 1000$ case. In contrast, the quasi-ML estimates of measurement noise variances showed lower estimated and MC SEs when $T = 300, N = 100$ than when $T = 1000$ and $N = 10$, possibly due to the larger N in the former case. Underestimation of the SEs of two of the noise variance parameters in the $T = 1000$ case has to be verified further in more extensive simulations, however.

In sum, unless the interindividual differences in initial conditions were appropriately accounted for, for instance, by using mixed effects modelling or other related techniques (e.g., Icaza & Jones, 1999), it is safer to collect more observations from each individual over time (and of course, from more individuals if possible) to ensure more accurate factor score and parameter estimations both at the individual level and at the group level. Thus, even if certain assumptions are violated (e.g., the assumption that the individuals are independent and identical replicates of one another with subject-invariant parameters), sufficient measurement occasions are still available from each person to permit model fitting at the individual level.

5.5 DISCUSSION

Much of the contemporary modelling techniques in social sciences has been developed to analyze cross-sectional or panel data with relatively few measurement occasions. The present chapter serves to present and summarize several alternative techniques that are used primarily to capture complex nonlinear dynamics using time series data. As illustrated in one of the simulation examples, generalization to multiple-subject settings can be readily accomplished in cases wherein all subjects are characterized by the exact same parameters and sufficient information is available at the individual level. Extending the techniques presented herein to the more "challenging" involving panel data is still a possibility, but the message the present article seeks to convey is as follows. If time series data are available from multiple subjects, the modelling difficulties one has to face are substantially reduced. Admittedly, collecting intensive time series data is not always feasible or even possible in certain content areas. However, what I hope to have accomplished here is to introduce the reader to the potential utility of some contemporary techniques for fitting nonlinear dynamical systems models. A few other relevant modeling techniques are discussed briefly below.

The central concepts underlying the UKF and its different variations are by no means novel. They are used in many other data analytic techniques and the UKF itself has some key parallels with a few other techniques for fitting dynamical systems models in the statistics and engineering literature. For instance, one other sigma-point nonlinear Kalman filter that has close correspondence to the UKF is the central difference Kalman filter (CDKF) proposed independently by Ito and Xiong (2000) and Nørgaard, Poulsen, and Ravn (2000). Instead of solving for the analytic first (and for second-order EKF, second) derivatives of a nonlinear function as in the EKF, the CDKF capitalizes on polynomial interpolation (see Steffensen, 1927) to derive numerical first and second order derivatives of the function. For instance, first and second derivatives of the dynamic function are approximated as

$$\frac{\partial f(\eta_{it})}{\partial \eta_{it}}\Big|_{\eta_{i,t-t|t-1}} \approx \frac{f(\eta_{i,t-1|t-1} + h\delta_\eta) - f(\eta_{i,t-1|t-1} - h\delta_\eta)}{2h} \quad (45)$$

and

$$\frac{\partial f^2(\eta_{it})}{\partial \eta_{it}^2}\Big|_{\eta_{i,t-1|t-1}} \approx$$

$$\frac{f(\eta_{i,t-1|t-1} + h\delta_\eta) + f(\eta_{i,t-1|t-1} - h\delta_\eta) - 2f(\eta_{i,t-1|t-1})}{2h}, \quad (46)$$

where h is a user-defined half-step size or time interval between two successive state estimates, and δ_η represents a new η value a small distance away from the previous estimates, $\eta_{i,t-1|t-1}$ (Ito & Xiong, 2000; Nørgaard et al., 2000; Wan & Van der Merwe, 2001). The CDKF can be formulated as a sigma-point Kalman filter by considering $\eta_{i,t-1|t-1} + h\delta_\eta$ and $\eta_{i,t-1|t-1} - h\delta_\eta$ as sigma points whose criterion of inclusion is determined by the scaling constant h, as opposed to the three scaling constants (α, β, and κ) as in the case of the UKF. The CDKF has been proven to show comparable computational accuracy to the UKF. The reader is referred to the work of Wan and Van der Merwe (2001) for more thorough descriptions of the parallels between the two (see also Lefebvre et al., 2002).

Closely associated with both the EKF and the CDKF is a second-order local linearization method presented by Shoji and Ozaki (1997) for fitting nonlinear stochastic differential equations. Unlike the CDKF, analytic Jacobian matrices still have to be provided. Specifically, these researchers linearize the dynamic function (i.e., $f[.]$) in small discrete time steps to yield a linear function comprised of Jacobian matrices involving first- and second-order partial derivatives of $f[.]$ with respect to the latent states, and first derivatives of $f[.]$ with respect to time. Indeed, similar statistical interpolation procedures have found extensive applications in many other areas. For instance, Boker and Graham (1998) used a largely similar interpolation technique to linearize a function with respect to time and the resultant numerical derivatives are then used as manifest variables in a structural equation model for assessing linear differential equation models.

As a whole, estimation of all nonlinear, non-Gaussian state-space models revolves around one major goal; to estimate the statistical properties of some possibly non-Gaussian densities, including the transition density, $p(\eta_t|\eta_{t-1}, \theta)$, posterior density, $p(\eta_t|y_t, \theta)$, and likelihood density, $p(y_t|y_1, \ldots, y_T, \theta)$. At times, the distributions involved are multimodal and do not have known analytic forms. The well-known Gaussian sum filter approach approximates non-Gaussian densities using mixtures of different Gaussian densities. Developing extensions of this method for use with other Monte Carlo-based filtering methods—collectively known as particle filters—is very much an ongoing research topic (e.g., Liu & West, 2001). Instead of attempting to sample from analytically intractable distributions, particle filter approaches aim to generate a large number of points or *particles* from an alternative distribution—often termed the *proposal distribution*—from which one can easily sample. These particles are then weighted and the associated weights can be used to approximate non-normal prior, posterior densities and/or likelihood functions (e.g., Kitagawa, 1998; Pitt, 2002; Singer, 2002). One of the earliest versions of such particle filter approaches is the bootstrap filter proposed by Gordon, Salmond, and Smith (1993). Other newer particle filter approach includes the work of Singer (2002), who proposed using a functional integral method with importance sampling that uses estimates obtained from running multiple chains of EKF to form the proposal distribution, which is then used in a weight function to yield the final state and covariance estimates. Within the context of sigma-point Kalman filters, multiple (rather than one single) UKF or CDKF chains can also be run to improve estimation accuracy (e.g., Ito & Xiong, 2000; Van der Merwe et al., 2000). In practice, particle filter techniques are often used in conjunction with Markov chain Monte Carlo methods (e.g., Van der Merwe et al., 2000) to improve their respective estimation accuracy. Interested readers are referred to Doucet, de Freitas, and Gordon (2001) for a collection of such methods (see also Durbin & Koopman, 2001; Shumway & Stoffer, 2004).

5.6 CONCLUSION

Over the last few decades, applications of nonlinear dynamical system-related concepts to empirical studies in social and behavioral sciences are largely limited in prevalence to the area of perceptual-motor development (e.g., Haken et al., 1985). In other substantive areas, well-known nonlinear dynamical systems models such as the Lorenz system are often used to represent different psychological, behavioral, and developmental phenomena, but such models are rarely subjected to the appropriate model-fitting and model validation processes. Undoubtedly, several methodological issues remain in fitting and evaluating nonlinear, non-Gaussian state-space models. Nonetheless, the Kalman filters' general utility as a model-fitting tool is evident and, hopefully, can help inspire more research into alternative methods that are suited for the study of more complex changes—both within and between individuals.

REFERENCES

Alligood, K. T., Sauer, T. D., & Yorke, J. A. (1996). *Chaos: An introduction to dynamical systems.* New York: Springer.

Anderson, B. D. O., & Moore, J. B. (1979). *Optimal filtering.* Englewood Cliffs: Prentice-Hall.

Arminger, G. (1986). Linear stochastic differential equation models for panel data with unobserved variables. In N. Tuma (Ed.), *Sociological methodology 1986* (pp. 187–212). San Francisco: Jossey-Bass.

Arminger, G., & Muthén, B. (1998). A Bayesian approach to nonlinear latent variable models using the Gibbs sampler and the Metropolis–Hastings algorithm. *Psychometrika, 63,* 271–300.

Boker, S. M., & Graham, J. (1998). A dynamical systems analysis of adolescent substance abuse. *Multivariate Behavioral Research, 33,* 479–507.

Boker, S. M., Neale, M. C., & Rausch, J. (2004). Latent differential equation modeling with multivariate multi-occasion indicators. In K. van Montfort, J. Oud, & A. Satorra (Eds.), *Recent developments on structural equation models: Theory and applications* (pp. 151–174). Dordrecht: Kluwer.

Boomsma, A., & Hoogland, J. J. (2001). The robustness of LISREL modeling revisited. In R. Cudeck, S. du Toit, & D. Sörbom (Eds.), *Structural equation models: Present and future. A Festschrift in honor of Karl Jöreskog* (pp. 139–168). Chicago: Scientific Software International.

Bremer, C. L., & Kaplan, D. T. (2001). *Markov chain Monte Carlo estimation of nonlinear dynamics from time series.* Unpublished manuscript, Department of Mathematics and Computer Science, Macalester College.

Browne, M. W., & du Toit, H. C. (1991). Models for learning data. In L. M. Collins & J. L. Horn (Eds.), *Best methods for the analysis of change: Recent advances, unanswered questions, future directions* (pp. 47–68). Washington, DC: American Psychological Association.

Caines, P. E., & Rissanen, J. (1974). Maximum likelihood estimation of parameters. *IEEE Transactions on Information Theory, IT-20,* 102–104.

Chow, S.-M., Ferrer, E., & Nesselroade, J. R. (in press). An unscented Kalman filter approach to the estimation of nonlinear dynamical systems models. *Multivariate Behavioral Research.*

Cobb, L. (1981). Parameter estimation for the cusp catastrophe model. *Behavioral Science, 26*(1), 75–78.

Coleman, J. S. (1968). The mathematical study of change. In H. M. Blalock, Jr. & A. B. Blalock (Eds.), *Methodology in social research* (pp. 428–478). New York: McGraw-Hill.

Dolan, C. V., & Molenaar, P. C. M. (1991). A note on the calculation of latent trajectories in the quasi Markov simplex model by means of regression method and the discrete kalman filter. *Kwantitatieve Methoden, 38,* 29–44.

Doucet, A., de Freitas, N., & Gordon, N. (Eds.). (2001). *Sequential Monte Carlo methods in practice.* New York: Springer.

Durbin, J., & Koopman, S. J. (2001). *Time series analysis by state-space methods.* New York: Oxford University Press.

Frederickson, B. L., & Losada, M. F. (2005). Positive affect and the complex dynamics of human flourishing. *American Psychologist, 60*(7), 678–686.

Gelb, A. (1974). *Applied optimal estimation.* Cambridge, MA: MIT Press.

Gilks, W. R., & Berzuini, C. (2001). Following a moving target—Monte Carlo inference for dynamic Bayesian models. *Journal of the Royal Statistical Society B, 63,* 127-146.

Gordon, N. J., Salmond, D. J., & Smith, A. F. M. (1993). Novel approach to nonlinear/non–Gaussian Bayesian state estimation. *IEEE Proceedings–F, Radar and Signal Processing, 140*(2), 107–113.

Haken, H., Kelso, J. A. S., & Bunz, H. (1985). A theoretical model of phase transitions in human hand movements. *Biological Cybernetics, 51,* 347–356.

Hamblin, R. L., Hout, M., Miller, J. L. L., & Pitcher, B. L. (1977). Arm races: A test of two models. *American Sociological Review, 42*(2), 338–354.

Hamerle, A., Nagl, W., & Singer, H. (1990). Problems with the estimation of stochastic differential equation using structural equations models. *Journal of Mathematical Sociology, 16*(3), 201–220.

Hamilton, J. D. (1994). *Time series analysis.* Princeton, NJ: Princeton University Press.

Harvey, A. C. (1989). *Forecasting, structural time series models and the Kalman filter.* Princeton, NJ: Princeton University Press.

Icaza, G., & Jones, R. H. (1999). A state-space EM algorithm for longitudinal data. *Journal of Time Series Analysis, 20*(5), 537–550.

Ito, K., & Xiong, K. (2000). Gaussian filters for nonlinear filtering problems. *IEEE Transactions on Automatic Control, 45,* 910–927.

Jöreskog, K. G., & Yang, F. (1996). Nonlinear structural equation models: The Kenny-Judd model with interaction effects. In G. A. Marcoulides & R. E. Schumacker (Eds.), *Advanced structural equation modeling* (pp. 57–88). Mahwah, NJ: Lawrence Erlbaum Associates.

Julier, S. J., & Uhlmann, J. K. (1996). *A general method for approximating nonlinear transformations of probability distributions.* (Tech. Rep.). Department of Engineering Science, University of Oxford.

Julier, S. J., & Uhlmann, J. K. (2002). Reduced sigma point filters for the propagation of means and covariances through nonlinear transformation. In *Proceedings of the IEEE American Control Conference* (pp. 887–892). Anchorage, AK: IEEE.

Julier, S. J., Uhlmann, J. K., & Durrant-Whyte, H. F. (1995). A new approach for filtering nonlinear systems. In *Proceedings of the American Control Conference* (pp. 1628–1632). Seattle, WA: IEEE.

Kalman, R. E. (1960). A new approach to linear filtering and prediction problems. *Transactions of the ASME–Journal of Basic Engineering, 82*(Series D), 35-45.

Kenny, D. A., & Judd, C. M. (1984). Estimating the nonlinear and interactive effects of latent variables. *Psychological Bulletin, 96,* 201–210.

Kim, C.-J., & Nelson, C. R. (1999). *State-space models with regime switching: Classical and Gibbs-sampling approaches with applications.* Cambridge, MA: MIT Press.

Kitagawa, G. (1998). A self-organizing state-space model. *Journal of the American Statistical Association, 93*(443), 1203–1215.

Klein, A., & Moosbrugger, H. (2000). Maximum likelihood estimation of latent interaction effects with the LMS method. *Psychometrika, 65,* 457–474.

Lefebvre, T., Bruyninckx, H., & Schutter, J. D. (2002). Comment on "A new method for the nonlinear transformation of means and covariances in filters and estimators." *IEEE Transactions on Automatic Control, 47*(8), 1406–1408.

Li, F., Duncan, T. E., & Acock, A. (2000). Modeling interaction effects in latent growth curve models. *Structural Equation Modeling, 7*(4), 497–533.

Liu, J., & West, M. (2001). Combined parameter and state estimation in simulation–based filtering. In A. Doucet, N. de Freitas, & N. Gordon (Eds.), *Sequential Monte Carlo methods in practice* (pp. 197–223). New York: Springer.

Lorenz, E. N. (1963). Deterministic nonperiodic flow. *Journal of Atmospheric Science, 20,* 130–141.

Martelli, M. (1999). *Introduction to discrete dynamical systems and chaos.* New York: Wiley.

McArdle, J., & Epstein, D. B. (1987). Latent growth curves within developmental structural equation models. *Child Development, 58*(1), 110–133.

McArdle, J. J., & Ghisletta, P. (2000). The future of latent variable modeling with interactions and nonlinearity. *Contemporary Psychology, APA Review of Books, 45*(1), 91–95.

McArdle, J. J., & Hamagami, F. (2001). Latent difference score structural models for linear dynamic analysis with incomplete longitudinal data. In L. Collins & A. Sayer (Eds.), *New methods for the analysis of change* (pp. 139–175). Washington, D.C.: American Psychological Association.

Meredith, W., & Tisak, J. (1990). Latent curve analysis. *Psychometrika, 55,* 107–122.

Molenaar, P. C. M., & Raijmakers, M. E. J. (1998). Fitting nonlinear dynamical models directly to observed time series. In K. M. Newell & P. C. M. Molenaar (Eds.), *Applications of nonlinear dynamics to developmental process modeling* (pp. 269–297). Mahwah, NJ: Lawrence Erlbaum Associates.

Nesselroade, J. R., & Boker, S. M. (1994). Assessing constancy and change. In T. Heatherton & J. Weinberger (Eds.), *Can personality change?* (pp. 503–541). Washington, DC: American Psychological Association.

Newell, K. M., & Molenaar, P. C. M. (Eds.). (1998). *Applications of nonlinear dynamics to developmental process modeling.* Mahwah, NJ: Lawrence Erlbaum Associates.

Nørgaard, M., Poulsen, N. K., & Ravn, O. (2000). New developments in state estimation for nonlinear systems. *Automatica, 36,* 1627–1638.

Otter, P. (1986). Dynamic structure systems under indirect observation: Indentifiability and estimation aspects from a system theoretic perspective. *Psychometrika, 51*(3), 415–428.

Oud, J. H. L., & Jansen, R. A. R. G. (2000). Continuous time state space modeling of panel data by means of SEM. *Psychometrika, 65*(2), 199–215.

Oud, J. H. L., Jansen, R. A. R. G., van Leeuwe, J. F. J., Aarnoutse, C. A. J., & Voeten, M. J. M. (1999). Monitoring pupil development by means of the Kalman filter and smoother based upon SEM state space modeling. *Learning and Individual Differences, 11,* 121–136.

Oud, J. H. L., van den Bercken, J. H., & Essers, R. J. (1990). Longitudinal factor score estimation using the Kalman filter. *Applied Psychological Measurement, 14*(4), 395–418.

Pitt, M. K. (2002). *Smooth particle filters for likelihood evaluation and maximisation.* (Warwick Economic research papers no. 651.) Coventry, UK: University of Warwick.

Press, W. H., Teukolsky, S. A., Vetterling, W. T., & Flannery, B. P. (2002). *Numerical recipes in C.* Cambridge, UK: Cambridge University Press.

Schumacker, R. E., & Marcoulides, G. A. (Eds.). (1998). *Interaction and nonlinear effects in structural equation modeling.* Mahway, NJ: Lawrence Erlbaum Associates.

Schweppe, F. (1965). Evaluation of likelihood functions for Gaussian signals. *IEEE Transactions on Information Theory, 11,* 61–70.

Shoji, I., & Ozaki, T. (1997). Comparative study of estimation methods for continuous time stochastic time stochastic processes. *Journal of Time Series Analysis, 18,* 485–506.

Shumway, R. H., & Stoffer, D. S. (2004). *Time series analysis and its applications.* New York: Springer.

Singer, H. (1993). Continuous-time dynamical systems with sampled data, errors of measurement, and unobserved components. *Journal of Time Series Analysis, 14,* 527–545.

Singer, H. (2002). Parameter estimation of nonlinear stochastic differential equations: Simulated maximum likelihood vs. extended Kalman filter and Itô-Taylor expansion. *Journal of Computational and Graphical Statistics*, *11*, 972–995.

Sitz, A., Kurths, J., & Voss, H. U. (2002). Estimation of parameters and unobserved components for nonlinear systems from noisy time series. *Physical Review*, *66*, 016210-1–016210-9.

Sorensen, H. W., & Stubberud, A. R. (1968). Non-linear filtering by approximation of the a posteriori density. *International Journal of Control*, *8*(1), 33–51.

Steffensen, J. F. (1927). *Interpolation*. Baltimore, MD: Williams & Wilkins.

Vallacher, R. R., & Nowak, A. (Eds.). (1994). *Dynamical systems in social psychology*. San Diego, CA: Academic Press.

Van der Merwe, R., Doucet, A., Freitas, N., & Wan, E. (2000). *The unscented particle filter*. (Tech. Rep. CUED/F-INFENG/TR 380.) Cambridge University Engineering Department, Cambridge, UK.

Van Geert, P. (1998). Dynamic modelling of cognitive and language development: From growth processes to sudden jump and multimodality. In K. M. Newell & P. C. M. Molenaar (Eds.), *Applications of nonlinear dynamics to developmental process modeling* (pp. 129–160). Mahwah, NJ: Lawrence Erlbaum Associates.

Wan, E., & Nelson, A. T. (2001). Dual extended Kalman filter methods. In S. Haykins (Ed.), *Kalman filtering and neural networks* (pp. 123–173). New York: Wiley.

Wan, E., & Van der Merwe, R. (2001). The unscented Kalman filter. In S. Haykins (Ed.), *Kalman filtering and neural networks* (pp. 221–280). New York: Wiley.

Wen, Z., Marsh, H. W., & Hau, K.-T. (2002). Interaction effects in growth modeling: A full model. *Structural Equation Modeling*, *9*(1), 20–39.

Young, P. C., McKenna, P., & Bruun, J. (2001). Identification of non–linear stochastic systems by state dependent parameter estimation. *International Journal of Control*, *74*(18), 1837–1857.

Zarchan, P., & Musoff, H. (2000). *Fundamentals of Kalman filtering: A practical approach. Progress in Astronautics and Aeronautics*. Reston, VA: American Institute of Aeronautics and Astronautics.

Chapter 6

Growth Models for Categorical Response Variables: Standard, Latent-Class, and Hybrid Approaches

Jeroen K. Vermunt

Tilburg University, The Netherlands

6.1 INTRODUCTION

There are three main approaches to the analysis of longitudinal data (Diggle, Liang, & Zeger 1994):

1. Conditional, change-score, or transitional models.

2. Marginal or population-average models.

3. Subject-specific, random-effects, or growth models.

   Transitional models such as Markov-type models concentrate on changes between consecutive time points. Marginal models can be used to investigate changes in univariate distributions, and random-effects or growth models study development of individuals over time. These three approaches do not only differ in the questions they address, but also in the way they deal with the dependencies between the repeated measures. Because of their structure, transitional models take the bivariate dependencies between observations at consecutive occasions into account. Growth models capture the dependence by introducing one or more latent variables (random effects). In marginal models, the dependency is not explicitly modeled, but dealt with as found in the data and in general is taken into account in a more ad hoc way in the estimation procedure. Variants of transitional, growth, and marginal models have been developed for categorical response variables (Agresti, 2002), as well as hybrids combining these approaches (Vermunt, Rodrigo, & Ato, 2001).

Growth modeling is probably the most popular tool for dealing with longitudinal data in social and behavioral sciences. In econometrics, it is usually referred to as panel regression. Basically, growth models are regression models for two-level data—time points nested within individuals—in which time enters as one of the predictors. Here, we deal with growth models for categorical response variables, which implies using mixed-effects variants of the appropriate regression models from the generalized linear modeling (GLM) family, such as random-effects binary, ordinal, and multinomial logistic, and Poisson regression.

In standard growth models unobserved heterogeneity is captured by means of continuous latent variables, but it is also possible to work with discrete latent variables, which yield what is referred to as latent-class (LC) growth modeling. The purpose of this tool is to identify subgroups or clusters showing different developmental patterns or trajectories. As is shown, the LC growth model is a special case of the mixture GLM for two-level data, which makes it straightforward to deal with categorical response variables, such as binary, nominal, ordinal, and count variables. As in standard growth models, one may use continuous random effects to account for (part of) the unobserved heterogeneity, yielding hybrids between LC and standard mixed models.

Various interesting extensions of the standard LC growth model can be derived using the new multilevel LC methodology proposed by Vermunt (2003, 2004, 2005). For example, one could build a latent classification using multiple indicators and specify a growth model for these latent classifications. Another example is an LC growth model for multilevel data, in which groups may belong to latent classes with different growth patterns or in which groups may differ with respect to the growth class distribution of their members.

I first describe the standard random-effects growth model for categorical response variables. Subsequently, I discuss the LC-based growth modeling approach, as well as hybrid variants combining discrete and continuous random effects. Then, I present an empirical example in which the standard, latent-class, and hybrid methods are applied. Subsquently, I compare the obtained results with the ones that would have been obtained with a Markov model. In the last section, I present extensions of the basic models that involve the use of methods for three-level instead of two-level data.

6.2 GROWTH MODELS

Let y_{it} denote the response of case i at occasion t on the response variable of interest, and N and T the number of cases and time points, respectively, where $1 \leq i \leq N$ and $1 \leq t \leq T$. It is not necessary to assume that each case has observation at each time point, which means that the longitudinal data set at hand may be unbalanced and may contain missing values.

Growth modeling involves specifying a random-effects regression model for y_{it}, in which the time-specific responses are assumed to be a function of time (Hedeker, 2004). Depending on the scale type of the dependent variable the regression model will be another member of the GLM family (Agresti Booth, Hobert, & Caffo, 2000). More specifically, after an appropriate transformation $g(\cdot)$, the expected value of the response variable $E(y_{it})$ is assumed to be a linear function of a set of predefined functions of t. In the binary case, the transformation could, for example, be the logit transformation, yielding $g[E(y_{it})] = \log \frac{P(y_{it}=1)}{1-P(y_{it}=1)}$.

The linear model for $g[E(y_{it})]$ has the following form

$$g[E(y_{it})] = \beta_{0i} + \sum_{s=1}^{S} \beta_{si} \cdot f_s(t) = \sum_{s=0}^{S} \beta_{si} \cdot f_s(t), \tag{1}$$

in which $f_s(t)$ is a predefined function of time, and $f_0(t) = 1$ for a compact representation of the constant term. Typical special cases are the linear growth model with $S = 1$ and $f_1(t) = t - 1$, and the quadratic growth model with $S = 2$ and $f_1(t) = t - 1$ and $f_2(t) = (t - 1)^2$. The functions $f_s(t)$ could also take on the form of a set of dummy variables for time points 2 to T, in which case $S = T - 1$, and $f_s(t) = 1$ if $s = t + 1$ and 0 otherwise. For an extended discussion of possible functional forms for the time dependence, see Snijders & Bosker (1999).

The index i appearing in the subscript of each of the regression coefficients in Equation 1 indicates that these may be subject specific; that is, each individual may have its own growth curve. Note that with longitudinal data, we have to take into account that the observations of the same individual at the various time points are not independent of one another. In fact, we are dealing with a two-level data structure in which time points are nested within cases (Snijders & Bosker, 1999). Equivalent to multilevel analysis, in growth model, the dependence between observation is dealt with by assuming that some of the model parameters are "group-specific," where for parsimony, these coefficients are assumed to be random coefficients coming from a multivariate normal distribution; that is $\beta_i \sim N(\beta, \Sigma_\beta)$. It is, however, not necessary to assume that all unknown regression coefficients vary across individuals. A simpler variant of the model described in Equation 1 is obtained by assuming that only the intercept is a random effect, in which case $\beta_{is} = \beta_s$ for $1 \leq s \leq S$. Inclusion of a random intercept is the minimal requirement for claiming an appropriate treatment of the dependencies between the repeated measures within cases. It amounts to assuming that the association structure between the observations has the form of a compound symmetric covariance matrix. With random change parameters one can pick up autocorrelation structures and changing variances across occasions (Hedeker, 2004; Snijders & Bosker, 1999).

Mixed modeling, an alternative formulation of the growth model described in Equation 1, is obtained by using the reparameterization $\beta_{si} = \beta_s + u_{si}$ for $0 \leq s \leq S$, where $\mathbf{u}_i \sim N(\mathbf{0}, \mathbf{\Sigma}_\beta)$. This yields:

$$g[E(y_{it})] = \sum_{s=0}^{S} \beta_s \cdot f_s(t) + \sum_{s=0}^{S} u_{si} \cdot f_s(t), \qquad (2)$$

in which the β_s are called *fixed effects* and the u_{si} are called *random effects*.

In the case of categorical response variables, for parameter estimation by means of maximum likelihood (ML), it is useful to parameterize the mixed-effects model as a factor-analytic model with uncorrelated latent variables (random effects) with variances equal to 1. This is necessary to be able to solve the integrals appearing in the log-likelihood function by Gauss-Hermite quadrature. The factor-analytic formulation of the growth model described in Equations 1 and 2 equals:

$$g[E(y_{it})] = \sum_{s=0}^{S} \beta_s \cdot f_s(t) + \sum_{s=0}^{S} \sum_{s'=0}^{s} \lambda_{ss'} \cdot F_{s'i} \cdot f_s(t), \qquad (3)$$

where $\mathbf{F}_i \sim N(\mathbf{0}, \mathbf{I})$ and the $\lambda_{ss'}$ are elements of a $(S+1)$ by $(S+1)$ lower-diagonal "factor loadings" matrix $\mathbf{\Lambda}$. The connection between the mixed-effects and the factor-analytic parameterization is that $\mathbf{\Sigma}_\beta = \mathbf{\Lambda}\mathbf{\Lambda}'$, where $\mathbf{\Lambda}$ is the Cholesky decomposition of $\mathbf{\Sigma}_\beta$ (Skrondal & Rabe-Hesketh, 2004; Vermunt & Magidson, 2005).

To see how the Cholesky decomposition works, consider the special case that $S = 1$, yielding a factor-analytic model of the form

$$g[E(y_{it})] = \beta_0 + \beta_1 \cdot f_1(t) + \lambda_{00} \cdot F_{0i} + \lambda_{10} \cdot F_{0i} \cdot f_1(t) + \lambda_{11} \cdot F_{1i} \cdot f_1(t).$$

The connection between the λ parameters and the covariances of the random effects is the following: $\sigma_{00} = (\lambda_{00})^2$, $\sigma_{01} = \lambda_{00} \cdot \lambda_{10}$, and $\sigma_{11} = (\lambda_{10})^2 + (\lambda_{11})^2$.

The factor-analytic parameterization is not only useful for parameter estimation using ML, it offers additional flexibility in terms of constraints that can be imposed on the random effects. For example, assuming "factor loading" λ_{10} to be equal to 0 yields a model in which the random effects u_{0i} and u_{1i} are mutually uncorrelated; and assuming $\lambda_{11} = 0$ yields a model in which u_{0i} and u_{1i} are perfectly correlated. Restricted factor-analytic structures are especially useful in models containing many random coefficients as may, for instance, occur in growth models based on time dummies. With $T-1$ time dummies and an intercept, an unrestricted random part would contain T random coefficients, and as a consequence $(T + 1) \cdot T/2$ unknown parameters in the matrix Σ_β. A much simpler factor-analytic structure with say two factors and some λ elements equal to 0 will most probably do an equally good job in terms of model fit.

The mixed-effects GLM described in Equations 1, 2, and 3 can be used with response variables that are continuous, binary, or counts. For dealing with ordinal and nominal response variables, however, which from a GLM perspective are in fact multivariate responses, we need to extend somewhat the above models. Denoting a particular response category as m and the number of response categories as M, an ordinal mixed-effects GLM can be defined as

$$g[E_m(y_{it})] = \beta_{0m} + \sum_{s=1}^{S} \beta_s \cdot f_s(t) + u_{0im} + \sum_{s=1}^{S} u_{si} \cdot f_s(t).$$

Here, $g[E_m(y_{it})]$ may represent one of the $M - 1$ logits defining an adjacent-category or cumulative logit model, or the underlying latent variable in an ordinal probit model. The main difference with the dichotomous case is that there are $M - 1$ fixed (β_{0m}) and random (u_{0im}) effects associated with the intercept instead of only one. Rather that using an $M - 1$ dimensional multivariate normal distribution, Hedeker and Gibbons (1996) proposed restricting these $M - 1$ random intercept terms using a single factor, that is, as $u_{0im} = \lambda_{0m} \cdot F_{0i}$ (see also Vermunt & Magidson, 2005).

In the nominal case, we obtain

$$g[E_m(y_{it})] = \sum_{s=0}^{S} \beta_{sm} \cdot f_s(t) + \sum_{s=0}^{S} u_{sim} \cdot f_s(t).$$

where $g[E_m(y_{it})]$ will usually be one of the $M - 1$ baseline category logits in a multinomial logistic regression model. Note that there are $M - 1$ random effects associated with each term, thus not only with the intercept (Agresti et al., 2000). These can, however, again be restricted using a factor-analytic parametrization with a single factor per term: $u_{sim} = \lambda_{sm} \cdot F_{si}$ (Hedeker, 2003; Vermunt 2005; Vermunt & Magidson, 2005).

Thus far, we assumed that there were no other predictors than the time variable itself. Equivalent to standard random-effects models, growth models can easily be extended to include both time-constant (between-subject) and time-varying (within-subject) predictors, denoted as z_{pi} and z_{qit}, respectively. Suppose we have a single between-subject predictor z_{1i} indicating whether case i belongs to the treatment group ($z_{1i} = 1$) or the control group ($z_{1i} = 0$). If we assume that the treatment affects both the initial value y_{i1} and the single change term $f_1(t)$, in the mixed-effects model formulation we obtain

$$g[E(y_{it})] = \beta_0 + \beta_1 \cdot f_1(t) + \beta_2 \cdot z_{1i} + \beta_3 \cdot z_{1i} \cdot f_1(t) + u_{0i} + u_{1i} \cdot f_1(t).$$

In the alternative but equivalent two-level model formulation, one would specify that $\beta_{si} = \beta_s + \beta_{S+s} \cdot z_{1i} + u_{si}$.

The random-effects growth models presented in this section are extremely valuable tools for dealing with longitudinal data. There are, however, also several problematic aspects associated with the use of these methods.

- With categorical response variables, they may become computationally very intensive when there are more than two or three random effects. The reason for this is that the integrals appearing in the likelihood function must be solved using approximation methods, such as linearization methods, numerical integration methods, or (Bayesian) simulation techniques. A possible way out this problem is to reduce the dimensionality of the problem by using the more restricted factor-analytic specification introduced earlier. Although approximation methods usually perform very well, this not always the case (Lesaffre & Spiessens, 2001; Rabe-Hesketh, Skrondal & Pickles, 2002; Rodriguez & Goldman, 2001).

- They rely on the untestable assumption that random coefficients come from a multivariate normal distribution (Aitkin, 1999; Vermunt & Van Dijk, 2001). Results obtained with these methods may be biased when this rather strong distributional assumption is violated.

- It is not at all straightforward to interpret the parameters associated with the random effects (the variances and covariances of the u_{si} terms). A common solution to this problem is to depict selected estimated individual-specific curves, for example, the curves at 0, 1, and 2 standard deviations from the mean.

6.3 LATENT-CLASS BASED AND HYBRID GROWTH MODELS

Some of the problems associated with the parametric random-coefficients approach discussed in the previous section may be circumvented by adopting a latent-class based nonparametric random coefficients approach. This group-based approach is usually referred to as latent class (LC) or mixture regression analysis (Vermunt & Van Dijk, 2001; Wedel & DeSarbo, 2002). Using the LC regression framework, we obtain the following LC growth model:

$$g[E(y_{it}|k)] = \sum_{s=0}^{S} \beta_{sk} \cdot f_s(t), \qquad (4)$$

where k denotes a particular latent class, and again $f_0(t) = 1$. The transformed expected value of y_{it} given that case i belongs to latent class k is a function of time, where parameters may differ across latent classes. The output obtained from growth modeling using LC regression analysis is thus K class-specific growth curves, where K is the number of classes or mixture components. Nagin (1999) proposed using the mixture growth model for the analysis of developmental trajectories with the purpose to identify distinctive groups of individual trajectories. Vermunt and Van Dijk (2001) and Vermunt and Hagenaars (2004) applied the method in the context of panel studies with categorical response variables.

Although this may not be directly clear from Equation 4, also in this model we are assuming that the regression coefficients are random—that they differ across individuals according to some distribution. In fact, we assume that the individual-specific parameters come from a K-mass discrete distribution with unknown locations β_k and unknown weights π_k. By increasing the number of classes K until the log-likelihood function no longer increases, we obtain what is referred to as the nonparametric ML estimator for the random-effects model of interest (Aitkin, 1999; Skrondal & Rabe-Hesketh, 2004; Vermunt 2004). Nagin (1999) referred to the situation in which a smaller number of classes is retained than the maximum that can be identified as a semiparametric ML estimator.

The similarity with the parametric approach described in the previous section becomes even clearer if one sees that the means and covariances of the random effects can easily be obtained from the β_{sk} and π_k parameters; that is

$$\beta_s = \sum_{k=1}^{K} \beta_{sk} \cdot \pi_k, \ \sigma_{ss'} = \sum_{k=1}^{K} (\beta_{sk} - \beta_s) \cdot (\beta_{s'k} - \beta_{s'}) \cdot \pi_k.$$

In most applications, these numbers will be similar in terms of size to their parametric counterparts (fixed effects β_s and entries of Σ_β). It should also be noted that we could write β_{sk} in terms of a fixed and a random effect: $\beta_{sk} = \beta_s + u_{sk}$.

Similar to the parametric approach, it is possible to assume that certain growth parameters vary across (classes of) individuals, whereas others do not. Such a constraint amounts to equating a particular growth parameter across classes: $\beta_{sk} = \beta_{s.}$. This is, however, not the only type of constraint that can be imposed. It is also possible to equate parameters across selected classes and to fix growth parameters to 0 or some other value in selected classes. The latter options make it possible to specify LC models in which the functional form of the time dependency differs across classes. For example, in a 4-class model, in class 1 the time dependence may be quadratic, in class 2 unrestricted ($S = T - 1$ dummies), and in classes 3 and 4 there may be no time dependence ($S = 0$; no change), whereas in class 4, the intercept is fixed to a very high negative value, yielding a so-called mover-stayer or zero-inflated model. This flexibility of having class-specific models makes it possible to test very specific hypotheses about developmental trajectories.

As in the parametric case, small modifications are needed for dealing with ordinal and nominal response variables. For ordinal responses, we again have a model with category-specific intercept terms:

$$g[E_m(y_{it}|k)] = \beta_{0mk} + \sum_{s=1}^{S} \beta_{sk} \cdot f_s(t);$$

and for nominal responses a model with category-specific intercepts and slopes:

$$g[E_m(y_{it}|k)] = \sum_{s=0}^{S} \beta_{smk} \cdot f_s(t).$$

As in standard growth models, in LC-based growth models, one can include time-varying and time-constant predictors in the regression equation for the dependent variable. Whereas in the standard growth models, regressing a random effect on time-constant predictors is equivalent to including those predictors in the regression model for the outcome variable of interest, in the discrete random-effects models discussed in this section this is not the case. As a result, there are two alternative ways to deal with time-constant covariates: They can be used in the regression model for the response variable or in the regression model for the latent classes. The latter can be accomplished by means of a multinomial logistic regression model of the form

$$\log \frac{\pi_{k|\mathbf{z}_i}}{\pi_{1|\mathbf{z}_i}} = \gamma_{0k} + \sum_{p=1}^{P} \gamma_{pk} \cdot z_{pi}.$$

One could, for example, be interested in knowing whether belonging to the treatment group (say $z_{1i} = 1$) increases the probability of belonging to a latent class with a favorable trajectory. This is an alternative to a model in which treatment is assumed to have a direct effect on (changes in) the response variable.

The LC-based approach has various advantages compared to the parametric models discussed in the previous section:

- It is much less computationally intensive when applied with categorical response variables. The log-likelihood function contains a sum over K latent classes rather than a set of integrals that should be approximated by, for example, numerical integration methods. Since the log-likelihood can be computed exactly, no approximations are needed when applied with categorical responses. In fact, no special provisions are needed for dealing with such variables.

- It does not rely on nontestable assumptions about the distributions of the random effects.

- It yields much easier to interpret results. Rather than a set means, variances and covariances summarizing the N observed trajectories, one obtains K basic trajectories.

The LC-based approach not only has advantages compared to the standard approach, but also certain weak points:

- Researchers are confronted with additional model selection issues. One not only needs to decide about the functional form of the time dependence and about which parameters should be assumed to vary across individuals, but also about the necessary number of latent classes, as well as about the form for each of the class-specific time functions. A way to simplify the model selection is to 1) work with the same type of time dependence for all classes, 2) determine the number of classes using BIC (Bayesian information criterion), and 3) investigate whether the selected model can be simplified by equating parameters across classes or fixing certain coefficients to 0.

- Local maxima are more common in nonparametric random-effects models than in parametric models. However, current software has provision for dealing with the local maxima problem by using multiple sets of random starting values for the model parameters (Vermunt & Magidson, 2005).

- The LC approach has what is sometimes referred to the problem of overextraction (Bauer & Curran, 2003). It may occur that a large number of latent classes is needed to fully capture the variation in the growth parameters, and that these classes differ mainly with respect to the intercept. This can be seen as an artifact of the LC method because it is usually not what the analyst is looking for. Most likely, he is interested in finding groups with different change parameters rather than different intercepts. A way out of this problem is the hybrid methodology described later, which involves combining discrete with continuous unobserved heterogeneity (Muthén, 2004).

A simple hybrid growth model that in most applications will resolve the overextraction problem is obtained by expanding the LC regression model described in Equation 4 with a random intercept (Lenk & DeSarbo, 2000; Vermunt & Magidson, 2005). That is,

$$
\begin{aligned}
g[E(y_{it}|k)] &= \sum_{s=0}^{S} \beta_{sk} \cdot f_s(t) + u_{0i} \\
&= \sum_{s=0}^{S} \beta_{sk} \cdot f_s(t) + \lambda_{00} \cdot F_{0i},
\end{aligned}
\tag{5}
$$

Note that this model relaxes the basic assumption of the LC model that latent classes are homogenous with respect to all model parameters by allowing for within-class heterogeneity with respect to the intercept. Another way to see the random intercept is as a way to relax the assumption that the (time-specific) responses are independent within latent classes.

As far as the random part of the model described in Equation 5 is concerned, there are two possible extensions. One is to include random change parameters in addition to a random intercept. Another interesting extension is to allow the variance of u_{0i} to vary across latent classes or, equivalently, to replace λ_{00} by λ_{00k}, where $\sigma_{00k} = (\lambda_{00k})^2$. Such a model not only assumes that there is within-class heterogeneity, but also that the amount of within-class heterogeneity may differ across classes, an assumption that may be more realistic in certain applications.

Any of the extensions of the LC regression model discussed above—equality, zero and other fixed-value restrictions, class-specific time functions, ordinal and nominal responses, and explanatory variables affecting the responses and/or the classes—can also be used in hybrid models.

6.4 AN EMPIRICAL EXAMPLE

The empirical example I use to illustrate the various types of growth models discussed earlier is taken from Hedeker & Gibbon's (1996) MIXOR program. It concerns a dichotomous outcome variable "severity of schizophrenia" measured at 7 occasions (consecutive weeks). This binary outcome was obtained by collapsing a severity score ranging from 1 to 7 into two categories, where a 1 indicates that the severity score was at least 3.5 (severe), and 0 that is was smaller than 3.5 (nonsevere).

In total, there is information on 437 cases. However, for none of the cases the information is complete. For 42 cases, we have observations at 2, for 66 at 3, for 324 at 4, and for 5 at 5 time points. There are 434, 426, 14, 374, 11, 9, and 335 observations at the 7 time points.

Besides the repeated measures for the response variable, there is one time-constant predictor, treatment (0=control group; 1=treatment group). The treatment is a new drug that is expected to decrease the symptoms related to

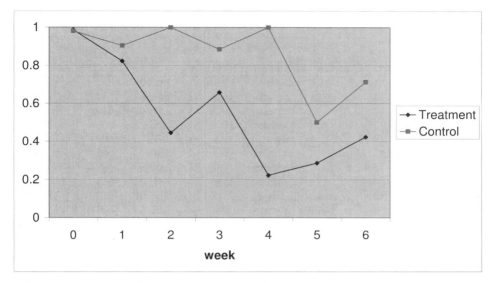

Figure 6–1. Observed trajectories for the treatment and control group.

schizophrenia. The main research question to be answered with this data set is whether the treatment reduces the symptoms related to schizophrenia.

Figure 6–1 depicts the observed probability of being in the severe state at each of the seven occasions for the treatment and control group. As can be seen, at the start of the study, almost all cases belong to the severe category in both the treatment and control group. At each of the next time points, the treatment group has a lower probability of having severe schizophrenia symptoms than the control group, showing that there is evidence for a treatment effect.

In the analysis of this data set, I followed Hedeker & Gibbon's (1996) suggestion to set $S = 1$, with $f_1(t) = \sqrt{t-1}$, and to use a binary logit model. This yields a model in which the logit of severity is a function of the square root of time. Although there is no strong theoretical motivation for using this functional form for the time dependence, there is a good empirical motivation: In a simple model without random effects, this model fits the time-specific response probabilities much better than a linear or a quadratic model, and almost as good as a model with an unrestricted time dependence. Table 6–1 reports the test results obtained by applying various of the models described in the previous two sections to the schizophrenia data set. Besides the log-likelihood value (LL), the number of parameters (# par), and the BIC value, the table provides information on the Wald test for the treatment effect (Wald value, df, and p-value). The latter is a test for the time-treatment interaction in Models 1–5 and for the treatment effect on class membership in Models 6–15.

As can be seen from Table 6–1, the estimated models differ in

TABLE 6–1
Test Results for the Growth Models Estimated With the Schizophrenia Data

Model	# Classes	Random	Treatment	Wald	df	p	LL	# par	BIC
1	1		response	2.7	1	1.0E-01	-681	4	1386
2	1	u_{0i}, u_{1i}	response	11.3	1	7.6E-04	-614	7	1270
3	2		response	9.5	1	2.1E-03	-619	7	1280
4	3		response	10.8	1	1.0E-03	-607	10	1275
5	4		response	17.5	1	2.9E-05	-602	13	1283
6	2		classes	9.5	1	2.1E-03	-625	6	1286
7	3		classes	12.4	2	2.0E-03	-608	10	1277
8	4		classes	11.2	3	1.1E-02	-601	14	1287
9	2	u_{0i}	classes	21.5	1	3.6E-06	-613	7	1268
10	3	u_{0i}	classes	12.0	2	2.5E-03	-604	11	1274
11	4	u_{0i}	classes	11.2	4	1.1E-02	-601	15	1293
12	2 (1 sqr)		classes	15.9	1	6.5E-05	-620	7	1282
13	3 (1 sqr)		classes	19.3	2	6.5E-05	-597	11	1261
14	2 (1 sqr)	u_{0i}	classes	24.8	1	6.2E-07	-601	8	1250
15	3 (1 sqr)	u_{0i}	classes	19.1	2	7.0E-05	-595	12	1263

- the way they capture unobserved heterogeneity. Model 1 contains no random effects, Model 2 is a standard growth model, Models 3–8 and 12–13 are LC-based models, and Models 9–11 and 14–15 are hybrid models

- how treatment enters in the equation. In Models 1–5 treatment affects the response, whereas in the other models, it affects class membership

- the assumed number of latent classes, ranging from 1 to 4.

- whether there is one latent class (the last one) with a different (quadratic) time dependence. This is specified by defining $f_2(t) = t - 1$ and $f_3(t) = (t - 1)^2$, and setting the parameters corresponding to these two terms to 0 in all but class K and the parameter corresponding to $f_1(t)$ to 0 in class K. This specification is used in Models 12–15.

For parameter estimation, I used version 4.0 of the Latent GOLD program (Vermunt & Magidson, 2005), which uses ML estimation. For numerical integration with Gauss-Hermite quadrature, I used the program's default setting of 10 quadrature points per dimension.

Model 1 without random effects served as a baseline model. Comparison of the log-likelihood and BIC values for Models 2–5 with the ones of Model 1 indicates clearly that it is necessary to take into account individual variation in the growth parameters. When using an LC-based approach, three latent

TABLE 6–2
Parameter Estimates Obtained with Model 14

Model for Responses	Class 1			Class 2		
	β or λ	s.e.	z-value	β or λ	s.e.	z-value
Intercept	8.79	1.17	7.54	6.76	0.88	7.64
StdDev Random Intercept	3.31	0.53	6.27	3.31	0.53	6.27
TIME			- 3.78	1.01	-3.75	
SQ-TIME				1.12	0.29	3.79
SQRT-TIME	-4.81	0.62	-7.80			

Model for Latent Classes	Class 1		
	γ	s.e.	z-value
Intercept	-0.65	0.31	-2.13
Treatment	1.78	0.36	4.98

classes seem to be needed. Whereas the log-likelihood value of the three-class model (Model 4) is clearly higher than of the standard growth model (Model 2), according to the BIC criterion the latter is somewhat better. What is most striking is that the treatment effect is not significant if we do not take unobserved heterogeneity into account (Model 1), but it turn out to be if we do so. It should be noted that Models 2 and 4 give similar answers concerning the significance and size of the treatment effect.

Models 6–8 differ from 3–5 in that treatment is assumed to affect class membership instead of having a direct effect on the outcome variable. The latter models fit somewhat worse (have lower log-likelihood and higher BIC values). Models 9–11 differ from 6–8 in that they contain a random intercept allowing for within-class heterogeneity. When using such a specification, no more than two latent classes are needed, and the Wald test for the treatment effect shows an even more significant result (see Model 9).

Models 12–15 are variants of Models 6–7 and 9–10 in which the time dependence in class K (the last class) is assumed to be quadratic instead of a function $\sqrt{t-1}$. It turns out that especially Model 14, which is a modified version of Model 9, does a very good job. It has a much lower log-likelihood value than Model 9, and despite the extra parameter, a much lower BIC value. Moreover, it indicates that there is even more evidence for a treatment effect.

Table 6–2 reports the parameter estimates obtained with Model 14. For each latent class, we have a set of parameters describing the time dependence of the logit of the probability of being in the severely schizophrenic state—Intercept and SQRT-TIME in class 1 and Intercept, TIME, and SQ-TIME in class 2—as well as the standard deviation of the random effect indicating how much the intercept varies within classes. The size of the latter parameter, which is assumed to be equal across latent classes, indicates that there is quite

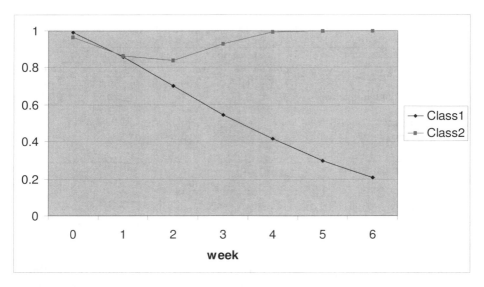

Figure 6–2. Class-specific trajectories obtained with Model 14.

some variation within classes. To get a better idea on what all these coefficients mean, Figure 6–2 depicts the estimated growth curves for the two latent
classes. The depicted time- and class-specific probabilities of being severely
depressed that are obtained by marginalizing over (integration out) the continuous random effects. The obtained figure is similar to Figure 6–1, with
the difference that the two development patterns are much smoother and more
different from one another. It can also be seen why the quadratic curve was
needed for class 2: After a small drop in weeks 1 and 2, the probability of a severe form of schizophrenia increased again, a pattern that cannot be described
by a monotonic function.

Out of the total sample, 65% is estimated to belong to latent class 1 and
35% to latent class 2. These numbers are 76% and 24% for the treatment group
and 34% and 66% for the control group. The treatment effect on class member
is given in terms of a logistic regression coefficient and its asymptotic standard
error in the lower part of Table 6–2—the odds of beginning in class 1 instead
of 2 is $\exp(1.78)$ higher for the treatment than for the control group. The encountered treatment effect shows, on the one hand, that there is a rather strong
relation between treatment and class membership, but, on the other hand, that
this relationship is far from perfect.

6.5 MARKOV MODELS

Whereas this chapter deals with growth models for repeatedly observed categorical response variables, as is already mentioned in the introduction, there are other alternatives for analyzing this type of data. The most important alternative is the standard Markov model or one of its variants (Collins & Wugalter, 1992; Langeheine & Van de Pol, 1994; Vermunt, Langeheine, & Böckenholt, 1999).

To understand the fundamental difference between a growth model and a Markov model, recall that in the former we try to describe and explain individual-level differences in the probability of being in a certain state at a particular time point. In the empirical example, we investigate whether this individual-level probability is time and treatment dependent. In Markov models on the other hand, we describe and explain aggregate transition probabilities; that is, the overall probability of being in a certain state given the state at the previous time point, possibly after controlling for covariates. In the empirical application, the question of interest could, for example, be whether the probability of experiencing a transition between schizophrenic and healthy is larger for the treatment than for the control group.

Mixed Markov and latent class Markov models are two important LC-based variants of the standard Markov model. In a mixed Markov model, individuals are assumed to belong to one of K classes that differ with respect to their transition probabilities. In the LC Markov model, the state variable is assumed to be measured with error, yielding a model in which transitions occur across time-specific *latent* states that are connected to observed states by means of a probabilistic mechanism.

I estimated a standard stationary first-order Markov model, a mixed Markov model with 2 latent classes, and an LC Markov model with 2 latent states per time point to the schizophrenia data set. The obtained log-likelihood values— -846, -844, and -844, respectively—show that these models fit as well as the best fitting growth models described previously. These log-likelihood values also show that the standard Markov model would suffice, indicating that there is no evidence for unobserved heterogeneity in the transition probabilities as assumed in the mixed Markov model, nor for measurement error in the time-specific schizophrenia state as assumed in the LC Markov model.

The estimated transition probabilities obtained with the stationary first-order Markov model indicate that the treatment group has a higher probability of a transition out of the schizophrenic state (0.23 v. 0.05 for control group) and a lower probability of a transition into the schizophrenic state (0.08 v. 0.16). This is in agreement with the evidence for a positive treatment effect as obtained with the growth modeling approach.

6.6 EXTENSIONS

Various interesting extensions of the growth models described and illustrated in the previous sections can be obtained using the multilevel LC framework that was recently proposed by Vermunt (2003, 2004, 2005). Two of these are growth models for multiple response variables and growth models for individuals nested within groups. Both applications yield data structures with three instead of two levels of nesting; that is, multiple responses nested within time points and time points nested within cases, and time points nested within cases and cases nested within groups.

Suppose that rather than with a single indicator we would measure the severity of schizophrenia using multiple indicators. Let $y_{it\ell}$ be the response of case i at occasion t on item ℓ and L the total number of items. A possible manner to deal with these multiple indicators is to construct a time-specific latent typology using a standard LC model (Goodman, 1974; Magidson & Vermunt, 2004). The time-specific LC model would be of the well-known form:

$$P(\mathbf{y}_{it} = \mathbf{m}) = \sum_{x=1}^{X} P(x_{it} = x) \prod_{\ell=1}^{L} P(y_{it\ell} = m_\ell | x_{it} = x),$$

where x_{it} denotes the class membership of case i at occasion t, x a particular latent class and X the number of latent classes. The growth model is no longer specified for the observed responses, but instead for the time-specific class memberships x_{it}. Depending on whether one uses a standard or an LC-based growth model, that part of the model would take the form of a mixed-effect multinomial logistic regression model

$$\log \frac{P(x_{it} = x)}{P(x_{it} = 1)} = \sum_{s=0}^{S} \beta_{sx} \cdot f_s(t) + \sum_{s=0}^{S} u_{sxi} \cdot f_s(t).$$

or an LC multinomial logistic regression model

$$\log \frac{P(x_{it} = x|k)}{P(x_{it} = 1|k)} = \sum_{s=0}^{S} \beta_{sxk} \cdot f_s(t).$$

This multilevel LC approach to multiple response growth modeling makes sense if the multiple responses are indicators of a single underlying latent variable. The proposed method is, in fact, similar to LC Markov modeling (Vermunt, Langeheine, & Böckenholt, 1999), but rather than modeling dependencies between the time-specific latent states using a transition structure, here these are modeled using random effects.

Nagin & Tremblay (2001) proposed an alternative growth modeling approach for multiple responses that makes more sense if these are *not* indicators of the same underlying variable. His approach amounts to specifying a separate LC growth structure for each response variable, where the multiple class memberships are allowed to be correlated with one another. Nagin's model can, in fact, be specified as standard LC regression model with specific equality constraints across the latent classes so that these can be interpreted as the categories of a joint discrete latent variable.

The three-level modeling approach cannot only be used to deal with multiple response variables, but also with situations in which individuals are nested within groups, such as children nested within schools, employees nested within firms, patients nested within therapists, or citizens nested within regions. In such situations, one may wish to investigate how the parameters of the specified growth model differ across groups. There are at least four types of hierarchical data extensions of the growth models discussed in the previous section that may be of interest:

1. Inclusion of group-level random effects in a standard growth model;

2. Inclusion of a group-level discrete latent variable affecting the response variable in a LC-based growth model;

3. Inclusion of group-level random effects in the model for the individual-level growth classes;

4. Inclusion of a group-level discrete latent variable affecting the individual-level growth classes.

Option 1 yields a standard three-level mixed-effects model, whereas option 2 yields its LC-based nonparametric counterpart (Vermunt, 2004). These models make it possible to assume that growth curves differ both across groups and individuals. Suppose that the patients participating in the schizophrenia study are nested within therapists, and that it makes sense to assume that there is a therapist effect on the outcome variable. In the standard random effects approach, this might give rise to a mixed-effects model of the form:

$$g[E(y_{jit})] = \sum_{s=0}^{S} \beta_s \cdot f_s(t) + \sum_{s=0}^{S} u_{sij} \cdot f_s(t) + \sum_{s=0}^{S} v_{sj} \cdot f_s(t),$$

where the index j refers to the therapist and v_{sj} are random therapist effects. Similarly, it is possible to expand the LC-based model with therapist effects by assuming that each therapist belongs to one of G classes of therapist. Denoting a particular group-level class by g, the three-level LC regression model can be defined as

$$g[E(y_{jit}|k,g)] = \sum_{s=0}^{S} \beta_{sk} \cdot f_s(t) + \sum_{s=0}^{S} v_{sg} \cdot f_s(t),$$

where v_{sg} are the group-level growth parameters.

Options 3 and 4 listed previously are variants of the multilevel LC models described by Vermunt (2003, 2005). The basic idea is that groups may differ with respect to the sizes of the growth classes. In the context of our schizophrenia application, this might mean that the probability of belonging to class 1—the class that showed a significant improvement over time—varies between therapists. Depending on whether one uses a standard or LC-based random-effects approach for this part of the model, one obtains

$$\log \frac{\pi_{k|\mathbf{z}_{ij},\mathbf{v}_j}}{\pi_{1|\mathbf{z}_{ij},\mathbf{v}_j}} = \gamma_{0k} + \sum_{p=1}^{P} \gamma_{pk} \cdot z_{pij} + v_{0kj},$$

where v_{0kj} is a group-level random intercept, or

$$\log \frac{\pi_{k|\mathbf{z}_{ij},g}}{\pi_{1|\mathbf{z}_{ij},g}} = \gamma_{0kg} + \sum_{p=1}^{P} \gamma_{pk} \cdot z_{pij},$$

where the index g in γ_{0kg} indicates that the intercept in the model for the individual-level classes differs across group-level classes. Whereas in these specifications only the intercept is assumed to be group specific, the covariate effects—for example, the treatment effect—can be assumed to differ across groups (therapists).

REFERENCES

Agresti, A. (2002). *Categorical Data Analysis*. New York: Wiley.

Agresti A., Booth, J. G., Hobert, J. P., & Caffo, B. (2000). Random-effects modeling of categorical response data. *Sociological Methodology, 30,* 27–80.

Aitkin (1999). A general maximum likelihood analysis of variance components in generalized linear models. *Biometrics, 55,* 218–234.

Bauer, D. J., & Curran, P. J. (2003). Distributional assumptions of growth mixture models: Implications for overextraction of latent trajectories. *Psychological Methods, 8,* 338–364.

Collins, L. M., & Wugalter, S. E. (1992). Latent class models for stage-sequential dynamic latent variables. *Multivariate Behavioral Research, 27,* 131-157.

Diggle, P. J., Liang, K.Y., & Zeger, S. L. (1994). *Analysis of longitudinal data.* Oxford: Clarendon Press.

Goodman, L. A. (1974). The analysis of systems of qualitative variables when some of the variables are unobservable: Part I. A modified latent structure approach. *American Journal of Sociology, 79,* 1179–1259.

Hedeker, D. (2003). A mixed-effects multinomial logistic regression model. *Statistics in Medicine, 22,* 1433–1446.

Hedeker, D. (2004). Introduction to growth modeling. In D. Kaplan (Ed.), *The Sage handbook of quantitative methodology for the social sciences* (215–234). Thousand Oaks, CA: Sage.

Hedeker, D., & Gibbons, R. D. (1996). MIXOR: A computer program for mixed-effects ordinal regression analysis. *Computer Methods and Programs in Biomedicine, 49,* 157–176.

Langeheine, R., & Van de Pol, F. (1994). Discrete-time mixed Markov latent class models. In A. Dale & R. B. Davies (Eds.), *Analyzing social and political change: A casebook of methods* (pp. 170–197). London: Sage.

Lenk, P.J., & DeSarbo, W.S. (2000). Bayesian inference for finite mixture models of generalized linear models with random effects. *Psychometrika, 65,* 93–119.

Lesaffre, E. & Spiessens, B. (2001), On the effect of the number of quadrature points in a logistic random-effects model: An example. *Applied Statistics, 50,* 325–335.

Magidson, J., & Vermunt, J.K. (2004). Latent class models. IN D. Kaplan (Ed.), *The Sage handbook of quantitative methodology for the social sciences* (175–198). Thousand Oaks, CA: Sage.

Muthén, B. (2004). Latent variable analysis: Growth mixture modeling and related techniques for longitudinal data. In D. Kaplan (Ed.), *The Sage handbook of quantitative methodology for the social sciences* (345–368). Thousand Oaks, CA: Sage.

Nagin, D. S. (1999). Analyzing developmental trajectories: A semiparametric group-based approach. *Psychological Methods, 4,* 139–157.

Nagin, D. S., & Tremblay, R. E. (2001). Analyzing developmental trajectories of distinct but related behaviors: A group-based method. *Psychological Methods, 6,* 18–34.

Rabe-Hesketh, S., Skrondal, A., & Pickles, A. (2002). Reliable estimation of generalised linear mixed models using adaptive quadrature. *The Stata Journal, 2,* 1–21.

Rodriguez, G. & Goldman, N. (2001). Improved estimation procedures for multilevel models for binary response: A case study. *Journal of the Royal Statistical Society, Series A, 164,* 339–355.

Skrondal, A. & Rabe-Hesketh, S. (2004). *Generalized latent variable modeling: Multilevel, longitudinal and structural equation models.* London: Chapman & Hall/CRC.

Snijders, T. A. B., & Bosker, R. J. (1999). *Multilevel analysis.* London: Sage.

Vermunt, J. K. (2003). Multilevel latent class models. *Sociological Methodology, 33,* 213–239.

Vermunt, J. K. (2004). An EM algorithm for the estimation of parametric and nonparametric hierarchical nonlinear models. *Statistica Neerlandica, 58,* 220–233.

Vermunt J. K. (2005). Mixed-effects logistic regression models for indirectly observed outcome variables. *Multivariate Behavioral Research, 40,* 281–301.

Vermunt, J. K., Langeheine, R., & Böckenholt, U. (1999). Latent Markov models with time-constant and time-varying covariates. *Journal of Educational and Behavioral Statistics, 24,* 178–205.

Vermunt, J. K., & Hagenaars, J. A. (2004). Ordinal longitudinal data analysis. In R. Hauspie, N. Cameron & L. Molinari (Eds.), *Methods in human growth research* (374–393). Cambridge, UK: Cambridge University Press.

Vermunt, J. K., & Magidson, J. (2005). *Technical guide to latent GOLD 4.0: Basic and advanced.* Belmont, MA: Statistical Innovations Inc.

Vermunt, J. K., Rodrigo, M. F., Ato, M. (2001) Modeling joint and marginal distributions in the analysis of categorical panel data. *Sociological Methods and Research, 30,* 170–196.

Vermunt, J. K., & Van Dijk. L. (2001). A nonparametric random-coefficients approach: The latent class regression model. *Multilevel Modelling Newsletter, 13,* 6–13.

Wedel, M., & DeSarbo, W. (2002). Mixture regression models. In J. Hagenaars & A. McCutcheon (Eds.), *Applied latent class analysis* (366–382). Cambridge, UK: Cambridge University Press.

Chapter 7

Dynamic Structural Equation Modeling in Longitudinal Experimental Studies

John J. McArdle

University of Southern California, Los Angeles

7.1 INTRODUCTION

In this research, we present contemporary statistical models useful for testing dynamic hypotheses using longitudinal experimental data. The statistical models described here come from recent research on using latent variable *structural equation modeling* (SEM) for longitudinal data, especially those proposed by McArdle and Nesselroade (1994, 2003). We use models with latent variables to represent group and individual changes in a bivariate dynamic system across different variables at different occasions of measurement. These dynamic structural equation models have been used before as the basis of a developmental interpretation of the sequential influences of one variable on another over time (e.g., Coleman, 1968; Cook & Campbell, 1979; Rogosa, 1978). However, this chapter emphasizes the use of these kinds of models in situations where individuals have been randomly assigned to one or more treatment groups in a randomized experiment (e.g., a clinical trial). Several standard ANOVA-based assumptions, including tests of mean differences over time between groups are possible to mimic using SEM. This chapter goes further with SEM analyses focused on isolating aspects of experimental manipulation that alter the dynamic processes, both within and between variables.

This dynamic SEM approach used here offers a practical approximation of dynamic interpretations for traditional experimental data with a standard collection of repeated measures. To illustrate this approach, we use data from the *Berlin Age Training Study* (*BATS*; Baltes, Dittmann-Kohli, & Kliegl, 1986). These data come from a cognitive experiment on older individuals who were randomly assigned to groups where they were either trained or not trained on specific cognitive tasks. All participants were repeatedly measured on several cognitive tasks on up to four occasions over a short period of time, and the data used here are presented in Figure 7-1. The first set of analyses are based on a univariate latent change score model to evaluate the *impacts of training over time*, and the second set of analyses use a bivariate latent difference score method to evaluate the *transfer of learning* (see Ellis, 1965; Kling & Riggs, 1971). Previous SEM using these data have been presented by Raykov (1997a, 1997b), but our new dynamic models have a different basis and yield different substantive conclusions. The results also highlight a key technical aspect of experimental and non-randomized analyses: the dynamic results of treatments are not only found in the group means.

Figure 7-1. BATS data for two groups on two tasks over four occasions

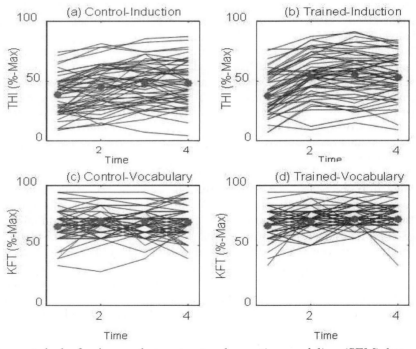

A great deal of prior work on *structural equation modeling* (SEM) has been devoted to the problems of longitudinal analyses and a complete overview will not be presented here (but see McArdle & Nesselroade, 2003). The well-known work of Jöreskog and Sörbom formalized and tested

auto-regressive simplex models using latent variables (Jöreskog, 1970, 1977; Jöreskog & Sörbom, 1979; Sörbom, 1975). These new models also provided a practical way to deal with the complex issue of measurement error estimation from panel data (e.g., McArdle & Woodcock, 1997; Sörbom, 1975; Wiley & Wiley, 1970). With a similar focus on longitudinal research, Meredith and Tisak (1990) showed how the "Tuckerized curve" models (after Tucker, 1958; cf. Rao, 1958) could be represented and fitted using structural equation modeling based on restricted common factors. This stimulated further work on this topic (e.g., McArdle, 1986, 1988, 1989), including advanced work on multivariate time series and differential equations structural modeling (e.g., Arminger, 1986; Boker, 2000; Molenaar, 1985; Oud & Jansen, 2000). The longitudinal models presented here are based on the use of latent difference scores (after McArdle, 2001; McArdle & Hamagami, 2004).

It is well known that *random assignment to treatment groups* permits key statistical assumptions about unobserved variables to be assured. That is, group assignment is assumed to be uncorrelated with all residual terms (in large samples) and this leads to unambiguous attribution of the treatment impacts in size and direction (e.g., Fisher, 1920). The SEM approach can be used to consider more general possibilities for experimental impacts and for evaluating non-random confounds and subsequent causal inference. The classic compilation of Blalock (1985), included key papers by Miller, Costner, and Alwin and Tessler. The main message in these papers was that SEM should be used together with sound experimental designs to clarify the relationship between model assumptions and related causal inferences. This was not surprising because these ideas are a reflection of the long history of creating powerful experimental designs in the behavioral sciences (e.g., Fisher, 1920; Healy, Proctor, & Weiner, 2003; Kling & Riggs, 1971; Subedi, 2004). However, this mixture of SEM and experimental design was not always part of the SEM-based search for causal structure (e.g., Glymour et al, 1987; Heise, 1975; James, Muliak, & Brett, 1982; Kenny, 1979; Shaffer, 1992). It is not surprising that SEM with stronger causal inference has become a key feature of contemporary statistical modeling (e.g., Holland, 1993; Pearl, 2000).

A *multiple group SEM approach* (MG-SEM) is used here. This also follows the seminal work of Jöreskog (1971) and Sörbom (1974, 1978; also see Horn & McArdle, 1992; McArdle, 1994; McArdle & Cattell, 1994; Muthen & Curran, 1997). The use of MG-SEM allows us to consider differences between groups in many different ways. We use these models to write the set of expectations for the means, variances, and covariances for all observed scores. We can then use these expectations to identify, estimate, and examine the goodness-of-fit of latent variable models representing change over time. Most of the models discussed here are based on fitting observed raw-score longitudinal growth data to a theoretical model using *maximum likelihood estimation* (MLE, as in Little & Rubin, 1987; McArdle & Bell, 2000).

These theoretical restrictions will not hold exactly in any real data, and this leads to the general issues of model testing and goodness-of-fit. A few available SEM computer programs (e.g., LISREL, Jöreskog & Sörbom, 1999; Mx, Neale et al, 1999; AMOS, Arbuckle & Wotke, 1999; Mplus, Muthen & Muthen, 2002) can be used to estimate the parameters of all analyses described herein.

7.2 METHODS

The data used here come from the *Berlin Age Training Study* (with the permission of the authors; Baltes, Dittmann-Kohli, & Kliegl, 1986). The general purpose of this data collection was to evaluate theory of "cognitive plasticity" that suggests that older adults have untapped cognitive resources that can be stimulated by cognitive training (for overview, see Baltes & Mayer, 1999). This specific data collection was intended to replicate and extend the training paradigm used earlier (Willis, Blieszner, & Baltes, 1981), and this experiment was carried out at the Max Planck Institute in Berlin (when the author was a visiting scientist). Details about this study are presented in detail in other published articles (e.g., Baltes et al., 1986; Raykov, 1997a, 1997b), so only essential details of the experiment are presented here.

Longitudinal Participants and Procedures

The study participants were N=248 individuals (188 females and 60 males) who were about 72 years of age (60-86) living in Berlin (West Germany) in the early 1980s. All of the participants were volunteers, of average educational level but with high cognitive functioning, and in good health (rated subjectively) and physically able to visit a cognitive laboratory. Persons were randomly assigned to one of two groups where they were either (a) trained on one of two cognitive tasks ($n = 161$), or (b) a no-contact (not trained) control group ($n = 87$). No significant demographic (age, gender, education) or health differences were found among these groups.

   The cognitive training program consisted of 10 sessions conducted in the first month. The sessions each dealt with training specifically focused on the improvement of aspects of "fluid intelligence" or "reasoning in novel situations" (see Horn, 1988) using training methods developed in earlier research (the ADEPT project; Willis et al, 1981). A cognitive measurement design included four rounds of repeated cognitive testing: (t = 0) A pre-test measurement followed by one-month of training of no-contact, (t = 1) a one week post-test measurement, (t = 2), a one month post-test measurement (t = 3), and a six-month post-test (t = 4) measurement. These time points were chosen because they were thought to represent critical junctures in the learning of these cognitive tasks.

At each measurement session, a battery of eight cognitive tests was repeatedly administered to everyone. Data from two of these eight tests are included in the analyses here:

Induction (IND). The score at each occasion is a weighted composite based on Letter Sets, Number Series, and Letter Series (see Willis et al, 1981). This was described by Baltes et al. (1986) as a "near-transfer" test and is expected to be directly impacted by the specific training.

Vocabulary (VOC). The score at each occasion is based on the German form of the KFT (from Beltz) and is similar to the vocabulary found in standard tests (e.g., the ETS-Kit test). This was described by Baltes et al. (1986) as a "far-transfer" test and is not expected to be directly impacted by the specific training.

Longitudinal Data and Previous Analyses

The repeated measures data on these two tasks are presented for the two groups in the longitudinal plots in Figure 7-1. The Induction scores are plotted in the upper half, with the control group measured (upper left hand) compared to the trained group (upper right half). The Vocabulary scores are plotted in the lower half, with the control group measured (upper left hand) compared to the trained group (upper right half).

Table 7-1 is a listing of the means, variances, and correlations of these two measures over time for both groups. The means and standard deviations for two composite variables show early increases followed by less change in the later months, and the trained group appears to exhibit higher cognitive scores. The variance generally increases, but not uniformly, and the Control group appears slightly more variable than the Experimental group. The correlations of these measures over four occasions are positive and high within each variable over time (e.g., $r > 0.8$-$.0.9$) and lower between variables over time (e.g., $r > 0.3$-$.05$). These summary statistics of Table 7-1 are used in the MG-SEM to follow.

TABLE 7-1a

Means for the two Groups on two Variables at four Occasions

	IND[0]	IND[1]	IND[2]	IND[3]	VOC[0]	VOC[1]	VOC[2]	VOC[3]
Untrained	38.60	44.94	47.87	48.00	65.77	69.73	69.92	69.22
Trained	37.47	53.28	54.80	52.62	66.05	69.84	71.39	71.39

TABLE 7-1b

Deviations for the two Groups on two Variables at four Occasions

	IND[0]	IND[1]	IND[2]	IND[3]	VOC[0]	VOC[1]	VOC[2]	VOC[3]
Untrained	17.86	20.25	20.22	20.80	15.22	13.17	13.36	13.23
Trained	17.53	19.42	19.80	19.41	15.09	13.55	11.18	12.57

TABLE 7-1c

Correlations for the two Groups on two Variables at four Occasions

Correlations for the Untrained Group ($n=87$)

	IND[0]	IND[1]	IND[2]	IND[3]
IND[0]	1.000			
IND[1]	0.902	1.000		
IND[2]	0.882	0.925	1.000	
IND[3]	0.896	0.923	0.928	1.000
VOC[0]	0.529	0.554	0.527	0.496
VOC[1]	0.466	0.473	0.439	0.449
VOC[2]	0.584	0.594	0.565	0.579
VOC[3]	0.511	0.439	0.443	0.446

	VOC[0]	VOC[1]	VOC[2]	VOC[3]
VOC[0]	1.000			
VOC[1]	0.753	1.000		
VOC[2]	0.699	0.765	1.000	
VOC[3]	0.584	0.626	0.702	1.000

Correlations for the Trained Group ($n=161$)

	IND[0]	IND[1]	IND[2]	IND[3]
IND[0]	1.000			
IND[1]	0.871	1.000		
IND[2]	0.849	0.949	1.000	
IND[3]	0.855	0.944	0.932	1.000

VOC[0]	0.339	0.365	0.356	0.338
VOC[1]	0.438	0.467	0.458	0.463
VOC[2]	0.424	0.395	0.390	0.420
VOC[3]	0.427	0.416	0.410	0.460

	VOC[0]	VOC[1]	VOC[2]	VOC[3]
VOC[0]	1.000			
VOC[1]	0.517	1.000		
VOC[2]	0.573	0.486	1.000	
VOC[3]	0.521	0.658	0.584	1.000

7.3 MODELS

Previous researchers have considered the application of standard multivariate models to repeated measures data (e.g., Harris, 1963; Horn, 1972). The original analyses by Baltes et al. (1986) used a Repeated Measures (Between x Within) ANOVA to examine the questions of group differences in trends over trials. All eight measures were rescaled into a common mean and variance, and these eight measures were compared against one another as a factor in the ANOVA. This ANOVA resulted in significant effects for main effects of group, time, and test, and for the interactions of group and test, and also for some tests and times. The differences in the means over variables were also aligned in a plot (see Figure 7-1, p. 160) showing that the ordering of the impacts was closely aligned with an *apriori* "spectrum of transfer."

Raykov (1997a, 1997b) reanalyzed one subset of these data using a model for multiple indicators of an Induction factor. The SEMs were based on factor analysis in multiple groups with correlated growth curves (as in McArdle, 1989). Raykov concluded that "The results indicate (a) group equivalence in the pattern of temporal development of ability variances, and (b) training effects in the experimental group that are stronger than the practice/experience effects in the control group, whereby both types of effects are maintained over the 6-month testing period." (1997a, p. 283). We do not use the same data or SEM models here, but the specific questions about group differences due to training are relevant to our analyses.

A few traditional models in the literature used for this purpose are now described in SEM terms. We then present more recent variations of SEM models based on latent difference scores. These new models are designed to highlight group and individual differences in the dynamic patterns of results that can be attributed to the training.

Initial Equality Across Treatment Groups

These longitudinal data of Figure 7-1 are assumed (a) to be measured on the same persons, (b) under the same conditions, (c) to represent the same constructs, and (d) are scored in the same units at each occasion. Assume we observe a constant set of persons (subscript n), split into at least two groups (G), and measured on multiple scores at multiple occasions over time (brackets t), so we can write

$$Y[t]_n, \ X[t]_n, \ t=0 \ \text{to} \ T, \ \text{and} \ G_n \tag{1a}$$

We can now further assume we have randomly assigned persons to one or more independent groups (G) and that membership in these groups is fixed over time. If the initial values ($Y[0]$ and $X[0]$) represent a measurement made as a "pre-test," we can add the assumption that the groups are the same at this pre-test. Most commonly, the means of the two groups are assumed to be identical, and this is symbolized here as

$$E\{G, Y[0]\}=0 \ \text{and} \ E\{G, X[0]\}=0. \tag{1b}$$

This expression uses the expectation operator ($E\{*\}$) to summarize the assumption that the group membership is independent of the initial values. Given, that we have multiple groups, these assumptions can be evaluated using standard SEM to both: (a) to find out if the groups do differ at the initial time point, and (b) to correct potential biases about changes that would occur if the groups do differ. The SEM constraints of Equation 1b are designed to provide a reasonable statistical answer to the key experimental question, "What treatment differences would appear if the groups were identical at the pre-test?"

Group Differences in Autoregressive Change Models
The description of the model for subsequent time points can take on any of several alternative forms. One popular model for longitudinal data with groups can be written as a structural regression model for a single outcome variable as

$$Y[t]_n = \beta_0 + \beta_1 \ Y[t-1]_n + \beta_2 \ G_n + e[t]_n, \tag{2a}$$

where the observed scores at any time ($Y[t]$) are a linear function of the score at the previous time ($Y[t-1]$), plus a shift in the intercept due to group membership (G), a group by score interaction ($G \ x \ Y[t-1]$), plus an independent residual error component (e). If a different treatment of the groups was carried out between time t-1 and time t, then this model is a form of an *analysis of covariance* model where the score at the previous time is the covariate (β_1), the group differences in the intercepts at the post-test (β_2) are independent of the initial status at the previous time

A path diagram of this ANCOVA model is depicted in Figure 7-2a. Following the rules for SEM diagrams (see McArdle, 2005), we draw observed variables as squares ($Y[0]$ and $Y[1]$), unobserved or latent variables as circles (e), fixed variables as triangles (the unit constant and the group code), and we include all the model parameters as either one-headed or two-headed arrows. The diagram matches the equation and it is clear that the score at the post-test ($Y[1]$) is a function of the pre-test score ($Y[0]$), and the group membership (G).

In general, this regression model is flexible because the group variable may be coded in different ways depending on the specific contrasts of interest (i.e., dummy coded). The use of the pre-test covariate ($Y[0]$) is intended to rule out any spurious within group variation and to provide a more accurate assessment of group differences in means (i.e., intercepts), especially when the assumption of Equation 1b is not met because groups have different initial means. However, because there is only one slope coefficient (β_1) for both groups, we essentially assume the relationship of $Y[0]$ and $Y[1]$ does not differ over groups. To investigate this possibility, it is typical to add a parameter to define the group differences in the autoregressions – the interaction (β_3) – so equal within group slopes may be evaluated simultaneously or sequentially by simply adding a product variable (G x $Y[0]$; see Cohen et al., 2003).

Figure 7-2a. A single group auto-regression model with fixed group differences

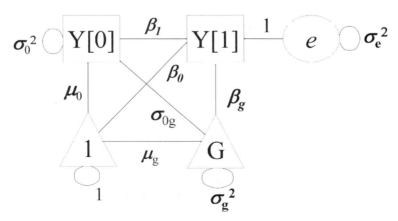

An alternative way of writing this model is to use a *multiple group* equation (following Sörbom, 1978). In this approach, the data are split into separate and independent groups and any parameter of the model may vary

over groups or may be equal over groups (i.e., invariant) To write this model, we eliminate the group variable but add a group coding (g) as a superscript on both the variables and the model parameters. In the simple case of autoregression we write

$$Y[t]_n^{(g)} = \beta_0^{(g)} + \beta_1^{(g)} \; Y[t-1]_n^{(g)} + e[t]_n^{(g)} \quad . \tag{2b}$$

This form of the model is also quite flexible and is depicted for two occasions and two groups in the path diagram of Figure 7-2b. In theory there are only a few differences between the two forms of this model. For example, the model of Equation 2a is used to ask questions about the intercept differences related to the group variable G (i.e., is $|\beta_2| > 0$?), while the model of Equation 2b is used to ask whether there is equality or invariance of the intercepts over groups (i.e., is $\beta_0^{(c)} = \beta_0^{(e)}$?). The model in Figure 2a includes a product term (G-by-$Y[1]$) and allows a test of equal slope assumption (i.e., is $|\beta_3| > 0$?) whereas in Figure 7-2b we would ask the same question in terms of the equality or invariance of the intercepts (i.e., is $\beta_1^{(c)} = \beta_1^{(e)}$?). The multiple group version (Figure 7-2b) does allow for different error variances over groups so homoskedasticity over groups can be examined. In practice, the multiple group model with invariance options offers an easy way to consider group differences in parameters.

Figure 7-2b. A multiple group autoregression model with fixed group differences.

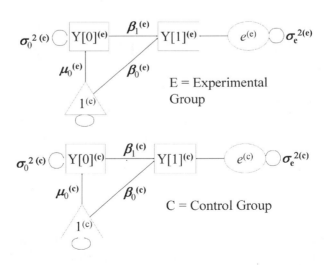

Group Differences in Difference Score Change Models

Another popular model for longitudinal data with groups can be written as

$$(Y[t]_n - Y[t\text{-}1]_n) = \alpha_0 + \alpha_1 \ G_n + d[t]_n \ , \tag{3a}$$

where the difference between observed scores at any two times ($Y[t]$ and $Y[t\text{-}1]$) is a linear function of some intercept (α_0) plus some shift in the intercept (α_1) due to group membership (G), plus some unique residual components (d). If we assume that some differential treatment of the groups was carried out between time t-1 and time t, then this is a form of a *repeated measures analysis of variance* model. As before, this regression model is flexible because the group variable may be coded in different ways depending on the specific contrasts of interest, the score at the previous time can be used as a covariate, and the group differences at the post-test are independent of the initial status at the previous time. In addition, group differences in these slopes may be evaluated by including a group by score product variable (i.e., $G \times Y[t\text{-}1]$; not included here).

In order to write this model following the basic rules of path analysis, we first rewrite Equation 3a as the

$$\Delta Y[t]_n = (Y[t]_n - Y[t\text{-}1]_n), \text{ or}$$
$$Y[t]_n = Y[t\text{-}1]_n + \Delta Y[t]_n \text{ or}$$
$$Y[t]_n = 1*Y[t\text{-}1]_n + 1*\Delta Y[t]_n, \tag{3b}$$

so the difference score ($\Delta Y[t]$) is represented as an indirectly observed linear combination (with unit weights) and appears as a variable in the model (from McArdle & Nesselroade, 1994). As the path diagram in Figure 7-3a shows, the use of this simple algebraic alternative allows us to write a model of the difference score without altering the position of the original observed variables. The comparison of Figure 7-2a and 7-3a directly shows how the two models use the same data under a different set of model assumptions. It should be noted that the interactions can be added to this model using product variables (as in Figure 7-2a), but this is hardly ever fitted. The differences between these well-known and widely used Equations 2a and 3a have led to "paradoxical" interpretations (e.g., Lord, 1969; Wainer, 1991).

Figure 7-3a. A latent difference score with fixed group differences.

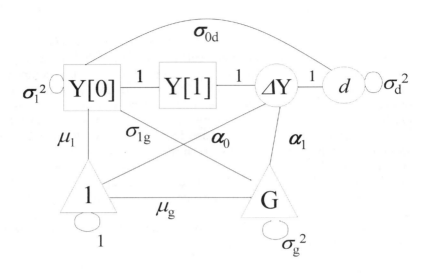

The difference model representation in Figures 3a and 3b naturally leads to a multiple group version written here simply as

$$\Delta Y[t]_n^{(g)} = \alpha_0^{(g)} + d[t]_n^{(g)} \quad , \tag{3c}$$

so the differences between groups are related to the shifts in the scores that may vary over groups. This kind of model is depicted for two variables and two groups in the path diagram of Figure 7-3b. In model 3a, questions about the intercept differences related to the group variable G (i.e., is $|\alpha_2| > 0$?) are equivalent to Equation 3c and Figure 7-3b questions about the equality or invariance of the intercepts (i.e., is $\alpha_0^{(c)} = \alpha_0^{(e)}$?). The multiple group version (Equation 3c) also allows for different residual variances over groups. As in the autoregressive case, the multiple group difference score model with invariance options offers an easy way to consider group differences.

Figure 7-3b. A more general multiple group latent difference score model with fixed group differences

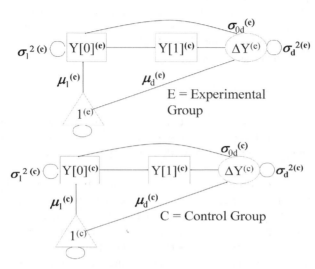

Group Differences in Latent Difference Score Models

In recent research, we recast the previous growth models using *latent difference scores* (McArdle, 2001). These models encompass the latent growth models just described, but they are formed in a different way and have properties that permit easy extensions to multivariate forms (after McArdle & Nesselroade, 1994, 2003). The key feature of this latent difference score approach is that we do not directly define the basis (*A*[t]) coefficients of a trajectory equation -- instead we directly define *changes as an accumulation of the first differences among latent variables*.

More formally, we first assume we have observed scores *Y*[t] and *Y*[t-1] measured over a defined interval of time (Δt), but we assume the latent variables are defined over an equal interval of time (Δt = 1). This definition of an equal interval latent time scale is nontrivial because it allows us to eliminate Δt from the rest of the equations. That is, in any model we can write

$$Y[t]_n = y[t]_n + e[t]_n \quad \text{and} \quad y[t]_n = y[t-1]_n + \Delta y[t]_n \ , \tag{4a}$$

with latent scores *y*[t] and *y*[t-1], residual scores *e*[t], possibly representing measurement error, and *latent difference scores* Δ*y*[t]. Even though this difference Δ*y*[t] is a theoretical score and not simply a fixed linear combination, we can write a structural model for *any latent change concept* without directly writing the resulting complex trajectory (as in McArdle, 2001; McArdle & Hamagami, 2001; McArdle & Nesselroade, 1994) as

$$Y[t]_n = y_{0,n} + (\Sigma_{i=1,t} \Delta y[t]_n) + u[t]_n .   \qquad (4b)$$

This simple algebraic device Equation 4a allows us to generally define the trajectory equation based on a summation ($\Sigma_{i=1,t}$) or accumulation of the latent changes ($\Delta y[t]$) up to time t, and these structural expectations are automatically generated using any standard SEM software (e.g., LISREL, Mplus, Mx, etc.; see Hamagami & McArdle, 2000).

This latent difference score approach makes it possible to consider any change model, including one where

$$\Delta y[t]_n = \alpha\, y_{1,n} + \beta\, y[t-1]_n + z[t]_n,   \qquad (4c)$$

where the y_1 is a latent slope score that is constant over time, and the α and β are coefficients that describe the change. This *dual change model* combines an additive change parameter (α) with a multiplicative change parameter (β; see McArdle, 2001).

To some degree, Equation 4c represents a simple combination of the autoregressive concepts of Equation 2 with the difference score equations 3a, 3b, and 3c. In general these dynamic coefficients (α and β) are not all re-quired to be invariant over time, and a family of more complex curves can result from fitting non-invariant coefficients ($\alpha[t]$ and/or $\beta[t]$) or adding the stochastic terms ($z[t]$). However, if the residual components of the latent change ($z[t]$) are not included, the expectations describe a more restricted set of latent curves that are required to be deterministic and smooth over time. This kind of a model is drawn as a path diagram in Figure 7-4a with all pa-rameters presumed to be equal over time. This deterministic approach is used to compare groups in the analyses presented here.

This approach leads to many ways of considering the treatment impacts in latent difference score models. One popular model is based on the use of extension variables added to Equation 4a as

$$y_{0,n} = v_0 + \kappa_0\, G + d_{0,n} , \quad and \quad y_{1,n} = v_1 + \kappa_1\, G + d_{1,n} ,   \qquad (5a)$$

so the variation in G indirectly impacts the observed scores through a regres-sion on the latent scores: (a) on the level with differences κ_0, and (b) on the slope with differences κ_1. This use of a group variable impacting the latent scores is the hallmark of the *mixed-effects* or *multilevel model* representation (e.g., Verbeke & Molenberghs, 2000).

A second alternative includes the group as a direct predictor of each dif-ference score. In this case we write

$$\Delta y[t]_n = \alpha y_{1,n} + \beta\, y[t-1]_n + \delta\, G_n + z[t]_n ,   \qquad (5b)$$

and this allow the other dynamic parameters to be adjusted for the group shift in the intercept term (δ).

As a third alternative, we can fit a multiple group model by eliminating the grouping variable and by writing each score and parameter with a group subscript. In this case we write

$$\Delta y[t]_n{}^{(g)} = \alpha^{(g)} y_{1,n}{}^{(g)} + \beta^{(g)} y[t-1]_n{}^{(g)} + z[t]_n{}^{(g)} \quad, \tag{5c}$$

and we use this model to evaluate the *invariance of the dynamic parameters over groups*. This model can easily be drawn as multiple group version of path diagram Equation 4a with all parameters readily accessible for evaluation across groups

Figure 7-4a. An LDS based on both additive (α) and proportional (β) changes with multilevel group effects

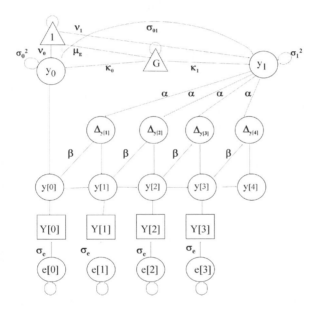

Group Differences in a Bivariate Latent Difference Score Model

The latent difference score approach is most useful when we start to examine time-dependent inter-relationships among multiple growth processes. As a final alternative model, we use an expansion of our previous latent difference scores logic to write a *bivariate dynamic change score* model as

$$\Delta y[t]_n = \alpha_y\, y_{1,n} + \beta_y\, y[t-1]_n + \gamma_{yx}\, x[t-1]_n + z_y[t]_n, \tag{6a}$$
and
$$\Delta x[t]_n = \alpha_x\, x_{1,n} + \beta_x\, x[t-1]_n + \gamma_{xy}\, y[t-1]_n + z_x[t]_n. \tag{6b}$$

In this model, each change is represented by dual changes (parameters α and β) but also includes *coupling* parameters (γ). The coupling parameter (γ_{yx}) represents the time-dependent effect of latent $x[t]$ on $y[t]$, and the other coupling parameter (γ_{xy}) represents the time-dependent effect of latent $y[t]$ on $x[t]$. This bivariate dynamic model is described in the path diagram of Figure 7-4b.

The key features of this model include the use of fixed unit values (unlabeled arrows) to define $\Delta y[t]$ and $\Delta x[t]$, and equality constraints within a variable (for the α, β, and γ parameters) to simplify estimation and identification. These latent difference score models can lead to more complex nonlinear trajectory equations (e.g., nonhomogeneous equations). These trajectories can be described by writing the implied basis coefficients ($A_j[t]$) as the linear accumulation of first differences for each variable ($\Sigma \Delta y[j]$, $j=0$ to t). Additional unique covariances within occasions ($u_y[t]\, u_x[t]$) are possible, but these will be identifiable only when there are multiple ($M > 2$) measured variables within each occasion.

Figure 7-4b. A bivariate latent difference score (LDS) model for one group.

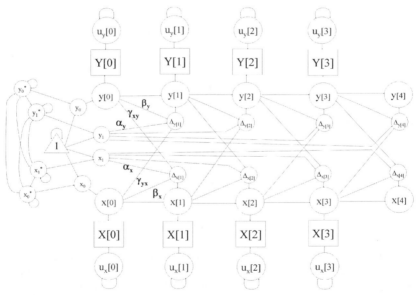

Group differences can also be added to the bivariate model in several ways. In a first alternative we assume the group variable does not impact the latent levels (due to randomization), but we can examine the group impact on the mean slopes of both sets (as in [6a]). In this kind of model, we can see if group membership accounts for variance and covariance of the latent slopes, and the other dynamic parameters might be altered when group membership is a covariate. A second alternative includes the group as a direct predictor of each difference score (as in Equation 5b). A third alternative is to use a multiple group framework to ask how the parameters differ over groups. The complete multiple group bivariate dual change model may be written as

$$\Delta y[t]_n^{(g)} = \alpha_y^{(g)} y_{1,n}^{(g)} + \beta_y^{(g)} y[t-1]_n^{(g)} + \gamma_{yx}^{(g)} x[t-1]_n^{(g)} + z_y[t]_n^{(g)} , \quad (7a)$$

and

$$\Delta x[t]_n^{(g)} = \alpha_x^{(g)} x_{1,n}^{(g)} + \beta_x^{(g)} x[t-1]_n^{(g)} + \gamma_{xy}^{(g)} y[t-1]_n^{(g)} + z_x[t]_n^{(g)} . \quad (7b)$$

This multiple group approach allows for differences in the latent means, slope variances, residual variance and dynamic coupling of the respective trajectories. The groups might have a different set of coupling parameters, and this would imply a more fundamental impact of the experiment -- *treatment alterations in the dynamic system.*

7.4 RESULTS

It is possible to fit all variations of the prior models using the data of Table 7-1 and standard SEM software. However, in order to focus in on the main results of this study we only describe multiple group models based on the latent difference score approach for univariate (Figure 7-4a) and bivariate (Figure 7-4b) data.

Results of Group Differences in Univariate Latent Difference Models

A set of latent difference score dynamic models were fitted and the parameters of these models are listed for the "Near-Transfer Induction" variable in Table 7-2 (i.e. the Mplus code is available upon request). Three alternative latent difference score models based on a multiple group version of Figure 7-4a and Equation 5b are considered in detail.

Two baseline models were first fitted (see Note to Table 7-2): (0a) A null baseline no-change model was fitted with only 3 parameters over all groups ($\chi^2 = 1619$ on $df = 26$), and (0b) a model with a "level only" constant covariance over time ($\chi^2 = 329$ on $df = 25$). The poor fit of the second baseline model suggests some changes are apparent over time or over groups.

The first substantive model fitted (Model 1) was a dual change score model with both additive (α) and proportional (β) changes possible, but all parameters are required to be invariant over groups The fit of this model ($\chi^2 = 88$ on $df = 21$) is a substantial improvement in fit over no changes at all ($\delta\chi^2 = 241$ on $\delta df = 4$). The parameters ($\alpha = 47.8$, $\beta = -.93$) yield an expected group curve that rises rapidly and then flattens out, but the individual differences around this curve are relatively large (e.g., $\sigma_1^2 = 325$). This is a reasonable description of both upper plots of Figure 7-1, but the fit is not yet acceptable (lower $\varepsilon_a = .127$, $> .05$).

One possible reason for this misfit is that the intervals of time do not represent an "equal spacing" of time (i.e., one week, one month, and six months), but this is the implied model of the use of constant dynamic parameters. To examine this issue the latent difference model was fit with a variety of other bases, including: (a), using a more precise counting of weeks between tests (i.e., A[t]=[0, 1, 4, 24]), (b) use of a power transformation (i.e., A[t]=[0,1,4,9]), and (c) free estimation of the latent basis (i.e., A[t]=[0, 1, 0.16, 0.04]; cf, Meredith & Tisak, 1990). These results suggested there may be some declines at later occasions but the dual change model based on a simple equal interval of time is a reasonable starting point for this variable.

This second substantive model (#2) from the table allowed the parameters representing the post-test mean changes to vary between the control and experimental group. The results show a clear improvement in fit ($\delta\chi^2 = 44$ on $\delta df = 2$), and group differences in the parameters of constant change ($\alpha^{(c)} = 39.5$, $\alpha^{(e)} = 51.5$) and proportional change ($\beta^{(c)} = -.84$, $\beta^{(e)} = -.95$). In this form, the changes are much greater for the Trained group but reach their asymptote earlier. However, there was still important misfit (lower $\varepsilon_a = .063$, > .05). First we examined the more typical statistical model of mean differences here only in the constant changes ($\alpha^{(c)} < \alpha^{(e)}$ but $\beta^{(c)} = \beta^{(e)}$) but there was still some misfit ($\delta\chi^2 = 5$ on $\delta df = 1$). Thus, as our third substantive alternative (#3, Table 7-2) we examined group differences in all the parameters representing changes over time. The result is an improvement in fit ($\delta\chi^2 = 12$ on $\delta df = 2$), and an acceptable overall model (lower $\varepsilon_a = .037$, <.05). The key difference here is that the Experimental group has much more variation in the constant slope ($\sigma_1^{2(c)} = 179$ but $\sigma_1^{2(e)} = 342$).

The trajectories of the best fitting latent difference model for the two groups on Induction scores can be written for both groups as

$$Y[t]_n = 37.8^* \{\pm 16.9^*\} + (\Sigma_{i=1,t} \Delta y[t]_n) + 0 \{\pm 5.1^*\}, \tag{8a}$$

where the fixed effects (group) are listed with their corresponding random effects (standard deviations) inside the brackets ($\{\pm\}$), and asterisks are used to indicate accuracy (at the .05 test level). In this model the latent changes for each group are defined as

$$\text{Control } \Delta y[t]_n = 32.1^* \{\pm 13.3^*\} y_{1,n} + -0.67^* y[t-1]_n , \tag{8b}$$
and
$$\text{Trained } \Delta y[t]_n = 52.6^* \{\pm 18.5^*\} y_{1,n} + -0.97^* y[t-1]_n , \tag{8c}$$

From these estimates, we calculate the expected group trajectories and a 5-year latent change accumulation as the combination. This increased mean and variance over time is an expected result if some people learn faster that others within the Experimental group (or else the variance would decrease over time), and seems to be a reasonable way to describe the impact of the experimental manipulation (e.g., Kling & Riggs, 1971; McArdle, 2001).

TABLE 7-2
Results for Alternative Dual Change Models Fitted to two Groups

Parameters	Model1: Invariant Over Groups Group C	Group E	Model 2: Free Fixed Dynamics Group C	Group E	Model 3: Free All Dynamics Group C	Group E
(a) *Change Components*						
Mean Slope α	47.8 (27)	==	39.5 (16)	51.5 (28)	32.1 (9)	52.6 (27)
Auto-Change β	-.927 (33)	==	-.843 (19)	-.952 (33)	-.673 (8)	-.972 (33)
Slope Variance σ_1^2	325 (9)	==	308 (19)	==	179 (4)	342 (9)
Slope Co-variance σ_{01}	279 (10) [.92]	==	277 (10) [.94]	==	216 (7) [.96]	289 (9) [.93]
(b) *Baseline Components*						
Initial Mean μ_0	37.8 (33)	==	37.8 (34)	==	37.8 (34)	==
Initial Variance σ_0^2	283 (10)	==	283 (10)	==	285 (10)	==
Unique Variance σ_u^2	26.7 (16) [.09]	==	26.2 (16) [.09]	==	25.9 (16) [.08]	==
(c) Goodness-of-Fit						
χ^2 / df	88 / 21		44 / 19		32 / 17	
ε_a (+90% bounds)	.161 (.127-.196)		.103 (.063-.143)		.084 (.037-.129)	

<u>Note.</u> Two group models fitted with the Mplus program with $N_c = 87$, $N_c = 161$;
Entries are MLE with t-values in parentheses (standardized in brackets);
Null Baseline → μ_0=47.8, σ_u^2=413, χ^2=1619 on df=26, ε_a=.703;
Level Baseline → μ_0=47.8, σ_0^2=329, σ_u^2=86 [.21], χ^2=751 on df=25, ε_a=.484.
Completely Free Groups → χ^2=27 on df=14, ε_a=.089;
Test of Non-Random Baselines → χ^2=5 on df=3.

Results From Fitting Bivariate Dynamic Models

In the next set of analyses, several bivariate models were fitted to the Induction-Vocabulary data of Table 7-1 and Figure 7-1. Six alternative models were considered based on a two-group version of the dynamic coupling model based on Figure 7-4 (i.e. the Mplus code is available upon request). The overall and comparative fit of these alternative models are presented in Table 7-3.

A first model (#0) included only the levels and unique components to represent a "no-change" hypothesis in both variables over time and over groups. Not surprisingly, this model fits very poorly ($\chi^2 = 878$ on $df = 80$). The next model (#1) required invariance over groups, but included all the bivariate change parameters, including six dynamic coefficients (two each for α, β, γ), four latent means (μ), six latent deviations (σ), and six latent correlations (ρ). This model represented a clear improvement in fit ($\delta\chi^2 = 720$ on $\delta df = 13$), and the overall parameters are available upon request.

The last four models present a sequence of group differences in the dynamic parameters. The first of these (#2) allows both constant slope means (termed α here) to vary over groups and the fit is improved substantially ($\delta\chi^2 = 39$ on $\delta df = 2$). The next model (#3) additionally allows group differences in proportional change and the fit is improved another small bit ($\delta\chi^2 = 6$ on $\delta df = 2$). The next model (#4) additionally allows the coupling parameters to change over groups and the fit is not improved ($\delta\chi^2 = 1$ on $\delta df = 2$). The next model (#5) additionally allows all slope variances and covariances to change over groups, and the result is another improvement in fit ($\delta\chi^2 = 20$ on $\delta df = 5$). To be complete, the final model allows all pre-test parameters to change as well and the improvement is relatively small ($\delta\chi^2 = 15$ on $\delta df = 8$).

The results of these models suggest that a very good fit was found using Model #5 (lower $\varepsilon_a = .048$, $<.05$). The MLE parameters and (t-values) of this bivariate model are listed in Table 7-4. The basic model for Induction ($Y[t]$) and Vocabulary ($X[t]$) scores can for both groups can now be written as

$$Y[t]_n = 37.8^* \{\pm 16.9^*\} + (\Sigma_{i=1, t} \Delta y[t]_n) + 0 \{\pm 5.0^*\}, \text{ and}$$
$$X[t]_n = 66.0^* \{\pm 12.9^*\} + (\Sigma_{i=1, t} \Delta x[t]_n) + 0 \{\pm 7.7^*\}, \text{ with}$$
$$\sigma_{y0,x0} = +0.48^*, \tag{9a}$$

These results suggest that the Vocabulary scores exhibit proportionally more unique variance (i.e., at pre-test, 26% vs only 8%) and, hence, are less reliable (i.e., at pre-test, 74% vs 92%), but the correlation among the latent levels is positive ($+.48^*$). In terms of the group differences, the results for the latent change scores are now interpreted for the Control (Un-Trained) group as

$$\Delta y[t]_n = 6.9^* \{\pm 13.9^*\} y_{1,n} + -0.83^* y[t-1]_n + 0.47^* x[t-1]_n, \text{ and}$$
$$\Delta x[t]_n = 35.9^* \{\pm 8.2^*\} x_{1,n} + -0.31 x[t-1]_n + -0.31^* y[t-1]_n, \text{ with}$$

$$\sigma_{yl,xl} = 0.78^*. \tag{9b}$$

In contrast, the latent changes for the Experimental (Trained) group are written as

$$\Delta y[t]_n = 51.4^* \{\pm 13.9^*\} y_{l,n} + -0.98^* y[t\text{-}1]_n + 0.02\, x[t\text{-}1]_n \text{ , and}$$
$$\Delta x[t]_n = 63.3^* \{\pm 8.2^*\} x_{l,n} + -0.92^* x[t\text{-}1]_n + 0.04\, y[t\text{-}1]_n \text{ , with}$$
$$\sigma_{yl,xl} = 0.54^*. \tag{9c}$$

One clear training impact is that the constant slopes are much higher in the Trained group for both variables. This is interesting because the second variable (Vocabulary) is a "Far-Transfer" variable, and no real training differences were expected. This interpretation of mean changes for different variables is often characterized as a "transfer of training" (e.g., Baltes et al, 1986), but we soon focus on a different set of parameters here. Also we see that the correlation among the latent slopes are high (+.78*) in the Control group and lower in the Experimental group (+.54*), but this is not what we expected as an impact where training is transferred.

Further group differences include parameters with different signs, so their total impacts are hard to interpret directly and individually. These parameters are one part of a system of dependent equations where seemingly small differences can accumulate over longer periods of time or over age. However, when we look at the set of parameters as a whole we do see a more interesting pattern emerge. In Equations 9b all fixed parameters were accurately different than zero, so the Control group equations can be described as a *coupled system* of latent scores. In contrast, the results presented in Equation 9c suggest the Experimental group equations have higher auto-proportions and no accurate coupling parameters, so this group can be described as an *un-coupled system* of latent scores. That is, the net result of the experimental training manipulation was that it both raised up and also un-coupled the scores on the two variables. This result could be due to the fact that training helped focus the persons on all tasks, and especially focused on the Induction-like tasks (near-transfer). At the same time the pattern of individual differences apparent here suggest the specific training seems to have set the Induction variable farther away from the Vocabulary variable than it was before.

The expected values from these parameters are displayed in Figure 7-5 (from Equation 9a, 9b). The expected values turn out to be an interpretable and unique set of bivariate trajectories. The two figures (7-5a and 7-5b) are *vector field plots for each group* (for details, see Boker & McArdle, 1995, 2005; McArdle et al., 2001). Within each group, any pair of coordinates is a starting point ($y[t]$, $x[t]$) and the ellipse gives the symmetric 95% confidence boundary around the actual data at t=0. The directional arrows are a way to display the expected pair of $\Delta t=1$ visit changes (Δy, Δx) from this point.

Both figures show an interesting dynamic property --- *the change expectations of a dynamic model depend on the starting point.*

From this perspective, we can also interpret the high level-level correlation ($\rho_{y0,x0} \sim 0.6^*$), which describes the placement of the individuals in the vector field, and the positive slope-slope correlation ($\rho_{y1,x1} = +0.78^*, +.54^*$), which describes the location of the subsequent change scores for individuals in the vector field. The resulting "flow surface" for the Control group shows that Induction abilities may have a tendency to impact score changes on the Vocabulary scores, but the most important result is that there is not such coupling effect in the Trained group. Instead the Trained group vectors appear to be headed for a common point of asymptote ($y[t]=50$, $x[t]=80$). Although much could be made of these specific points, it appears that the Training did have a direct dynamic impact of de-coupling the existing system. This specific result is certainly not strong evidence of a transfer of training across these variables. In contrast, the Training seems to have isolated the abilities that were trained, and possibly moving these scores towards other unmeasured variables. Needless to say, these dynamic differences due to training are not easy to see in the typical comparison of changes in the means.

Figure 7-5. Dynamic vector field plots for the Untrained and the Trained groups with 95% confidence intervals (arrows = direction of changes).

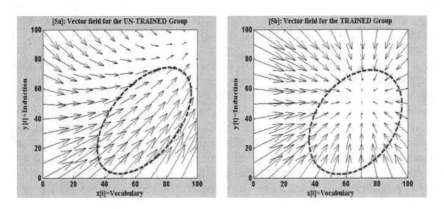

7.5 DISCUSSION

These SEM analyses were intended to describe contemporary longitudinal alternatives for the standard mean comparisons so prevalent in analyses of randomized experiments. Whereas the use of a fully randomized design is a critical benefit to clear causal inference, the reliance on tests of means differences is not. Indeed, one key result here is that the impact of experiments may not always be found in the mean changes between groups. This point of view seems to be well understood in longitudinal studies where randomization to groups is often not possible (i.e., quasi-experiments) and comparative trends are looked for as dynamic evidence (see Cook & Campbell, 1977; Rogosa, 1978). Nevertheless, the issues of group differences in dynamics seem to be overlooked in much of the important literature on randomized clinical trials (see Cnaan, Laird, & Slasor, 1997) and only the group differences in the means of the slopes are considered the essential evidence of treatment.

We have embraced the general treatment of the multiple group issue uses concepts derived from multiple-group factor analysis (e.g., Jöreskog & Sörbom, 1999). Indeed, all models were fit in a sequence that conforms to the logic of models of factorial invariance of measurement --- relaxing the latent variable means first, then the latent variable covariances, and so on (e.g., Horn & McArdle, 1992; McArdle & Cattell, 1994). The multiple group growth model permits the examination of the presumed invariance of the latent basis functions and the rejection of these constraints (based on χ^2/df) implies that some independent groups have a different basic shape of the growth curve. Multiple group models can also be a useful way to express problems of incomplete data (as in McArdle & Hamagami, 1992). Longitudinal data collections often include different numbers of data points for different people and different variables, and one way to deal with these kinds of statistical problems is to consider multiple group model strategies (e.g., McArdle, 1994; McArdle & Bell, 2000; McArdle & Hamagami, 1992).

There are many unresolved issues in employing a multiple group strategy in randomized experiments. In this analysis we started by forcing all parameters to be invariant across groups, suggesting no impact of training at all, and we progressively relaxed parameters and examined changes in fit to answer key substantive questions. However, it is not assured that the substantive results would be the same if we started with a more relaxed model (e.g., all parameters free over groups) and added constraints until we lost acceptable fit. Another reasonable variation on both approaches would be to start with the Control group data and, after fit was deemed acceptable, move to the Experimental group data to look for differences. At some phases of analysis, the results (i.e., likelihood surfaces) would be identical, but when this is not true the specific answers to the training questions might change with the parametric context.

In this analysis the invariance of the groups at the initial time of measurement (i.e., the pre-test) was also considered essential (see Equation 1b). In the data studied here comparisons at baseline are examined, but the relaxation of the baseline parameters does not change the fit very much; (e.g., Table 7-2; $\delta\chi^2 = 5$ on $\delta df = 3$). Given the basic theory of randomized experiments, however, a reasonable case can be made that the parameters of the pre-test scores should not be allowed to vary over groups. Of course, there can be some lack of balance across groups yielding differences at the pre-test, and this possibility increases as the samples become smaller. Nevertheless, if inferences about subsequent changes require invariance at baseline, it follows that we should allow this form of misfit to retain a proper interpretation of the changes from a common set of baseline parameters. This SEM opportunity to insure an invariant statistical starting point can be used to account for any "cross-over" controversy (e.g., Lord, 1969; Wainer, 1991). This is a somewhat odd "benefit of misfit" but it is commonly used in the MAR corrections for incomplete data (e.g., Little & Rubin, 1987; McArdle & Bell, 2000; McArdle & Hamagami, 1992).

As in any substantive analysis, there may be many additional variables that are randomly related to the group membership but that can have an impact on the results within groups and between groups. Initial group differences within groups may have contributed to the high initial level variance and level-slope correlations. In this experiment the selection of persons was designed to examine older ages with different educational levels, and previous experiments have found age and education effects can impact outcomes of learning new tasks. To examine these possibilities, we need to fit additional models not fully detailed here. In the first model, we could include group invariant regressions of latent levels and slopes on the measured age variable. Additional degrees-of-freedom will come from the model restriction that all age effects can be accounted for at the latent variable level. We do not allow the {age+ education}→level regressions to vary over groups to keep the inferential baseline, but we can examine group differences in the {age+ education}→slope relationships. In alternative models, we can also examine direct {age+ education}→$\Delta y[t]$ relationships, and we allow these to vary over groups. These kind of dynamic models reflect a statistical balance that is not often found in the current literature. However, these models are relatively easy to fit and may have direct consequences on the other estimates and interpretations of the simpler dynamic models.

The latent difference score approach used here is designed to be a natural extension on standard repeated measures ANOVA/ANCOVA model. One practical advantage is that these types of models can be easily fitted using standard structural modeling software. The structural path diagrams illustrate how fundamental change score concepts can be directly represented using standard longitudinal structural equation models. As in other latent growth models (e.g., Meredith & Tisak, 1990), the numerical values of the parameters (α, β and γ) can now be combined to form many different kinds of individual and group trajectories over age or time, including the addition of covariates. All these features are apparent without directly specifying an integral equation for the trajectory over time. Variations on any of these models can be considered by adding more factors or by adding structure to the specific factors but we did not investigate these possibilities here. But it is also important to recognize the well-known divergence between the difference score approach used here and the differential structural equation models proposed by others (e.g., Arminger, 1987; Boker, 2000; Oud & Jansen, 2000).

In future research, the focus will be on the discrimination of (a) models of multiple curves for a single group of subjects from (b) models of multiple groups of subjects with different curves. These substantive issues are based on heterogeneity within groups, and can benefit from models that test hypotheses about *latent curves between latent groups*. The recent series of models termed *growth mixture models* have been developed for this purpose (Hagenaars & McCutcheon, 2002; Muthen & Muthen, 2002; Nagin, 1999), and these are easily extended to latent difference score forms. These analyses provide a test of the invariance of growth model parameters without knowing exactly the group membership of each individual. By combining some aspects of the previous sections, we can consider a *group difference dynamic change score* model in different ways. In one model, we add the group contrasts as a covariate in the difference model. In another model we add a multilevel prediction structure of the dynamic slopes. In general, we can always consider that a model where multiple groups are independent or probabilistic, and where the group dynamics are different.

The dynamic analyses presented here represent only one subset of a much larger family of dynamic possibilities. Although a complete historical perspective on dynamic models was not presented, the current models seem to meet many of the essential goals of most longitudinal-experimental data analyses (e.g., Baltes & Nesselroade, 1979; Horn & McArdle, 1980; McArdle & Bell, 2000; Wohwill, 1973). To reflect true impacts of cognitive training on people using longitudinal sequences, we surely need to expand the standard models of analysis to include more individual differences variables. In recent research we have examined four variables in a dynamic system over the adult part of the life span and concluded that the network of cognitive dynamic relationships is far more complex than the one portrayed herein (McArdle, et al., 2001). In this sense, the models highlighted here mainly point out new opportunities to understand the dynamic complexities of behavioral trajectories and the potentially important impacts of experimental training.

REFERENCES

Arminger, G. (1986). Linear stochastic differential equation models for panel data with unobserved variables. In N. Tuma (Ed.), *Sociological methodology*, pp. 187–212. San Francisco: Jossey-Bass.

Arbuckle, J. L., & Wotke, W. (1999). *AMOS 4.0 User's Guide*. Chicago: Smallwaters.

Baltes, P. B., Dittmann-Kohli, F., & Kliegl, R. (1986). Reserved capacity of the elderly in aging-sensitive tests of fluid intelligence: Replication and extension. *Psychology and Aging, 1* (2), 172–177.

Baltes, P. B., & Mayer, K. U. (Eds.). (1999). *The Berlin aging study: Aging from 70 to 100.* New York: Cambridge University Press.

Baltes, P. B., & Nesselroade, J. R. (1979). History and rationale of longitudinal research. In J.R. Nesselroade. & P.B. Baltes (Eds.). *Longitudinal research in the study of behavior and development* (pp. 1–40). New York: Academic Press.

Blalock, H. M. (Ed.). (1985). *Causal models in panel and experimental designs.* New York: Aldine.

Boker, S. M. (2001). Differential structural equation models. In L. Collins & A. Sayer (Eds.). *Methods for the analysis of change* (3–28). Washington, DC: APA Press.

Boker, S. M., & McArdle, J. J. (1995). A statistical vector field analysis of longitudinal aging data. *Experimental Aging Research, 21,* 77–93.

Boker, S. M, & McArdle, J .J. (2005). Vector field plots. In P. Armitage & P. Colton (Eds). *Encyclopedia of biostatistics* (2nd ed., pp. 5700–5708). Chichester, England: Wiley.

Coleman, J. (1968). The mathematical study of change. In H. M. Blalock & A.B. Blalock (Eds.), *Methodology in social research* (pp. 428–475). New York: McGraw-Hill.

Cnaan, A., Laird, N. M., & Slasor, P. (1997). Using the general linear mixed model to analyse unbalanced repeated measures and longitudinal data. *Statistics in Medicine, 16,* 2349–2380.

Cohen, J., Cohen, P., West, S., & Aiken, L. (2003). *Applied multiple regression/correlation analysis for the behavioral sciences* (3rd ed.). Hillsdale, NJ: Lawrence Erlbaum Associates.

Cook, T. D., & Campbell, D. T. (1979). *Quasi-experimentation design and analysis issues for field settings.* Skokie, IL: Rand-McNally.

Ellis, H. C. (1965). *The transfer of learning.* New York: MacMillian.

Fisher, R. A. (1920), *The design of experiments.* Oxford, England: Oxford University Press.

Glymour, C., Scheines, R., Spirtes, P., & Kelly, K. (1987). *Discovering causal structure: artificial intelligence, philosophy of science, and statistical modeling.* Orlando: Academic Press.

Hagenaars, J.A., & McCutcheon, A. L. (2002). *Applied latent class analysis.* Cambridge, UK: Cambridge University Press.

Hamagami, F., & McArdle, J. J. (2000). Advanced studies of individual differences linear dynamic models for longitudinal data analysis. In G. Marcoulides & R. Schumacker (Eds.), *Advanced structural equation modeling: issues and techniques* (pp. 203–246). Mahwah, NJ: Lawrence Erlbaum Associates.

Harris, C. W. (1963). *Problems in measuring change.* Madison, WI: University of Wisconsin Press.

Healy, A., Proctor, R. W., & Weiner, I. B. (2003). *Handbook of psychology: experimental psychology* (vol. 4). New York: Wiley.

Heise, D. R. (1975). *Causal analysis.* New York: Wiley.

Holland, P. W. (1993). Which comes first, cause or effect? In G. Keren & C. Lewis (Eds.), *A handbook for data analysis in the behavioral sciences: methodological issues* (pp. 273–282). Hillsdale, NJ: Lawrence Erlbaum Associates.

Horn, J. L. (1972). The state, trait, and change dimensions of intelligence. *British Journal of Educational Psychology, 2, 159-185.*

Horn, J. L. (1988). Thinking about human abilities. In J. R. Nesselroade (Ed.), *Handbook of multivariate psychology* (pp. 645–685). New York: Academic Press.

Horn, J. L., & McArdle, J. J. (1980). Perspectives on mathematical and statistical model building (MASMOB) in research on aging. In L. Poon (Ed.), *Aging in the 1980's: psychological issues* (pp. 503–541). Washington: American Psychological Association.

Horn, J. L., & McArdle, J. J. (1992). A practical guide to measurement invariance in research on aging. *Experimental Aging Research, 18 (3),* 117–144.

James, L. R., Mulaik, S. A., & Brett, J. M. (1982). *Causal analysis: Assumptions, models, and data.* Beverly Hills, CA: Sage.

Jöreskog, K. G. (1970). Estimation and testing of simplex model. *British Journal of Mathematical and Statistical Psychology, 23,* 121–145.

Jöreskog, K. G. (1971). Simultaneous factor analysis in many populations. *Psychometrika, 36* (4), 409–426.

Jöreskog, K. G. (1977). Statistical models and methods for the analysis of longitudinal data. In D. V. Aigner & A. S. Goldberger (Eds). *Latent variables in socioeconomic models* (pp. 77–102). Amsterdam: North Holland Publishers.

Joreskog, K. G., & Sorbom, D. (1979). *Advances in factor analysis and structural equation models.* In J. Magdson (Ed.), Cambridge, MA: Abt Books.

Jöreskog, K. G., & Sörbom, D. (1999). *LISREL 8.30: LISREL 8: Structural equation modeling with the SIMPLIS command language.* Hillsdale, NJ: Scientific Software International.

Kenny, D. A. (1979). *Correlation and causality.* New York: Wiley.

Kling, J. W., & Riggs, L. A. (1971). *Woodworth & scholsberg's experimental psychology.* New York: Holt, Rinehart & Winston.

Lord, F. M. (1967) A paradox in the interpretation of group comparisons. *Psychological Bulletin, 68,* 304–305.

Little, R. T. A., & Rubin, D.B. (1987). *Statistical analysis with missing data.* New York: Wiley.

McArdle, J. J. (1986). Latent variable growth within behavior genetic models. *Behavior Genetics, 16* (1), 163–200.

McArdle, J. J. (1988). Dynamic but structural equation modeling of repeated measures data. In J. R. Nesselroade & R .B. Cattell (Eds.), *The handbook of multivariate experimental psychology* (vol. 2, pp. 561–614). New York, Plenum Press.

McArdle, J. J. (1989). Structural modeling experiments using multiple growth functions. In P. Ackerman, R. Kanfer & R. Cudeck (Eds.), *Learning and individual differences: abilities, motivation, and methodology* (pp. 71–117). Hillsdale, NJ: Lawrence Erlbaum Associates.

McArdle, J. J. (1994). Structural factor analysis experiments with incomplete data. *Multivariate Behavioral Research, 29*(4), 409-454.

McArdle, J. J. (2001). A latent difference score approach to longitudinal dynamic structural analyses. In R. Cudeck, S. du Toit, & D. Sörbom (Eds.). *Structural equation modeling: present and futur* (pp. 342–380). Lincolnwood, IL: Scientific Software International.

McArdle, J.J. (2005). The development of RAM notation for structural equation modeling. In A. Madeau & J. J. McArdle, (Eds.). *Contemporary advances in psychometrics* (pp. 225–273) Mahwah, NJ: Lawrence Erlbaum Associates.

McArdle, J. J., & Bell, R. Q. (2000). Recent trends in modeling longitudinal data by latent growth curve methods. In T.D. Little, K.U. Schnabel, & J. Baumert (Eds.). *Modeling longitudinal and multiple-group data: practical issues, applied approaches, and scientific examples* (pp. 69–108). Mahwah, NJ: Lawrence Erlbaum Associates.

McArdle, J. J., & Cattell, R .B. (1994). Structural equation models of factorial invariance in parallel proportional profiles and oblique confactor problems. *Multivariate Behavioral Research, 29*(1), 63–113.

McArdle, J. J., & Hamagami, E. (1992). Modeling incomplete longitudinal and cross-sectional data using latent growth structural models. *Experimental Aging Research, 18*(3), 145–166.

McArdle, J. J., & Hamagami, F. (2001). Linear dynamic analyses of incomplete longitudinal data. In L. Collins & A. Sayer (Eds.). *Methods for the analysis of change* (pp. 137–176). Washington, DC: APA Press.

McArdle, J. J., & Hamagami, F. (2004). Longitudinal structural equation modeling methods for dynamic change hypotheses. In K. van Montfort, J. Oud & A. Satorra (Eds.), *Recent developments in structural equation models* (pp. 295–336). London: Kluwer Academic Publishers.

McArdle, J. J., Hamagami, F., Meredith, W., & Bradway, K. P. (2001). Modeling the dynamic hypotheses of Gf-Gc theory using longitudinal life-span data. *Learning and Individual Differences, 12* (2000), 53–79.

McArdle, J. J., & Nesselroade, J. R. (1994). Structuring data to study development and change. In S. H. Cohen & H. W. Reese (Eds.), *Life-span developmental psychology: methodological innovations* (pp. 223–267). Hillsdale, N.J.: Lawrence Erlbaum Associates.

McArdle, J. J., & Nesselroade, J. R. (2003). Growth curve analyses in contemporary psychological research. In J. Schinka & W. Velicer (Eds.), *Comprehensive handbook of psychology, Volume II. Research Methods in Psychology* (pp. 447–480). New York: Pergamon.

McArdle, J. J., & Woodcock, J. R. (1997). Expanding test-rest designs to include developmental time-lag components. *Psychological Methods, 2* (4), 403–435.

Meredith, W., & Tisak, J. (1990). Latent curve analysis. *Psychometrika, 55*, 107–122.

Molenaar, P. C. M. (1985). A dynamic factor model for the analysis of multivariate time series. *Psychometrika, 50*, 181–202.

Muthen, B. O., & Curran, P. (1997). General longitudinal modeling of individual differences in experimental designs: A latent variable framework for analysis and power estimation. *Psychological Methods, 2*, 371–402.

Muthen, L. K., & Muthen, B. O. (2002). *Mplus, the comprehensive modeling program for applied researchers user's guide.* Los Angeles, CA: Muthen & Muthen.

Nagin, D. (1999). Analyzing developmental trajectories: Semi-parametric. Group-based approach. *Psychological Methods, 4*, 139–177.

Neale, M. C., Boker, S. M., Xie, G., & Maes, H. H. (1999). *Mx statistical modeling* (5th Ed.), Unpublished program manual, Virginia Institute of Psychiatric and Behavioral Genetics, Medical College of Virginia, Virginia Commonwealth University, Richmond, VA.

Oud, J. H. L., & Jansen, R. A. R. G. (2000). Continuous time state space modeling of panel data by means of SEM. *Psychometrika, 65*, 199–215.

Pearl, J. (2000). *Causality: Models, reasoning, and inference.* Cambridge: Cambridge University Press.

Rao, C.R. (1958). Some statistical methods for the comparison of growth curves. *Biometrics, 14*, 1–17.

Raykov, T. (1997a). Disentangling intervention and temporal effects in longitudinal designs using latent curve analysis. *Biometric Journal, 39*, 239–259.

Raykov, T. (1997b). Growth curve analysis of ability means and variances in measures of fluid intelligence of older adults. *Structural Equation Modeling, 4*(4), 283–319.

Rogosa, D. (1978). Causal models in longitudinal research: Rationale, formulation, and interpretation. In J. R. Nesselroade & P. B. Baltes (Eds.), *Longitudinal research in the study of behavior and development* (pp. 263–302). New York: Academic Press.

Shaffer, J. P. (1992). *The role of models in nonexperimental social science: Two debates.* Washington, DC: American Educational Research Association and the American Statistical Association.

Sörbom, D. (1975). Detection of correlated errors in longitudinal data. *British Journal of Mathematical and Statistical Psychology, 28,* 138–151.

Sörbom, D. (1978). An alternative to the methodology for analysis of covariance. *Psychometrika, 43,* 381–396.

Subedi, B. S. (2004). Emerging trends in research on the transfer of learning. *International Education Journal, 5* (4), 591–599.

Tucker, L. R. (1958). Determination of parameters of a functional relation by factor analysis. *Psychometrika, 23,* 19–23.

Verbeke, G., & Molenberghs, G. (2000). *Linear mixed models for longitudinal data.* New York: Springer.

Wainer, H. (1991). Adjusting for differential base rates: Lord's paradox again. *Psychological Bulletin, 109* (1), 147–151.

Wiley, D. E. & Wiley, J.A. (1970). The identification of measurement errors in panel data. *American Sociological Review, 35,* 112–117.

Willis, S. L., Blieszner, R., & Baltes, P.B. (1981). Intellectual training research in aging: Modification of performance on the fluid ability of figural relations. *Journal of Educational Psychology, 73,* 41–50.

Wohwill, J. F. (1973). *The study of behavioral development.* New York: Academic Press.

Chapter 8

A Second Order Structured Latent Curve Model for Longitudinal Data

Shelley Blozis

University of California, Davis

8.1 INTRODUCTION

Popular approaches to the analysis of longitudinal data include the latent curve model. The model simultaneously characterizes change in a variable at the population and individual level, providing descriptions of average change as well as individual differences in change characteristics (Laird & Ware, 1982; Meredith & Tisak, 1984, 1990). A special aspect of the model is that it may be applied to unequally spaced data where times of measurement may be completely unique to each individual, as well as to data that are unbalanced due to a different number of observations for different individuals (Bryk & Raudenbush, 1987; Jennrich & Schluchter, 1986; Laird, 1988; Mehta & West, 2000). Estimation of the model may rely on the observed mean vector and covariance matrix (usually when data are complete and balanced) or on the raw data directly (often required when data are incomplete or unbalanced). Estimation yields parameter estimates of the population-level characteristics of change and elements that define the covariance structure describing both within- and between-individual variation in responses over time.

Standard use of a latent curve model for a single population considers a single manifest variable as a function of time, where time may be measured in a variety of ways, such as by subject age, calendar time, grade level, or number of years following a significant onset (e.g., disease diagnosis). A common form of the model is one that assumes linear change and includes an intercept

189

and linear time effect, both of which may be unique to the individual. The individual-level coefficients (e.g., intercept and slope) are often referred to as random effects or random coefficients (Laird & Ware, 1982; Raudenbush & Bryk, 2002). The model for the response as a function of time constitutes the first level of the model. At the second level, one or more of the individual-level coefficients from the first level may simply vary across individuals (often expressed as a linear sum of a fixed and random effect) or be treated as criterion variables regressed on person-level characteristics, such as sex or treatment status (Browne, 1993; Willett & Sayer, 1994). Also at the second level are the population-level coefficients that characterize change across individuals.

In a two-level model, there are two sources of random error. At the first level, error represents a combination of measurement and time-specific error, assuming the response is measured with error as is often the case in practice. Without person-level predictors of the random coefficients at the second level, the random coefficients represent individual-level deviations about the population-level characteristics of change. With the addition of person-level variables as predictors, the errors at the second level are the result of the regressions.

As noted earlier, the error at the first level of the model often represents a combination of time-specific and measurement error. To partition this error into unique components, the latent curve model may be extended to include multiple indicators of a latent variable at each measurement occasion (Chan, 1998; Duncan & Duncan, 1996; McArdle, 1988; Sayer & Cumsille, 2001). McArdle (1988) referred to this model as a curve-of-factors model. At each occasion, a common factor is assumed to account for the linear dependencies among a set of manifest variables, with the remaining variance in the manifest variables assumed due to measurement error. The latent variable on which the manifest variables depend is then targeted as the variable whose form of change is of interest. In this model formulation then, it is a latent variable that is studied as a function of time, with the error associated with change in the latent variable representing time-specific error without the confounding influence of measurement error.

Thus, a second-order latent curve model yields three sources of random variation. First is the measurement error directly related to the manifest variables. This source of error refers to the fallible nature of manifest variables as indicators of a latent variable. Second is the time-specific error in characterizing the latent variable as a function of time. Unlike the standard latent curve model, this error is not confounded by measurement error. Finally, the third source of random variation concerns the latent person-level change characteristics (e.g., intercept and slope) on which the latent repeated measures depend.

8.1.1 Measurement Invariance

In a standard latent curve model in which observed scores are studied directly, with a single score assumed to represent the construct, the validity of the assessment of change in scores is dependent on the assumption that the same construct has been measured across time (McArdle & Epstein, 1987; Meredith & Horn, 2001), although in this particular case the assumption cannot be formally tested. This property of the scores is known as measurement invariance. A common means of testing measurement invariance is by confirmatory factor analysis when multiple indicators of a latent variable are available at each occasion (see Millsap & Meredith, in press, for a more general discussion concerning factorial invariance). Using this approach, a series of models are typically compared, each differentiated by increasing equality constraints on model parameters across groups in multiple-group, cross-sectional comparisons and across occasions in longitudinal analyses (Meredith, 1993). Issues concerning factorial invariance are briefly reviewed here in the context of longitudinal studies, although these ideas generally apply to multiple-group analyses. Readers are referred to Widaman and Reise (1997) for an illustration in methods for evaluating factorial invariance.

Factorial invariance in longitudinal investigations generally concerns the comparability of factor structure across measurement occasions. In the case of longitudinal investigations, it is common to allow some degree of autocorrelation between the same indicators across occasions when evaluating these models. The least restrictive form of factorial invariance is configural invariance. This level of invariance implies that the pattern of zero and nonzero factor loadings are identical across occasions with no additional constraints made on model parameters (Thurstone, 1947). While informative about the factor patterns, this level of invariance provides no supporting evidence of measurement invariance across time because the regressions of the manifest variables on the latent variables may differ across time. If configural invariance holds across measurement occasions, three additional models may be fitted that represent varying levels of invariance of specific model parameters across time.

The first of these three, termed "metric invariance" (Horn & McArdle, 1992; Thurstone, 1947), hereafter referred to as weak factorial invariance (Widaman & Reise, 1997), implies that the factor loadings are equivalent across occasions. Although the regression slopes relating the factors and indicators are equal across time, this level of factorial invariance is not a sufficient condition for the study of change in a latent variable over time. This is because the latent intercept could vary across time, implying possibly parallel regressions with unequal intercepts. Assuming weak factorial invariance holds, strong factorial invariance is then typically evaluated by assuming that both the factor loadings and the latent intercepts are equal across time (Meredith, 1993). This level of factorial invariance assumes equivalent regressions of indicators on their respective factors, thus allowing for meaningful comparisons of factors across time (however, see Lubke & Dolan, 2003). Assuming strong factorial invariance holds, a more restrictive model may then be considered. Strict factorial invariance assumes that the factor loadings, the latent intercepts, and the unique variances are invariant across time (Meredith, 1993). Assuming strict factorial invariance, meaningful comparisons of factors means, variances, and covariances may be made.

8.1.2 Addressing Form of Change

Similar to a first-order latent curve model, a second-order latent curve model is flexible in terms of how the form of change in the latent variable may be specified. Forms of change may range from simple linear trends to higher order polynomial trends (e.g., quadratic and cubic) to linear piecewise and spline models (e.g., Sayer & Cumsille, 2001). Some nonlinear models are possible. That is, the only restriction for a latent curve model in terms of its parameters is that coefficients that vary across individuals must enter the model in a linear fashion. Those that enter nonlinearly are strictly fixed. Thus, various nonlinear forms of change may be handled by this general framework. Estimation of the model is often straightforward using techniques commonly employed to fit linear models, such as those used to estimate linear factor models (e.g., EQS, CALIS, MPlus, and LISREL).

An alternative to directly specifying a form of change, such as by a linear or piecewise linear spline, is to consider a latent basis curve model. In this model, the general form of change in the response variable is not specified in advance, but instead is determined by the data. That is, the intervals characterizing change in the response are considered unknown coefficients to be estimated (McArdle, 1988; McArdle, 1998; Meredith & Tisak, 1990). The latent basis curve model is appropriate for situations in which individuals have been observed at the same times, though naturally there is allowance for missing data. A shortcoming of the model, however, is that a relatively large number of parameters is needed to characterize change given a large number of measurement occasions.

8.1.3 Structured Latent Curve Models

The structured latent curve model proposed by Browne (1993; see also Browne & Du Toit, 1991) is a nonlinear factor model in which the observed variables are nonlinear functions of latent characteristics of change. A brief overview of the model is given here, with a more thorough treatment given in the following section. In a structured latent curve model, the mean response may follow a specific function, possibly nonlinear in its parameters. A factor matrix is then defined by a set of basis curves determined by the first-order partial derivatives of the mean function taken with regard to its coefficients. Thus, a basis curve may be a function of parameters that enter nonlinearly, with fixed and and possibly unknown coefficients. Similar to a latent curve model, the basis curves determine the shape of the common response curve. The factors, known as person weights, represent different characteristics of change that may vary across individuals.

The factor matrix and person weights linearly combine to yield individual latent trajectories. That is, the individual curves are a linear weighted combination of the basis curves, where the weights are unique to the individuals. Estimation of the model may proceed using methods used for linear models because the coefficients of the basis curves (that may enter in a nonlinear manner) are strictly fixed, and the factors that are stochastic variables enter the model in a linear manner (Blozis & Cudeck, 1999). In contrast to the latent basis curve model where the form of change is not directly specified, a structured latent curve model relies on a specific function. This often results in a reduction in the number of parameters necessary to describe change. An advantage of the latter approach is that it may be possible to choose a nonlinear function with coefficients that are directly relevant to the behavior under study, leading to improved model interpretation. Similar to the first-order latent curve model, the structured latent curve model makes no explicit provision for measurement error in the manifest variables. That is, error in the manifest variables represents a combination of time-specific error and measurement error, as in most cases where the observed measures are measured with error. This issue is addressed here.

This chapter builds on existing work by extending the second-order latent curve model to handle nonlinear response functions for the latent variables by allowing model parameters to enter nonlinearly (Blozis, 2004a). This work also represents an extension of the structured latent curve model (Browne, 1993) to handle multiple indicators of a latent variable whose mean may follow a nonlinear function. This formulation of the structured latent curve model extends it from a two-level to a three-level random-effects model, treating random variation in the manifest variables, the first-order latent variables, and the second-order latent variables. Manifest variables need not be measured according to the same measurement occasions for all individuals and randomly missing data are allowed. It is important to note, however, that when data are observed at very different measurement occasions across individuals, standard methods for evaluating the invariance of a factor structure across time may not apply, and so assumptions of measurement invariance would need to hold for valid inference about change in the latent variable means.

In a second-order structured latent curve model, where multiple manifest variables are linearly dependent on one or more latent variables at each occasion, a nonlinear function is chosen to characterize mean change in the latent variable. Individual latent curves are also nonlinear functions but not necessarily of the same form as the mean curve. The model may be considered within a class of partially nonlinear mixed-effects models because parameters that enter the model nonlinearly are strictly fixed (Davidian & Giltinan, 1995; also referred to as a conditionally linear mixed-effects model (Blozis & Cudeck, 1999). Parameters that enter linearly may be either fixed or random. The interpretation of the structured latent curve model differs, however, from a partially nonlinear mixed model in that the former specifies a function of change at the population level and the latter at the individual level. The benefits of the structured latent curve model are that it provides a nonlinear model of true change in a latent variable, as well as a means for testing factorial invariance across measurement occasions. Development of the model is presented, followed by an example. For convenience, the model is presented assuming complete data with measures assessed according to the same points in time across individuals. In the example that follows, this assumption is relaxed.

8.2 MODEL SPECIFICATION

First, consider a single point in time, t, where a latent variable, η_i^*, is assumed to be measured by a set of observed variables, $\mathbf{Y}_{ti}^* = (Y_{1ti}, \ldots, Y_{kti})'$, where k is the number of observed variables at time t, and i is an individual. For example, $\mathbf{Y}_i^*$ may be a set of manifest variables that serve as indicators of a single construct, such as self-esteem. In the first stage of formulating the second-order latent curve model, a common factor model for $\mathbf{Y}_{ti}^*$ is specified (cf. Lawley & Maxwell, 1971):

$$\mathbf{Y}_{ti}^* = \tau_t^* + \lambda_t^* \eta_{ti}^* + \varepsilon_{ti}^*,$$

where at time t, τ_t^* is a $k \times 1$ set of latent intercepts, λ_t^* is a $k \times 1$ factor loading vector, η_{ti}^* is a common factor, and ε_{ti}^* is a $k \times 1$ set of uniquenesses, or measurement errors, associated with the regressions of the manifest variables on the latent variable. Assuming the factors and errors are independent, it is assumed that the errors will be mutually independent given that the linear dependencies among the manifest variables are accounted for by the factors.

Next, assume that repeated measures of the set of observations, $\mathbf{Y}_i^*$, have been observed on multiple occasions, $t = 1, \ldots, T$, where T is the total number of measurement occasions. Let $\mathbf{Y}_i = (\mathbf{Y}_{1i}^{*'}, \ldots, \mathbf{Y}_{Ti}^{*'})'$ represent a stacked collection of manifest variable sets for an individual observed according to t. The response vector is of length $q = T * k$. Similar to stacking the observed variables to create the multiple-occasion response set $\mathbf{Y}_i$, a common factor model for $\mathbf{Y}_i$ is formed by stacking model components relating to each measurement occasion:

$$\mathbf{Y}_i = \tau + \mathbf{\Lambda}\eta_i + \varepsilon_i, \tag{1}$$

where τ is a $q \times 1$ stacked vector of latent intercepts,

$$\tau = \begin{bmatrix} \tau_1 \\ \vdots \\ \tau_T \end{bmatrix};$$

Λ is a $q \times T$ block diagonal matrix,

$$\Lambda = \begin{bmatrix} \lambda_1 & 0 & 0 \\ 0 & \ddots & 0 \\ 0 & 0 & \lambda_T \end{bmatrix};$$

η_i is a $T \times 1$ stacked factor vector,

$$\eta = \begin{bmatrix} \eta_{1i} \\ \vdots \\ \eta_{Ti} \end{bmatrix};$$

and ε_i is a $q \times 1$ stacked vector of measurement errors,

$$\varepsilon = \begin{bmatrix} \varepsilon_{1i} \\ \vdots \\ \varepsilon_{Ti} \end{bmatrix}.$$

In a structured latent curve model, an observation is assumed to be the sum of a common score and error, denoted here as c_i and ϵ_i, respectively. The means of the common scores over repeated occasions are assumed to follow a smooth function, $f(\theta, t)$ (Browne, 1993). That is, $E[c_i] = f(\theta, t)$. The target function, $f(\theta, t)$, is a function of a fixed parameter vector, θ, where θ may contain one or more parameters that enter the model nonlinearly, and discrete times of measurement, $t = 1, ..., T$.

In the current model development,[1] the first-order factor across occasions, $\eta_i = (\eta_{1i}, ..., \eta_{Ti})'$, is assumed to be a sum of a common score and error, denoted here by $\pi_i = (\pi_{1i}, ..., \pi_{Ti})'$ and $\zeta_i = (\zeta_{1i}, ..., \zeta_{Ti})'$, respectively:

$$\begin{bmatrix} \eta_{1i} \\ \vdots \\ \eta_{Ti} \end{bmatrix} = \begin{bmatrix} \pi_{1i} \\ \vdots \\ \pi_{Ti} \end{bmatrix} + \begin{bmatrix} \zeta_{1i} \\ \vdots \\ \zeta_{Ti} \end{bmatrix} \qquad (2)$$

---

[1] A change in notation from that appearing in Browne (1993) is done here to emphasize that it is a common factor whose mean is assumed to change over time and not the mean of the common score as presented in Browne.

The mean of the common score, $E[\pi_i] = \mu_\pi$, is assumed to follow a smooth function, $\mathbf{g}(\varphi, t)$:

$$
E \begin{bmatrix} \pi_{1i} \\ \vdots \\ \pi_{Ti} \end{bmatrix} = \begin{bmatrix} \mu_{\pi 1} \\ \vdots \\ \mu_{\pi T} \end{bmatrix} = \begin{bmatrix} g_1(\varphi, 1) \\ \vdots \\ g_T(\varphi, T) \end{bmatrix}, \tag{3}
$$

where $\varphi = (\varphi_1, ..., \varphi_R)'$ is a set of R fixed coefficients that represent specific features of change in the population curve. For example, $g(\varphi, t)$ may be an exponential function, such as that presented in Meredith and Tisak (1990, p. 117). See also Browne (1993). The common score, π_i, and the error, ζ_i, are assumed to be independent such that $\mathrm{cov}(\pi_i, \zeta_i') = \mathbf{0}$. The error is assumed to have a mean of zero and symmetric covariance matrix $\boldsymbol{\Psi}$.

In a second-order structured latent curve model, the common score, π_i, is assumed to follow a first-order Taylor polynomial taken with respect to the mean function:

$$
\pi_{ti} = g(\varphi, t) + \xi_{1i}^* g_1'(\varphi, t) + ... + \xi_{Ri}^* g_R'(\varphi, t), \tag{4}
$$

where $g_r'(\varphi, t)$ is the first-order partial derivative of the mean function $g(\varphi, t)$ with respect to the r-th parameter in φ :

$$
g_r'(\varphi, t) = \frac{\partial g(\varphi, t)}{\partial \varphi_r}.
$$

The coefficient ξ_{ri}^* is an individual-level deviate with expected value equal to zero, for $r = 1, ..., R$. Similar to that in Browne (1993), setting the means of the individual-level coefficients in Equation 4 to zero means that the expected value of the common score π_i, $E[\pi_i]$, will be equal to the mean function, as in Equation 3.

The partial derivatives of the mean function in Equation 3 are used to make up the columns of a factor matrix, denoted here as $\boldsymbol{\Gamma}$:

$$
\boldsymbol{\Gamma} = \begin{bmatrix} g_1'(\varphi, 1) & \cdots & g_R'(\varphi, 1) \\ \vdots & \ddots & \vdots \\ g_1'(\varphi, T) & \cdots & g_R'(\varphi, T) \end{bmatrix}.
$$

Then, assuming the common score π_i is expressed as a first-order Taylor polynomial, the latent score vector η_i, expressed earlier in Equation 2 may be reexpressed as

$$
\eta_i = \mathbf{g}(\varphi, t) + \boldsymbol{\Gamma}\xi_i^* + \zeta_i \tag{5}
$$

where $\xi_i^* = (\xi_{1i}^*, ..., \xi_{Ri}^*)'$ and $\mathbf{g}(\varphi, t) = (g(\varphi, 1), ..., g(\varphi, T))'$ is the mean function evaluated across occasions, $\mathbf{t} = (1, ..., T)'$. The expression in Equation 5 does not yet follow the form of a structured latent curve model in which the latent score is a linear combination of basis curves and person weights. Given that the mean function is invariant to a constant scaling factor, the mean function may be decomposed into a matrix composed of its basis curves and a vector containing the means of the person weights (see Browne, 1993, p. 177). Assuming this scaling invariance, $\mathbf{g}(\varphi, \mathbf{t}) = \boldsymbol{\Gamma}\kappa$, where κ may be obtained by solving the linear equation $\mathbf{g}(\varphi, \mathbf{t}) = \boldsymbol{\Gamma}\kappa$ (see Browne, 1993). It follows that the model for the first-order factor η_i in Equation 5 may be reexpressed as

$$\eta_i = \boldsymbol{\Gamma}\kappa + \boldsymbol{\Gamma}\xi_i^* + \zeta_i.$$

Assuming $\xi_i = \kappa + \xi_i^*$, where $\kappa = E[\xi_i^*]$, the model for η_i simplifies to

$$\eta_i = \boldsymbol{\Gamma}\xi_i + \zeta_i. \tag{6}$$

In the model specified in Equation 6, a set of second-order factors, ξ_i, is assumed to be a combination of a set of fixed effects, κ, and a person-level weight vector, ξ_i^*, that depends on the basis curves in $\boldsymbol{\Gamma}$. Elements of ξ_i represent different characteristics of change unique to the individual. Analogous to ξ_i in interpretation are the coefficients contained in φ that characterize different aspects of change in the population curve. Based on the model in Equation 6, the mean vector and covariance matrix for the first-order factor η_i are $\boldsymbol{\Gamma}\kappa$ and $\boldsymbol{\Gamma}\boldsymbol{\Phi}\boldsymbol{\Gamma}' + \boldsymbol{\Psi}$, respectively.

In the final stage of formulating the model, the first-order common factor model for manifest variables in Equation 1 and the model for the first-order factors in Equation 6 are expressed jointly:

$$\mathbf{Y}_i = \tau + \boldsymbol{\Lambda}(\boldsymbol{\Gamma}\xi_i + \zeta_i) + \varepsilon_i, \tag{7}$$

where the model in Equation 7 is a reexpression of the model in Equation 1 in which η_i, the first-order factor, is replaced by the second-order factor model, $\boldsymbol{\Gamma}\xi_i + \zeta$. Based on the second-order structured latent curve model, the mean value and covariance matrix of the response $\mathbf{Y}_i$, are

$$\mu_Y = \tau + \boldsymbol{\Lambda}\boldsymbol{\Gamma}\kappa \tag{8}$$

and

$$\boldsymbol{\Sigma}_Y = \boldsymbol{\Lambda}(\boldsymbol{\Gamma}\boldsymbol{\Phi}\boldsymbol{\Gamma}' + \boldsymbol{\Psi})\boldsymbol{\Lambda}' + \boldsymbol{\Theta}_\varepsilon. \tag{9}$$

In Equation 9, the matrix $\boldsymbol{\Phi}$ is an $R \times R$ symmetric covariance matrix for the second-order factors corresponding to change characteristics of the first-order factors. The elements contained in the diagonal of the matrix $\boldsymbol{\Phi}$ are the variances of the change characteristics, and thus, describe the extent to which individuals vary in terms of each characteristic. The off-diagonal elements of the matrix are the covariances of the change characteristics. These values characterize the direction and magnitude of the linear associations among the change features.

The matrix $\boldsymbol{\Theta}_\varepsilon$ is a $q \times q$ symmetric covariance matrix for the measurement errors corresponding to the common factor model of the repeated measures. The diagonal elements of this matrix are the variances of the measurement errors. The off-diagonal elements represent the covariances of these errors at this level. In longitudinal studies, it is common to provide an autocorrelation structure among the errors. For example, an error covariance structure for $\boldsymbol{\Theta}_\varepsilon$ that assumes temporally adjacent errors relating to the same measures are mutually correlated is

$$
\boldsymbol{\Theta}_\varepsilon =
\begin{bmatrix}
\theta_{11} & & & & & & \\
0 & \ddots & & & & & \\
0 & 0 & \theta_{k1} & & & & \\
\vdots & \vdots & \vdots & \ddots & & & \\
\rho_1 & 0 & 0 & \cdots & \theta_{1T} & & \\
0 & \ddots & 0 & \cdots & 0 & \ddots & \\
0 & 0 & \rho_k & \cdots & 0 & 0 & \theta_{kT}
\end{bmatrix},
$$

where $\rho_1, \dots, \rho_k$ are autocorrelation coefficients that may differ according to the different indicator variables.

8.2.1 Missing and Unbalanced Data

The model developed here allows for missing data. Statistical inference of maximum likelihood estimates is valid under the assumption that data are missing at random in the sense that the missingness is independent of the missing data (Little & Rubin, 2002; Rubin, 1976). At the level of the observed variables for a given measurement occasion, data need not be complete for each individual because a common factor model, in general, may be estimated given incomplete data (Finkbeiner, 1979). Across measurement occasions, data also need not be complete. For example, an individual may have data for only one measurement occasion. The ability of the latent curve model to handle missing data is very important, particularly in the context of longitudinal studies where data are often incomplete. In cases where data are not missing at random, it becomes especially important to take steps to include what data are available and to take into account the missing data patterns to avoid biased results.[2] Unbalanced data are also common in longitudinal studies because individuals are often observed at different times or at unequally spaced intervals. The model presented here could naturally handle different times of measurement across

---

[2]This issue of nonrandomly missing data is not addressed here as it is beyond the scope of the current chapter. Readers are referred to Rubin (1976) and Little and Rubin (2002), for issues relating to this problem in general, as well as an application of a pattern-mixture random effects model for longitudinal data presented in Hedeker and Gibbons (1997) as one possible method for addressing such data.

individuals and estimates would be unbiased assuming the patterns of measurement occasions were unrelated to the response measures. Tests of factorial invariance using standard methods, however, could not be performed in cases where data are observed at very different times across individuals. This limitation is shared by the latent curve model in general.

8.2.2 Model Identification

Model identification concerns the uniqueness of a solution for a given model. To help identify the current model, certain constraints must be placed on model parameters. At the first level of the model in which a common factor model is specified for the manifest variables, the model may be identified by selecting particular response variables to serve as reference variables of the latent variables. For example, assuming the same set of response variables have been measured at each occasion, the same variable may be selected as the reference variable for all occasions. This may then involve setting to zero the intercept of the common factor model that corresponds to the reference variable and setting to one the factor loading that also corresponds to the reference variable. Further, the errors of measurement need not be constrained. At the second level of the model, the first-order factor is assumed to be a function of a factor loading matrix (composed of basis curves that may be functions of time and fixed parameters that may be unknown), second-order factors corresponding to characteristics of change in the latent variable, and the error of the second-level regression. Given the constraints on the factor loading matrix, the variance and covariance matrix for the second-order factors would typically not be constrained. Additional constraints, however, are often necessary to solve identification problems.

8.3 EXAMPLE

To illustrate the utility of the proposed method, an example is provided based on data from the Seattle Longitudinal Study.[3] Accessible to researchers are data for individuals who participated in the first four waves of data collection in the years 1956, 1963, 1970, and 1977. Assessments of mental ability were included as part of the longitudinal battery. Participants included 10 cohorts that were based on year of birth in 7-year increments, with cohort membership

---

[3]The example relied on data from the Seattle Longitudinal Study (SLS), 1956–1977, made accessible in 2003 through the SLS website, *http://geron.psu.edu/sls/datasets.html*. Data were collected by K. Warner Schaie and Sherry L. Willis of The Pennsylvania State University, University Park, Pennsylvania in cooperation with the Group Health Cooperative of Puget Sound and the University of Washington, Seattle, Washington. Funding for these data was provided by a grant from the National Institute of Aging (AG00480, 1973–1979; AG03544, 1982–1986; AG04770, 1984–1989) (R037 AG08055, 1989–2006). A summary of the study is provided in Schaie (2005).

remaining consistent throughout the study. Age of subjects was represented by the midpoint of a 7-year age group range. For example, the age group identified as 46 years contained individuals who ranged in age from 43 to 49 years. Actual age is not included in the dataset. Age blocks ranged from 25 to 88 years.

Mental ability was assessed by the Primary Mental Abilities, Ages 11–17—Form AM (Copyright 1948, by L. L. Thurstone and Thelma Gwinn Thurstone) that contains five timed subtests and is administered in a group testing session. Readers can access descriptions of these subtests at the SLS website. The subtests include (1) Verbal-Meaning, (2) Space, (3) Reasoning, (4) Number, and (5) Word Fluency. Thurstone and Thurstone (1949) suggested a composite of these five subtests as an index of a conventional measure of intelligence, with this score included in the dataset described earlier. Plots of this index suggested a relatively stable level of mental ability across age, with a slow decrease in scores at older ages. The five measures of mental ability are considered here as indicators of a latent measure of mental ability. Here, only scores during the latter ages are considered. Data are presented for 1994 adults who completed the mental ability battery and who fell within the age block 46 up through age block 74 at any time of measurement. This span included five age blocks (46, 53, 60, 67 and 74) with a single individual providing data for up to four occasions, with complete data within age blocks. Cohort effects are not considered in this analysis but could be considered in future explorations. The data help illustrate the usefulness of a second-order structured latent curve model, because the model handles multiple indicators of a latent variable whose mean pattern of change is nonlinear.

8.3.1 Testing Factorial Invariance

Prior to fitting a second-order structured latent curve model, four factor models distinguished by varying levels of factorial invariance were fitted to the data. Evaluation of model fit was done by evaluating and comparing normal theory chi-square statistics, estimates of the root mean squared error of approximation (RMSEA), the Akaike information criterion (AIC), the comparative fit index (CFI), and the Tucker Lewis index (TLI) [a.k.a. the nonnormed fit index (NNFI)]. Indices of fit for the model series are summarized in Table 8–1. For the current sample, strict factorial invariance provided a good fit to the data with the fewest parameters. Based on the RMSEA, all four models provided a close fit to the data (RMSEA ranged from .040 to .042). The AIC favored the most complex model. The CFI and TLI were both highest under configural invariance, although values associated with the remaining models are not appreciably different. Without information about the behavior of these fit indices under the current sampling conditions, it may be difficult to draw with great confidence conclusions about which model is preferred given the comparabil-

TABLE 8–1

Model Comparisons for Varying Levels of Factorial Invariance

Model	-2lnL	p	df	χ^2	RMSEA	AIC	CLI	TLI
1	102661	105	245	1047.84	.0405	102871	.903	.881
2	102719	89	261	1106.23	.0403	102897	.898	.882
3	102826	73	277	1213.34	.0412	102972	.887	.877
4	102965	53	297	1351.78	.0422	103071	.872	.871

Note. Model 1 is configural invariance; Model 2 is weak factorial invariance with equal factor loadings and unequal latent intercepts and measurement error variances; Model 3 is strong factorial invariance with equal factor loadings and latent intercepts and unequal measurement error variances; Model 4 is strict factorial invariance with equal factor loadings, latent intercepts, and measurement error variances. p is the number of parameters for a given model. The baseline model on which the CLI and TLI are based is a model for which the covariances between the manifest variables are zero.

ity of many of the indices across models. Given that all models seem to provide reasonable fits to the data, strong factorial invariance was provisionally taken as an acceptable model. This model represents the minimum level of factorial invariance generally considered necessary for meaningful comparisons of means. Further analyses were based on this model but caution must be taken in the interpretation. A consequence of failure to have invariance of the factor structure over time is that differences in means may be attributable at least in part to differences in a factor's scale.

A common factor model was specified for the manifest variables. Latent measures of mental ability were assumed to be indicated by the five test scores at each age block, with blocks coded as $t = -2, -1, 0, 1, 2$. The common factor model for $\mathbf{Y}_i^*$ at time t, $\mathbf{Y}_{ti}^*$, was specified as

$$\mathbf{Y}_{ti}^* = \tau^* + \lambda^* \eta_{ti}^* + \varepsilon_{ti}^*.$$

The vector τ^* was a 5×1 set of intercept values, with the first element set equal to zero ($\tau_1 = 0$) so that the first indicator could arbitrarily serve as the reference for the latent variable. The remaining elements $\tau_2, ..., \tau_5$ were considered fixed but unknown and not unique to the measurement occasion:

$$\tau^* = \begin{bmatrix} 0 \\ \tau_2 \\ \tau_3 \\ \tau_4 \\ \tau_5 \end{bmatrix}.$$

The coefficient λ^* was a 5×1 vector of factor loadings, with the first element set equal to 1 ($\lambda_1 = 1$) so that again the first indicator variable could serve as the reference for the latent variable. Elements $\lambda_2, \ldots, \lambda_5$ were considered fixed but unknown and also not unique to the measurement occasion:

$$\lambda^* = \begin{bmatrix} 1 \\ \lambda_2 \\ \lambda_3 \\ \lambda_4 \\ \lambda_5 \end{bmatrix}.$$

The latent variable η_{ti}^* represents the common mental ability score at time t. The vector ε_{ti}^* was a 5×1 set of unique measurement errors associated with the regression of the five manifest variables, $Y_{1ti}, \ldots, Y_{5ti}$ and on the latent variable at time t:

$$\varepsilon_{ti}^* = \begin{bmatrix} \varepsilon_{1ti} \\ \varepsilon_{2ti} \\ \varepsilon_{3ti} \\ \varepsilon_{4ti} \\ \varepsilon_{5ti} \end{bmatrix}.$$

A multivariate response vector, $\mathbf{Y}_i$, was formed by stacking across occasions the response sets within waves to create a single response vector. Given that each individual contributed data for at most four occasions, $\mathbf{Y}_i$ for a given individual was at most of length 20. The model is initially presented based on an assumption that measures were taken across all five age blocks. Thus, the multivariate response vector is tentatively taken to be $\mathbf{Y}_i = (\mathbf{Y}_{1i}^*, \ldots, \mathbf{Y}_{5i}^*)$. Following development of the model, a method is described that allows for model specification that is unique to the individual. Based on an earlier discussion, strong factorial invariance was taken as an acceptable model in which the factor loadings and latent intercepts but not the measurement error variances were invariant across age blocks. A common factor model for $\mathbf{Y}_i$ was formed by stacking model components relating to each of the five occasions:

$$\mathbf{Y}_i = \tau + \mathbf{\Lambda}\eta_i + \varepsilon_i. \tag{10}$$

The vector τ was a stacked set of intercept values of length 25;

$$\tau = \begin{bmatrix} \tau^* \\ \tau^* \\ \tau^* \\ \tau^* \\ \tau^* \end{bmatrix};$$

The matrix Λ_i was a 25 x 5 block diagonal matrix; for example,

$$\Lambda = \begin{bmatrix} \lambda^* & 0 & 0 & 0 & 0 \\ 0 & \lambda^* & 0 & 0 & 0 \\ 0 & 0 & \lambda^* & 0 & 0 \\ 0 & 0 & 0 & \lambda^* & 0 \\ 0 & 0 & 0 & 0 & \lambda^* \end{bmatrix},$$

where the vector λ^* is as defined above; η_i was a 5 x 1 stacked factor vector of latent responses,

$$\eta_i = \begin{bmatrix} \eta_{1i} \\ \vdots \\ \eta_{5i} \end{bmatrix};$$

and ε_i was a 25 x 1 stacked vector of measurement errors across the five age blocks,

$$\varepsilon_i = \begin{bmatrix} \varepsilon_{1i}^* \\ \varepsilon_{2i}^* \\ \varepsilon_{3i}^* \\ \varepsilon_{4i}^* \\ \varepsilon_{5i}^* \end{bmatrix}.$$

At the second level, the latent mental ability scores across occasions, η_i, were assumed to be the sum of a common score, $\pi_i = (\pi_{1i}, \ldots, \pi_{5i})'$, and error, $\zeta_i = (\zeta_{1i}, \ldots, \zeta_{5i})'$. The means of the common factor over time were assumed to follow a variation of an exponential function (cf. Meredith & Tisak, 1990, p. 117):

$$\mu_\pi = g(\varphi, t) = \varphi_1 - \exp\{\varphi_2(t)\} \tag{11}$$

where $\varphi = (\varphi_1, \varphi_2)'$ contains the characteristics of change in the latent response. The coefficient φ_1 represents the population upper asymptote, and φ_2 represents the population rate of change. As population characteristics, the coefficients φ_1 and φ_2 are fixed across members of the population. Also note that φ_1 enters Equation 11 in a linear manner and φ_2 enters nonlinearly. Finally, the common score vector, π_i, and the error vector, ζ_i, were assumed to be independent. Additionally, the error at the second level was assumed to be normally distributed with mean zero and covariance matrix Ψ: $\zeta_i \sim N(\mathbf{0}, \Psi)$.

The common response, π_{ti}, was then assumed to be a linear, weighted combination of a set of basis curves based on a first-order Taylor polynomial taken with regard to the mean function, $g(\varphi, t)$:

$$\pi_{ti} = g(\varphi, t) + \xi_1^* g_1'(\varphi, t) + \xi_2^* g_2'(\varphi, t). \tag{12}$$

The quantity $g'_r(\varphi, t)$ is the first-order derivative of the target function $g(\varphi, t)$ in Equation (11) taken with regard to the r-th parameter in φ, $r = 1, 2$:

$$g'_r(\varphi, t) = \frac{\partial g(\varphi, t)}{\partial \varphi_r}.$$

With the target function $g(\varphi, t)$ defined in Equation (11), the partial derivatives of $g(\varphi, t)$ with regard to elements in φ are

$$g'_1(\varphi, t) = \frac{\partial g(\varphi, t)}{\partial \varphi_1} = 1 \qquad (13)$$

and

$$g'_2(\varphi, t) = \frac{\partial g(\varphi, t)}{\partial \varphi_2} = -t \exp\{\varphi_2(t)\}. \qquad (14)$$

The basis curves in Equations 13 and 14 define the shape of the population curve for the common score, π_i, as a function of age blocks. The first basis curve, given in Equation 13, corresponds to the upper asymptote. The second, given in Equation 14, relates to the rate of change in the latent measure of mental ability. With regard to the common score model defined in Equation 12, the coefficients in $\xi^* = (\xi_1^*, \xi_2^*)'$ are individual-level effects assumed to have means equal to zero. Each coefficient represents a specific characteristic of change unique to the individual and has an interpretation analogous to that of the corresponding population effect in φ.

The first-order factor η_{ti} was then assumed to be a linear combination of the factor loading matrix and person weights. The factor loading matrix was defined by the partial derivatives in Equations 13 and 14. The second-order factor loading matrix, $\boldsymbol{\Gamma}$, was thus defined as:

$$\boldsymbol{\Gamma} = \begin{bmatrix} g'_1(\varphi, 1) & g'_2(\varphi, 1) \\ \vdots & \vdots \\ g'_1(\varphi, 5) & g'_2(\varphi, 5) \end{bmatrix}.$$

The set of second-order factors, denoted by ξ_i, was assumed to be a sum of population effects, denoted by κ, and the individual-level effects, ξ_i^*, defined in Equation 12, where the population effect, κ, was assumed to be the expected value of ξ_i. With the target function defined by the exponential function in Equation 11, the population effect, κ, was obtained by solving the equation $\mathbf{g}(\varphi, \mathbf{t}) = \boldsymbol{\Gamma}\kappa$, where $\kappa = (\varphi_1, 0)'$.

The repeated measures of Equation 10 are reexpressed by combining the models for the first- and second-order factors:

$$\mathbf{Y}_i = \tau + \boldsymbol{\Lambda}(\boldsymbol{\Gamma}\xi_i + \zeta_i) + \varepsilon_i, \qquad (15)$$

where η_i in Equation 10 is substituted with $\Gamma\xi_i + \zeta_i$. Assuming independence among the second-order factors, ξ_i, and the errors at both levels (i.e., ζ_i and ε_i), the mean vector and covariance matrix of the response set, $\mathbf{Y}_i$, are

$$\mu_Y = \tau + \mathbf{\Lambda}\mathbf{\Gamma}\kappa$$

and

$$\mathbf{\Sigma}_Y = \mathbf{\Lambda}(\mathbf{\Gamma}\mathbf{\Phi}\mathbf{\Gamma}' + \mathbf{\Psi})\mathbf{\Lambda}' + \mathbf{\Theta}_\varepsilon$$

where the orders of μ_Y and $\mathbf{\Sigma}_Y$ are both 25. The matrix $\mathbf{\Phi}$ is a 2×2 symmetric covariance matrix for the second-order factors corresponding to the change characteristics of the first-order factors:

$$\mathbf{\Phi} = \left[\begin{array}{cc} \phi_{11} & \\ \phi_{21} & \phi_{22} \end{array} \right],$$

where the diagonal elements, ϕ_{11}, and ϕ_{22}, are the variances of the random coefficients corresponding to upper asymptote and rate of change in responses, respectively. The off-diagonal element in $\mathbf{\Phi}$ is the covariance between the random change characteristics. The matrix $\mathbf{\Psi}$ was a 5×5 symmetric covariance matrix for the regression errors at the second level. Assuming constant error variance across age blocks, the matrix $\mathbf{\Psi}$ was diagonal with a unique element, ψ, where ψ denotes the variance of the latent regression error, ζ_i:

$$\mathbf{\Psi} = \left[\begin{array}{ccc} \psi & & \\ & \ddots & \\ & & \psi \end{array} \right].$$

The matrix $\mathbf{\Theta}_\varepsilon$ was a 25×25 symmetric covariance matrix for the measurement errors corresponding to the common factor model of the repeated response times. The diagonal elements of this matrix are the variances of the measurement errors. The off-diagonal elements are their covariances. Assuming strong factorial invariance, the measurement error variances could vary across scales and age blocks. Further, the covariances between the same scales at different occasions were allowed to covary with no equality constraints on these values. A path diagram of the model is given in Figure 8–1.

8.3.2 Handling Missing and Unbalanced Data

Given that individuals had data for occasions ranging between one and four time points, the order of the mean vector and covariance matrix relating to the response set, $\mathbf{Y}_i$, varied across individuals, with a minimum order of 5 and a maximum of 20. To handle the various patterns of observed data, an index, denoted by w, is specified with values corresponding to the age blocks. Let $w = (w_1, ..., w_5)'$ represent a set of index values corresponding to the five age

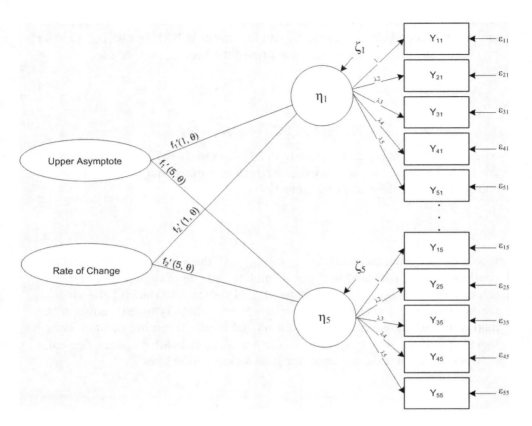

Figure 8–1.Second-order structured latent curve model path diagram. Not shown are the correlations between the latent change characteristics and the measurement errors corresponding to
temporally adjacent values for the same indicators.

blocks. For individual i, the index w_i is a subset of w with length that varies
from 1 to 4 depending on the number of occasions on which individual i was
measured. For example, for an individual with complete data on the first, third,
and fourth measurement occasions, the index is equal to $w_i = (1, 3, 4)$. The
multivariate response vector is now specifically given as

$$\widetilde{\mathbf{Y}}_i = [\mathbf{Y}_i]_{w_i}$$

with mean vector and covariance matrix

$$\widetilde{\mu_Y} = [\mu_Y]_{w_i} = \tau_i + \mathbf{\Lambda}_i \mathbf{\Gamma}_i \kappa$$

and

$$\widetilde{\mathbf{\Sigma}_Y} = [\mathbf{\Sigma}_Y]_{w_i} = \mathbf{\Lambda}_i (\mathbf{\Gamma}_i \mathbf{\Phi} \mathbf{\Gamma}_i' + \mathbf{\Psi}_i) \mathbf{\Lambda}_i' + \mathbf{\Theta}_{\varepsilon i}.$$

TABLE 8–2

Maximum Likelihood Estimates for Population- and Individual-Level Change Characteristics

Parameter	MLE	Lower[a]	Upper[a]
Change characteristic			
Upper asymptote, φ_1	33.1	24.5	33.6
Rate of change, φ_2	.480	.362	.656
Change characteristics variances and covariance matrix[b]			

$$\begin{bmatrix} 93.5 & .104 \\ 1.35 & 1.81 \end{bmatrix}$$

Note. [a] "Lower" and "Upper" refer to lower and upper limits, respectively, for 90% confidence intervals.

[b] The lower diagonal element is the covariance between the two random coefficients and the upper diagonal element is the corresponding correlation.

Maximum likelihood estimates were obtained using Mx (Neale, Boker, Xie, & Maes, 2003). Script used to obtain these estimates is given in the appendix. Parameter estimates relating to the coefficients that characterized change in the response at the population level and the variances relating to individual differences in these coefficients are presented in the Table 8–2. The estimated upper asymptote representing potential level prior to decline was 33.1 with a 90% CI of (24.5, 33.6). The estimated mean rate of change was .480 with a 90% CI of (.362,.656). Evidence for individual differences in change features in the latent responses are given by the variances of the random effects corresponding to the basis curves. The estimated variances corresponding to the upper asymptote and change rate indicated individual differences in levels before decline as well as in the rate of change.

8.4 DISCUSSION

A version of the structured latent curve model is presented that allows for measurement error in a set of manifest variables observed on multiple occasions, where the latent variable means follow a function that may be nonlinear in its parameters. The model addresses the imperfect nature of measured variables as indicators of latent variables and allows for tests of the assumption of factorial invariance across time. The former benefits studies where a variable of interest is not directly observed but can be indicated by a small number of manifest variables. The latter benefit is that it provides a means for direct assessment of the tenability of the assumption that the same factor has been measured across occasions. Further, the model allows for the study of change in latent variables that can be described by a function nonlinear in its parameters, such as an exponential or logistic function.

The distinction between latent variables and latent characteristics of change is important in the context of latent curve models in general. A latent variable may be considered an attribute that is not directly observable (see McDonald, 1985), such as self-esteem or intelligence. Multiple measurable variables that serve as indicators of an unobservable variable may be available, and a common factor model may then serve to represent the linear dependencies of observed variables on the common latent measure. In a latent curve model, the factors represent unobservable change characteristics, such as true rate of change, and so have a different interpretation from the standard definition of a latent variable. McArdle and Epstein (1987) refer to latent growth features as chronometric factors. In a second-order latent curve model, this difference in interpretation is clearly highlighted by the separate model components that address measurement error in the observed repeated measures and the change features that characterize the latent variable over time.

The current model was developed for a single latent repeated measure, although the model may be extended to handle multiple latent variables. The structured latent curve model has been considered for multiple repeated measures to allow for the study of two or more observed variables, where each variable is assumed to follow a structured latent curve model (Blozis, 2004b; MacCallum, Kim, Malarkey, & Kiecolt-Glaser, 1997). The model presented in this chapter, like its predecessors, may also include a common factor model for covariates observed at either the level of the measurement occasion or at the level of the individual. Time-varying latent variables whose values change from one occasion to another may be related to the outcome of interest, and it may be important to statistically partial out the effects of these variables to better understand change in the primary variable of interest. For time-varying covariates, concerns about factorial invariance may also be relevant. Latent variables measured at the individual level are typically variables that are either considered to be time-invariant, such as those variables that are stable characteristics of an individual, or measures taken at a particular point in time, such as at the start of a study. Finally, selection of a suitable model for change in a variable should take careful consideration. Several different functions may give reasonable descriptions of the data. Researchers are encouraged to consider not only alternative functional forms to describe data but also to consider other potentially useful modeling frameworks.

REFERENCES

Blozis, S. A. (2004a, June). *Second-order structured latent curve model for normal repeated measures.* Paper presented at the International Meeting of the Psychometric Society, Pacific Grove, CA.

Blozis, S. A. (2004b). Structured latent curve models for the study of change in multivariate repeated measures. *Psychological Methods, 9,* 334–353.

Blozis, S. A., & Cudeck, R. (1999). Conditionally linear mixed-effects models with latent variable covariates. *Journal of Educational & Behavioral Statistics, 24,* 245–270.

Browne, M. W. (1993). Structured latent curve models. In C. M. Cuadras & C. R. Rao (Eds.), *Multivariate analysis: Future directions 2* (pp. 171–197). Amsterdam: Elsevier Science.

Browne, M. W., & Du Toit, S. H. C. (1991). Models for learning data. In L. M. Collins & J. L. Horn (Eds.), *Best methods for the analysis of change* (pp. 47–68). Washington, DC: American Psychological Association.

Bryk, A. S., & Raudenbush, S. W. (1987). Application of hierarchical linear models to assessing change. *Psychological Bulletin, 101,* 147–158.

Chan, D. (1998). The conceptualization and analysis of change over time: An integrative approach incorporating longitudinal mean and covariance structures analysis (LMACS) and multiple indicator latent growth modeling (MLGM). *Organizational Research Methods, 1,* 421–483.

Davidian, W., & Giltinan, D. M. (1995). *Nonlinear models for repeated measurement data.* London: Chapman & Hall.

Duncan, S. C., & Duncan, T. E. (1996). A multivariate growth curve analysis of adolescent substance use. *Structural Equation Modeling, 3,* 323–347.

Finkbeiner, C. (1979). Estimation for the multiple factor model when data are missing. *Psychometrika, 44,* 409–420.

Hedeker, D., & Gibbons, R. D. (1997). Application of random-effects pattern-mixture models for missing data in longitudinal studies. *Psychological Methods, 2,* 64–78.

Horn, J. L., & McArdle, J. J. (1992). A practical and theoretical guide to measurement invariance. *Experimental Aging Research, 18,* 117–144.

Jennrich, R. I., & Schluchter, M. D. (1986). Unbalanced repeated measures models with structured covariance matrices. *Biometrics, 42,* 805–820.

Laird, N. M. (1988). Missing data in longitudinal studies. *Statistics in Medicine, 7,* 305–315.

Laird, N. M., & Ware, J. H. (1982). Random-effects models for longitudinal data. *Biometrics, 38,* 963–974.

Lawley, D. N., & Maxwell, A. E. (1971). *Factor analysis as a statistical method.* New York: American Elsevier.

Little, R., & Rubin, D. (2002). *Statistical analysis with missing data* (2nd ed.). New York: Wiley.

Lubke, G. H., & Dolan, C. V. (2003). Can unequal residual variances across groups mask differences in residual means in the common factor model? *Structural Equation Modeling, 10,* 175–192.

MacCallum, R. C., Kim, C., Malarkey, W. B., & Kiecolt-Glaser, J. K. (1997). Studying multivariate change using multilevel models and latent curve models. *Multivariate Behavioral Research, 32,* 215–253.

McArdle, J. J. (1988). Dynamic but structural equation modeling of repeated measures data. In J. R. Nesselroade & R. B. Cattell (Eds.), *Handbook of multivariate experimental psychology* (pp. 561–614). New York: Plenum Press.

McArdle, J. J. (1998). Modeling longitudinal data by latent growth curve methods. In G. Marcoulides (Ed.), *Modern methods for business research* (pp. 359–406). Mahwah, NJ: Lawrence Erlbaum Associates.

McArdle, J. J., & Epstein, D. (1987). Latent growth curves within developmental structural equation models. *Child Development, 58,* 110–133.

McDonald, R. P. (1985). *Factor analysis and related methods.* Hillsdale, NJ: Lawrence Erlbaum Associates.

Mehta, P. D., & West, S. G. (2000). Putting the individual back into individual growth curves. *Psychological Methods, 5,* 23–43.

Meredith, W. (1965). Some results based on a general stochastic model for mental tests. *Psychometrika, 30,* 419–440.

Meredith, W. (1993). Measurement invariance, factor analysis, and factorial invariance. *Psychometrika, 58,* 107–122.

Meredith, W., & Horn, J. (2001). The role of factorial invariance in modeling growth and change. In L. M. Collins & A. G. Sayer (Eds.), *New methods for the analysis of change (*pp. 203–240). Washington, DC.: American Psychological Association.

Meredith, W., & Tisak, J. (1984, June). *Tuckerizing curves.* Paper presented at the Annual Meeting of the Psychometric Society, Santa Barbara, CA.

Meredith, W., & Tisak, J. (1990). Latent curve analysis. *Psychometrika, 55,* 107–122.

Millsap, R. E., & Meredith, W. (in press). Factorial invariance: Historical perspectives and new problems. In R. Cudeck & R. C. MacCallum (Eds.) *Factor analysis at 100.* Mahwah, NJ: Lawrence Erlbaum Associates.

Neale, M. C., Boker, S. M., Xie, G., Maes, H. H. (2003). *Mx: Statistical modeling* (6th ed.). Richmond, VA: VCU, Department of Psychiatry.

Raudenbush, S. W., & Bryk, A. S. (2002). *Hierarchical linear models.* Thousand Oaks, CA: Sage.

Rubin, D. B. (1976). Inference and missing data. *Biometrika, 63,* 581–592.

Sayer, A. G., & Cumsille, P. E. (2001). Second-order latent growth models. In L. M. Collins, & A. G. Sayer (Eds), *New methods for the analysis of change* (pp. 179–200). Washington, DC: American Psychological Association.

Schaie, K. W. (2005). *Developmental influences on adult intelligence: The Seattle Longitudinal Study.* New York: Oxford University Press.

Thurstone, L. L. (1947). *Multiple factor analysis.* Chicago: University of Chicago.

Thurstone, L. L. (1949). *Examiner manual for the SRA Primary Mental Abilities Test.* Chicago: Science Research Associates.

Widaman, K. F., & Reise, S. P. (1997). Exploring the measurement invariance of psychological instruments: Applications in the substance use domain. In K. J. Bryant, M. Windle, & S. West (Eds.), *The science of prevention: Methodological advances from alcohol and substance abuse research* (pp. 281–324). Washington, DC: American Psychological Association.

Willett, J., & Sayer, A. (1994). Using covariance structure analysis to detect correlates and predictors of individual change over time. *Psychological Bulletin, 116*, 363–380.

Appendix

Mx script

```
#ngroups 3
Group 1:
Calculation
Matrices;
Q zero 1 1
R full 1 1 free
S full 1 1 free
T full 5 1
U unit 5 1
V full 25 1
W full 25 5
X symm 5 5
Y symm 2 2 free
Z symm 25 25
End Matrices
! Set model constraints and provide starting values
! Target function parameters
ST 36 R 1 1
```

ST .4 S 1 1
! AGE BLOCKS
VA -2 T 1 1
VA -1 T 2 1
VA 0 T 3 1
VA 1 T 4 1
VA 2 T 5 1
! Tau
VA 0 V 1 1 V 6 1 V 11 1 V 16 1 V 21 1
FR V 2 1 V 7 1 V 12 1 V 17 1 V 22 1
EQ V 2 1 V 7 1 V 12 1 V 17 1 V 22 1
ST 1 V 2 1 V 7 1 V 12 1 V 17 1 V 22 1
FR V 3 1 V 8 1 V 13 1 V 18 1 V 23 1
EQ V 3 1 V 8 1 V 13 1 V 18 1 V 23 1
ST 1 V 3 1 V 8 1 V 13 1 V 18 1 V 23 1
FR V 4 1 V 9 1 V 14 1 V 19 1 V 24 1
EQ V 4 1 V 9 1 V 14 1 V 19 1 V 24 1
ST 1 V 4 1 V 9 1 V 14 1 V 19 1 V 24 1
FR V 5 1 V 10 1 V 15 1 V 20 1 V 25 1
EQ V 5 1 V 10 1 V 15 1 V 20 1 V 25 1
ST 1 V 5 1 V 10 1 V 15 1 V 20 1 V 25 1
! Lambda
VA 1.0 W 1 1 W 6 2 W 11 3 W 16 4 W 21 5
FR W 2 1 W 7 2 W 12 3 W 17 4 W 22 5
EQ W 2 1 W 7 2 W 12 3 W 17 4 W 22 5
ST .7 W 2 1 W 7 2 W 12 3 W 17 4 W 22 5
FR W 3 1 W 8 2 W 13 3 W 18 4 W 23 5
EQ W 3 1 W 8 2 W 13 3 W 18 4 W 23 5
ST .7 W 3 1 W 8 2 W 13 3 W 18 4 W 23 5
FR W 4 1 W 9 2 W 14 3 W 19 4 W 24 5
EQ W 4 1 W 9 2 W 14 3 W 19 4 W 24 5
ST .7 W 4 1 W 9 2 W 14 3 W 19 4 W 24 5
FR W 5 1 W 10 2 W 15 3 W 20 4 W 25 5
EQ W 5 1 W 10 2 W 15 3 W 20 4 W 25 5
ST .7 W 5 1 W 10 2 W 15 3 W 20 4 W 25 5
! Phi
ST 10 Y 1 1
ST 1 Y 2 1
ST 1 Y 2 2
! Theta Epsilon
FR Z 1 1 Z 6 6 Z 11 11 Z 16 16 Z 21 21
ST 41 Z 1 1 Z 6 6 Z 11 11 Z 16 16 Z 21 21

```
FR Z 6 1 Z 11 6 Z 16 11 Z 21 16
FR Z 2 2 Z 7 7 Z 12 12 Z 17 17 Z 22 22
ST 63 Z 2 2 Z 7 7 Z 12 12 Z 17 17 Z 22 22
FR Z 7 2 Z 12 7 Z 17 12 Z 22 17
FR Z 3 3 Z 8 8 Z 13 13 Z 18 18 Z 23 23
ST 12 Z 3 3 Z 8 8 Z 13 13 Z 18 18 Z 23 23
FR Z 8 3 Z 13 8 Z 18 13 Z 23 18
FR Z 4 4 Z 9 9 Z 14 14 Z 19 19 Z 24 24
ST 69 Z 4 4 Z 9 9 Z 14 14 Z 19 19 Z 24 24
FR Z 9 4 Z 14 9 Z 19 14 Z Z 24 19
FR Z 5 5 Z 10 10 Z 15 15 Z 20 20 Z 25 25
ST 102 Z 5 5 Z 10 10 Z 15 15 Z 20 20 Z 25 25
FR Z 10 5 Z 15 10 Z 20 15 Z 25 20
! Psi
FR X 1 1 X 2 2 X 3 3 X 4 4 X 5 5
EQ X 1 1 X 2 2 X 3 3 X 4 4 X 5 5
ST 1 X 1 1 X 2 2 X 3 3 X 4 4 X 5 5
End Group
Group 2:
Data NI=25 NO=1994
VLENGTH file=C:\IQ.dat
Labels v46 s46 r46 n46 w46
v53 s53 r53 n53 w53
v60 s60 r60 n60 w60
v67 s67 r67 n67 w67
v74 s74 r74 n74 w74;
Begin Matrices = Group 1;
End Matrices;
Begin Algebra;
G = U;
I = -T.(\exp(S@T));
J = G|I;
C = R_Q;
End Algebra;
Mean V + W*J*C /
Covariance W*(J*Y*J' + X)*W' + Z /
End Group
Group 3:
Data Calculation
MATRIX
P FULL 59 1
COMPUTE P /
```

SPECIFY P
1 2 6 11 16 21 26 31 36 41 91 3 4 5 46 55 64 73 82 51 47 60 56 69 65 78
74 87 83 52 48
61 57 70 66 79 75 88 84 53 49 62 58 71 67 80 76 89 85 54 50 63 59 72 68
81 77 90 86
End group

Chapter 9

Patterns of Persistence of Abnormal Returns: A Finite Mixture Distribution Approach

Juan Carlos Bou

Universitat Jaume I, Spain

Albert Satorra

Universitat Pompeu Fabra, Spain

9.1 INTRODUCTION

Abnormal returns, that is, profits well above or below the competitive or equilibrium level, have been studied extensively in strategic management research. They are usually interpreted as a measure of the relative ability of firms to avoid competitive forces and achieve sustained competitive advantage.

Numerous theories in strategic management research and in related fields, such as industrial organization economics and organizational ecology, have proposed alternative explanations of the dynamical behavior of abnormal returns. For example, Neoclassical Economics (Arrow & Hahn, 1971) and the Austrian School of Economics (Jacobson, 1992) predict that abnormal returns are transitory and they vanish when markets reach an equilibrium, or when factors such as imitation, substitution, and innovation erode or supersede all sources of competitive advantage. In contrast, other theoretical approaches including industrial organization economics (Bain, 1956) and the resource-based view of the firm (Barney, 1991; Wernerfelt, 1984) propose the existence of industry- and firm-specific factors that sustain competitive advantages and superior economic performance over time.

Differences in predictions are related not only to the persistence, but also to the presence of groups of firms that exhibit different patterns of abnormal returns, and to firms' characteristics in each group. For example, theoretical approaches such as industrial organization economics (Bain, 1956; Caves & Porter, 1977) and strategic group theory (Hunt, 1972; Porter, 1979) predict the existence of stable groups of firms that exhibit extremely abnormal returns due to entry and mobility barriers, respectively, whereas the Austrian School of Economics predicts turnover in the membership of firms in the high-performer group (Wiggings & Rueffli, 2002). Regarding the firms' characteristics, organizational ecology predicts stability of both high and low performers due to inertia that is greater for larger and older firms. However, resource-based theorists emphasize the stability of only high-performing firms with valuable, rare, imperfectly imitable, and nonsubstitutable resources (Barney, 1991; McGahan & Porter, 2003).

In summary, theoretical approaches differ in how abnormal returns evolve and in the type of firms that follow each path. The study of the patterns of evolution of abnormal returns can thus provide important insights into the relevance of predictions of theories in strategic management; further, it can also help in understanding the relationship between competitive advantage and abnormal returns.

With the exception of Mueller (1986) and the so-called *persistence of profit* line of research (Connolly & Schwartz, 1985; Geroski & Jacquemin, 1988; Odagiri & Yamawaki, 1986; Schohl, 1990), less attention has been paid to the dynamics of abnormal returns. In a regression-based time-series study, Mueller (1986, 1990) found evidence that abnormal profits vanish because profits tend to converge toward the mean. He found that high-performing firms tended to have a slower rate of convergence than did low performers.

More recently, the dynamics of abnormal returns has received additional attention. Using panel data of American corporations from 1981 through 1994, McGahan and Porter (1999) found differences in the persistence of industry, corporate-parent, and business-level effects, where the transient industry effect was more persistent than business-segment and corporate-parent transient effects. Based on these results, they highlight the importance of the industry in the dynamic behavior of abnormal returns. In a later study, McGahan and Porter (2003) explored the patterns in the emergence and sustainability of abnormal returns in high- and low-performer firms. They found evidence of differences in both, emergence and sustainability, across two groups of firms. For example, they found that low performance arises from business-specific factors, whereas for high performers, both industry and business-line factors are important. Wiggings and Ruefli (2002) also reported empirical evidence of the dynamics of above-normal returns in a sample of 40 industries. They found that at least one firm achieved 10 or more years of persistent superior economic performance in every industry, that large firms are more likely to achieve persistent superior performance, and that industry membership and market share were not always significant factors in persistent superior performance.

The present study continues the research on the dynamics of abnormal returns. The chapter has three objectives; (a) to establish the existence of alternative forms of how abnormal returns evolve, and to estimate the percentage of firms whose abnormal returns follow each path; (b) to describe each pattern of evolution and its implications for the predictions of alternative theoretical approaches; (c) to describe the characteristics of firms that form each group.

Two assumptions characterize our approach. First, we assume the existence of *dynamic heterogeneity* in abnormal returns; that is, the evolution of abnormal returns follows alternative paths. This assumption is in accord with previous empirical studies (Mueller, 1986; Odagiri & Yamawaki, 1986; Schohl, 1990), which, for example, found that high-performing firms exhibit a slower convergence of abnormal returns than did firms that obtain normal returns. The main implication of this assumption is that the evolution of firms' abnormal returns varies, not only across firms, corporations, and industries, as Waring (1996) and McGahan and Porter (1999) among others have reported, but also in the way they evolve. Under dynamic heterogeneity, time is an important dimension and is introduced into the study of abnormal returns as an additional source of variation. The second assumption is that the dynamic heterogeneity is *latent* or *unobserved*, that is, it is not possible to know a priori which path best describes the evolution of abnormal returns for each firm. In our approach, we assign firms into groups not with certainty, but based on the probability of belonging of each firm to a group.

We investigated the dynamical behavior of abnormal returns on $5,000$ Spanish firms in a 6-year period. We fit first a dynamic panel data model that decomposes abnormal returns into three components; static or permanent, transient, and firm-year specific. Each component corresponds to a different evolution of abnormal returns. In the second stage, we adopt a finite mixture approach to uncover various alternative paths of abnormal returns (classes) that compose the data set, obtaining for each firm its probability of belonging to each class.

Our research shares some of the assumptions of previous studies. We recognize that abnormal returns vary substantially across firms over time; that abnormal returns at any point in time provide only a snapshot of the type and the sustainability of competitive advantage; and that differences in abnormal returns can be studied in greater detail in longitudinal studies, in which abnormal returns are recorded over an extended period of time. But our research differs from previous work in three aspects. First, our objective is to explain how abnormal returns evolve over time, taking into account unobserved dynamic heterogeneity. Second, we employ a different statistical method, relying on multivariate normal mixture models. The finite mixture approach is adequate when the studied population (Spanish firms) comprises a small number of groups (patterns) with a relatively homogeneous distributions. As we do not assume that the abnormal returns of all the firms follow the same path, nor do we assign firms to classes based on the firms' levels of performance, our approach prevents bias that can arise in the analysis with an a priori classification of firms into groups. Finally, previous research is based mainly on data from the United States. and other large economies (Japan, U.K., Germany, Canada, etc.), so it will be interesting to investigate persistence in another country and compare our results with previous research.

9.2 MODEL

We use a dynamic model for panel data to examine the pattern of evolution of abnormal returns. This is Anderson and Hsiao's state-dependence model (1982), and Kenny and Zautra's trait-state-error model (1985, 2001). We extend the latter to mixture analysis in the next section.

The model decomposes firms' abnormal profits into a static, a dynamic, and an error term component,

$$Y_{it} = \lambda_t P_i + A_{it} + U_{it} \tag{1}$$
$$A_{it+1} = \beta_t A_{it} + D_{it}, \tag{2}$$

where Y_{it} is the mean deviation of profit rate of firm i at time t (Y_{it} is the difference of the firms' profit rates in year t minus the overall mean of the firms' profit rates in that year). P_{it} is the static or *permanent component*, and its variance captures long-run or sustainable differences across firms (i.e., the differences that persist in a period longer than the length of the series). A_{it} is the dynamic or *transient component*. Its variance captures short-run or nonsustainable rents that disappear over time as a result of the competitive process. As in previous studies (Geroski & Jacquemin, 1988; Jacobson, 1988; McGahan & Porter, 1999; Mueller, 1986), A_{it} is assumed to follow a first-order autoregressive process, AR(1). Component U_{it} is an idiosyncratic, unexplained, *firm-by-year component*. It encompasses all the specific and unstable circumstances that affect a firm's profit rate in one specific year, as well as measurement error (Benston, 1985; Demsetz, 1979; Fisher & McGowan, 1983). Finally, D_{it} is the *disturbance component* of the dynamic autoregressive part of the model. Here U_{it} and D_{it} are centered random variables, assumed to be independent across i and t, λ_t denotes the factor loading associated with the permanent component, and β_t is the so-called autoregressive parameter.

To better represent the nature of the model, Figure 9–1 shows a path diagram representation of the model, a representation used often in structural equation modeling (SEM).

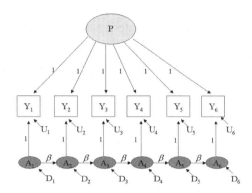

Figure 9–1. Path-diagram representation of the model.

Observable variables are represented in squares, while latent variables are shown in circles. An arrow leading from the predictor to the dependent variable indicates a loading or a regression effect. In the graph, the values of the loadings and regression effects are represented by the 1s and the βs respectively. Disturbance and error terms in the regression equations are represented by D_ts and U_ts respectively, the sub-index indicating the time point. This path diagram shows that the variance of firms' profit rates (Y_{it}) is decomposed into the "permanent" component (P) that exerts a (static) effect on Y_{it}, the "temporary" components (A_{it}) that have an autoregressive structure, and the "unexplained firm-by-year component" (U_{it}). These three components are assumed to be uncorrelated with different structures of correlations over time. The absolute value of the first-order autoregressive parameter β indicates a "memory effect" ($\beta = 0$, zero memory) of the time-dependent component of abnormal returns.

The model also assumes a stationary dynamic component. This implies that the autoregressive parameters (β_t), the variances of the disturbance terms (D_{it}), and the loadings λ_t are equal across t. For the model to be identified, we need to fix one of the loading parameters λ_t; all the loadings are set to 1. [1]

These conditions imply that

$$\mathrm{Var}\,(A_{it}) = \mathrm{Var}\,(A_{it-1}), \tag{3}$$

---

[1]This is a more restricted version of the model than is strictly needed, because identification is attained by just setting one of the λ_t to 1.

and hence

$$\text{Var}\,(A_{it}) = \frac{\text{Var}\,(D_{it})}{1 - \beta^2}. \tag{4}$$

This equality constrains the variance of the transient component on the first year, the variance of A_{i1}. It is easy to derive the identities

$$\text{Var}\,(Y_{it}) = \lambda^2 \text{Var}\,(P_i) + \frac{\text{Var}\,(D_{it})}{1 - \beta^2} + \text{Var}\,(U_{it}) \tag{5}$$

$$\text{Cov}\,(Y_{it}, Y_{is}) = \lambda_t \lambda_s \text{Var}\,(P_i) + \text{Cov}\,(A_{it}, A_{is}), \quad t \neq s, \tag{6}$$

and

$$\text{Cov}\,(A_{it}, A_{is}) = \beta^{|t-s|}\text{Var}\,(A_{it}). \tag{7}$$

Equation 4 is used to assign the value of the parameter variance of A_{it} at the initial condition $t = 1$.

By the stationarity assumption, β is smaller than one in absolute value, hence the correlation among A_{it} and A_{is} decreases to zero when the time distance $\mid t - s \mid$ increases. From Equations 6 and 7, it follows that different parameters of the model produce different variances and covariances of observed variables; hence the model is identified.

9.2.1 A Finite Mixture Model

In this section, we extend the previous model by allowing for several distinct patterns of evolution of abnormal returns. The finite mixture approach is suitable when the studied population is comprised of a small number of groups or classes with relatively homogeneous distributions within the classes and the groups into which a firm belongs is not known (see, e.g., Muthén, 2002). The objective is to carry out inferences accounting for such unobserved heterogeneity and, ultimately, to classify individuals (firms) into groups. To do this, mixture models incorporate a latent categorical variable with K classes, with the unknown marginal (unconditional) probability of membership π_k of a firm to be in latent class k. Conditional on the individuals being in class k ($k = 1, \ldots, K$), the T-dimensional (T is the number of time points) vector z of observed (mean centered) profit rates is assumed to be normally distributed with a mean vector μ_k and a covariance matrix Σ_k. Such a mean vector and covariance matrix are, as in a typical SEM analysis, functions of a vector of parameters ϑ_k, according to the dynamic model specification of the previous section. That is, we have $z \sim \mathcal{N}(\mu_k, \Sigma_k)$, with $\mu_k = \mu_k(\vartheta_k)$ and $\Sigma_k = \Sigma_k(\vartheta_k)$, ϑ_k being a vector of parameters that collects the regression coefficients, loading parameters, and the variances and covariances of stochastic components of the model. Given observed data $(z_1, \ldots, z_n)$, the log-likelihood function to be maximized is

$$\log \ell = \sum_{i=1}^{n} \log \left\{ \sum_{k=1}^{K} \pi_{ik} f_k(z_i \mid \vartheta_k) \right\} \tag{8}$$

where f_k is the density function of $\mathcal{N}(\mu_k, \Sigma_k)$. We define the parameter vector $\psi = (\pi, \vartheta)'$, where $\pi = (\pi_1, \ldots, \pi_K)$ is the vector of mixing proportions (i.e., the probabilities of class membership) and ϑ is a vector that collects all the distinct elements of the class-specific ϑ_k. In this approach, we allow parameters of the model to vary across latent classes. So, we consider a specific structure of the mean and the variance and covariance matrix in each class; each class has a characteristic pattern of evolution of abnormal returns. Estimation of the model is carried out using the approach made explicit in Muthén (2002) and implemented in the software Mplus of Muthén and Muthén (2004); (see also McLachlan & Peel, 2000).

9.3 PATTERNS OF THE DYNAMICS OF ABNORMAL RETURNS

The decomposition of abnormal returns into permanent, temporary, and unexplained components introduces the time dimension into the analysis and allows alternative patterns of evolution to be formulated. Each pattern is a particular case of the model of the previous section where different components are absent. Firms whose abnormal returns follow a similar pattern are assigned to the same class. In this section, we introduce the alternative paths that firms can follow, and discuss the implications of each path for the efficiency of the competitive process and the sustainability of firms' abnormal returns. Next, we propose various models with a different number of classes as alternative hypotheses about the evolution of abnormal returns.

In the simplest pattern of evolution, abnormal returns are completely random, that is, they correlate neither across time nor across firms. This corresponds to no systematic differences between firms for abnormal returns and no time dependence. In this pattern, abnormal returns (and the potential sources that generate them) are eroded instantly or over a period shorter than the time sequence of the observations. Firms' competitive advantages are not sustainable and markets are always in equilibrium. The model that represents this path constrains the variance of the permanent and temporary components to be zero, as the firm-by-year component is the only one in the model ($Y_{it} = U_{it}$). The evolution of abnormal returns has the properties of a random shock model, where abnormal returns fluctuate around zero, and the variance of U_{it} determines the size of the heterogeneity in profit rates.

Abnormal returns evolve in a different way if we assume that firms' profit differences vanish completely, but only after some time. This occurs, for example, when abnormal returns are the result of long-lived assets with appropriable values (Barney, 1991; Williams, 1992), when there are impediments to imitation as *isolation mechanism* (Rumelt, 1984), or when the structure of the industry may promote persistence (Bain, 1956). Such a pattern of evolution, consistent with the empirical research in *persistence of profit research line*, is also a particular case of the model of the previous section. As profit differences are only transitory, the permanent component is absent, var $(P) = 0$. In this case, the time dependence of the abnormal returns can be modeled as a first-order autoregressive process, AR(1). The speed of convergence (i.e., the sustainability of abnormal returns) is governed by the value of the autoregressive parameter (β). The higher the β, the more persistent the abnormal returns will be, and consequently, the lower the efficiency of the competitive process.[2]

An entirely different pattern of evolution of abnormal returns arises when the differences in profit rates are completely static, and do not vanish. In this case, abnormal returns persist, and firms that are more (less) profitable at the beginning of the period remains more (less) profitable at the end (i.e., abnormal returns are stable). This pattern of evolution is possible, for example, when the sources that sustain profit differences are not eroded by competitive forces, or the processes of imitation are not effective against them, at least, in the period of study. Winter (1987) focused on this type of rents and exemplifies this situation when there are Ricardian rents generated by an asset with fixed supply because replication and imitation processes are not effective.

In terms of the model in the previous section, this pattern of evolution implies that the autoregressive coefficient (β) and the variance of the disturbance term (D_{it}) of the dynamic part of the model are zero. Thus the evolution of abnormal returns has the properties of a static process $(Y_{it} = P_i + U_{it})$.

Finally, firms' abnormal returns can follow a combination of the previous patterns of evolution if we assume that they are partly permanent and partly transient. In this pattern, all the components of the model in the previous section are different from zero, and the same conclusions made earlier can be applied in the portion of abnormal returns that follow each path.

Having introduced the alternative patterns of evolution, various models with different number of classes are proposed. Table 9–1 shows the alternative hypotheses of the number of latent classes that we have considered, and the dynamics of abnormal returns in each class. Model 0 is the base model and assumes the same pattern of evolution of abnormal returns for all firms (i.e., there is no latent dynamic heterogeneity). It corresponds to a single-class model with abnormal returns formed by the three components of the model $(P, A, \text{ and } U)$. Both models 1 and 2 assume the existence of two classes,

---

[2]Abnormal returns converge toward the mean when $0 < \beta < 1$. We do not consider values of β out of this range because it is not in accordance with economic theory, and because of previous evidence of convergence of abnormal profits.

but in class 1 of Model 1 abnormal returns are static, whereas in class 1 of Model 2 they are partly permanent and partly transient. In Model 3, there are three classes; partly permanent and partly transient, permanent, and transient. Finally, Model 4 introduces a fourth class of firms with completely random abnormal returns.

TABLE 9–1

Description of Alternative Models with Their Associated Number of Free Parameters and Values of the Goodness of Fit Index BIC

	Class				No.	
Model	*1*	*2*	*3*	*4*	*param.*	*BIC**
	Components of variance			**		
0	P A U				9	207.26
1	P U	A U			29	188.83
2	P A U	A U			32	188.36
3	P A U	P U	A U		46	184.71
4	P A U	P U	A U	U	59	184.42

* $\times 10^3$

** P = Permanent, A = Autoregressive, U = Unexplained

Our objective is to find subgroups of firms whose abnormal returns follow a similar path. Because we do not know a priori how many different groups of firms there are, and which path best describes each group, we first choose the number of different paths (classes) by assessing the goodness of fit of various different models; see the goodness of fit value BIC (to be described below) shown in the last column of Table 9–1. Once we have chosen the number of latent classes, we fit the corresponding finite mixture model by maximum likelihood. At the end, we assign firms to classes based on the probability of class membership arising from the mixture analysis.

9.4 DATA AND ESTIMATION

The database is composed of 5,000 large Spanish firms, belonging to all sectors of the economy excluding financial and public companies. For each firm, financial data was collected for the 1995–2000 period. The dataset contained information about return on assets (ROA), sales, assets, and a four-digit standard industrial classification (SIC) code that characterizes industry membership. Our initial database contains 30,000 records, six annual records for each of the 5000 firms.

Like other databases usually used in previous studies in persistence (e.g., Compustat, FCT, *Fortune 500*, etc.), our database presents several advantages.

First, it captures a large portion of Spanish economy, including all sectors (agriculture and mining, manufacturing, wholesale and retail trade, transportation, lodging, entertainment, and other services) except for financial and government sectors. Second, our sample contains time series over the 6 years allowing for studying the dynamic behavior of profit rates over time, and separating the static, transient, and year-specific effects. Finally, it covers only large Spanish firms, although, compared with other databases, such as Compustat, or *Fortune 500*, the average size of the Spanish firm is smaller than for the American firms. The average firm in our database has assets of 62.9 million euros, with annual sales of 64.8 million euros.

A plot of the profiles of ROA for a sample of 15 firms is shown in Figure 9–2. In this plot we see a wide fluctuation of the profits across the years within each firm. This variation is what we want to model using a finite mixture model approach.

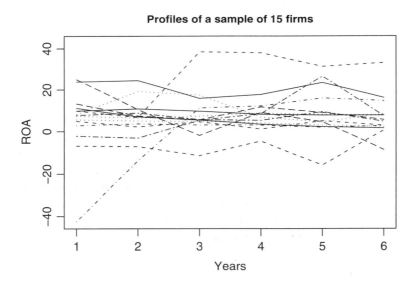

Figure 9–2. Profiles of ROA for a random sample of 15 firms.

9.4.1 Variables

Accounting return data was used in the analysis. As in previous studies (McGahan & Porter, 1999, 2003; Wiggings & Ruefli, 2002), we used ROA as the measure of business performance. This variable was constructed by dividing the annual income (before extraordinary items) by the total assets. ROA was recorded annually from 1995 to 2000. By subtracting ROA from its annual mean we constructed the observed variable Y_{it}, where the indices i and t denote firm and time, respectively. Annual sales, firm size (measured as firms' total assets), and industry membership was used to describe the classes emerging from the analysis.

9.4.2 Estimation

Estimation was conducted using structural equation model methodology. SEM permits a suitable approximation for most research designs for longitudinal data, as we can easily formulate relationships between latent variables, rather than directly between their fallible measures. In fact, within SEM, permanent and temporary components are modeled as latent factors, and the portion of the total variance accounted for by the different latent variables. Standard software can be used for fitting models within the SEM approach. However, when we turn to the mixture analysis, we found Mplus (Muthén & Muthén, 2004) to be the most suitable software. Mplus uses maximum likelihood (ML) estimation employing the EM algorithm (Muthén & Muthén, 2004).

9.5 RESULTS

9.5.1 Heterogeneity in the Evolution of Abnormal Returns

We fit first the conventional model in which all firms have the same pattern of evolution of abnormal returns (Model 0 in Table 9–1). We found a significant chi-square goodness-of-fit value of $\chi_{12}^2 = 62.878$, $p \leq 0.05$, indicating a poor fit. It may be interpreted as evidence of heterogeneity in the evolution of abnormal returns that the single-class model does not capture. To improve the fit, we fit the models 1 to 4 of Table 9–1, that assume several groups of firms with distinct patterns of persistence.

9.5.2 Number of Classes

In finite mixture analysis, the number of classes is typically assessed by goodness-of-fit indices such as the Bayesian information criterion (BIC; Schwartz, 1978) or the Akaike information criterion (AIC; Akaike, 1974). The recommendation is to choose a model with the smallest AIC or BIC. Here we use BIC. In our context, we have that $\text{BIC} = 2\log L - q\log n$, where L is the likelihood, q is the number of parameters in the model, and n is the number of firms.

In the last column of Table 9–1 we see the BIC values for models with different number of latent classes. The model with four classes yield the smallest BIC value; therefore, we choose the four-class model (Model 4 in Table 9–1) as our final model.

9.5.3 Description of Classes

Having assessed the number of classes, a description of the dynamics of the abnormal returns in each class is in order. This involves examination of the size of the components of the variances of abnormal returns as well as the ROA average within each latent class. Estimated parameters with standard errors for the four classes are shown in Table 9–2. Note that the covariance structure and the size of the components of variance vary among latent classes.

TABLE 9–2

Parameter Estimates of the Four-Class Mixture Model (standard errors in brackets)

	Class			
Parameter	*1*	*2*	*3*	*4*
Var(P)	5.45	550.477		
	(0.78)	(108.52)		
β	.67		.83	
	(0.04)		(0.01)	
Var(D)	3.48		23.28	
	(0.37)		(1.83)	
Var(A)	6.26		74.05	
Var(U)	0.60	642.66	5.23	142.56

Both classes 1 and 3 have a significant autoregressive component β (0.67 and 0.83, respectively), and their variances of the temporary components are also significant. Moreover, in class 1 the variance of the permanent component, Var(P), is also significant. It accounts for a higher proportion of variance than the transient component. These results indicate that, although abnormal returns persist in both classes, they evolve differently in them. In class 3, abnormal returns disappear completely over the 6 years, whereas in class 1, a significant proportion is permanent, and does not vanish completely over the observation time. The differences between classes 1 and 3 are analyzed in greater detail in the discussion section.

In class 2, abnormal returns are static (i.e., complete persistence), because no transient components are allowed. Table 9–2 shows that the permanent component has an extremely high variance (Var (P) = 550.48) indicating that firms in this class present stable high or low profitability. In class 2, we also see a very large variance for the atemporal component U (Var (U) = 142.56), indicating that in this class, profit rates fluctuate around zero with a high variability. The high variability across firms in classes 2 and 4 indicates that those firms are highly unstable in profitability, so they are firms of high risk. Finally, class 4 comprises firms whose abnormal returns are random. The only restriction that we have introduced in this class is that the variance of the firm-by-year specific component is constant across years to ensure that the process is stationary. We comment more about this in the discussion section.

9.5.4 Proportion of Firms in each Class

Table 9–3 shows the estimated number and proportions of firms in each of the four classes of Model 4. Classes 1 and 3 account for 90% of firms (39% and 51% respectively), representing the most common patterns of evolution. Classes 2 and 4 represent only 4% and 6% of the firms respectively, and they represent atypical patterns of the evolution of abnormal returns. In fact, these are patterns that depart markedly from the assumptions of the economic theory and from the previous empirical studies. We see that the firms in these minority classes have unusual extreme variances on the components of P and U. Later on we discuss the parameter estimates of the model of each of the four classes.

TABLE 9–3

Estimated Proportion and Number of Firms in Each Class (fitted model)

Class	Count	%
1	1969	39
2	174	4
3	2541	51
4	316	6
Total	5000	100

TABLE 9–4

The Average Probability of Belonging to the Classes for the Firms Classified in Each of the Four Classes (rows)

Class	1	2	3	4
1	0.903	0.000	0.096	0.000
2	0.000	0.912	0.029	0.060
3	0.057	0.003	0.909	0.031
4	0.000	0.074	0.104	0.822

Using the firms' posterior probabilities to belong to the different classes, we assign firms to the class with highest posterior probability. Table 9–4 shows the average probability to belong to each of the classes 1 to 4 (columns) for the firms that were classified in class 1 to 4 (the rows). Note that these average probabilities are relatively high, ranging from 0.822 to 0.912, indicating the suitability of the four-class solution.

9.5.5 Variance Decomposition

The decomposition of variance of abnormal returns by year for the four classes is given in Table 9–5. In class 1, temporary and permanent components represent 39% and 56% of the variance of abnormal returns, respectively. This means that more than half of the abnormal returns in firms in class 1 remains stable. In class 3, the autoregressive component of abnormal returns represents more than 86% of the variance of abnormal returns. Finally, 50% of the abnormal returns in class 2 are permanent, whereas in class 4 all abnormal returns are obviously random.

Table 9–5 also shows the means of the abnormal returns for each class, as estimated by the model. A comparison of the average of ROA shows differences in their evolution by classes. Class 1 shows low ROA averages ranging from 6.2 to 5.2%, with a trend of slowing decrease. Firms in class 3 achieve higher average profitability than class 1 and an upward trend. In this class, ROA ranges around 9.5%.

9.5.6 Characteristics of the Firms by Classes

To further characterize the four derived classes, Table 9–6 presents additional information about annual sales and assets by class and by year. As shown in Table 9–6, firms in four groups differ in their size. Classes 1 and 3 are formed by larger firms, with sales and assets significantly higher (almost twice), than the other two groups. Classes 1 and 3 also have differences between them. Firms in class 1 have average assets higher than class 3 (70.1 and 61.9 respectively), where as the average in sales in class 3 is 4.2 million euros higher that in class 1 (69.2 and 64.9 respectively). There are also differences in the evolution of sales and assets between groups. In all classes, sales and assets increase, but their rates of growth differ. Class 4 has the higher growth rate in assets, followed by classes 3, 2, and 1 in that order; and class 2 has the higher growth rate in sales, followed by class 4, 3, and 1. So, among the two most common patterns of abnormal returns, firms in class 3 not only are more profitable, but also have a higher growth rate in sales and in assets.

Finally, Table 9–7 shows the percent of firms in each class, grouped by one-digit SIC code. Class 1 contains relatively more transportation and communications firms (SIC = 4), and wholesale and retail trade firms (SIC = 5), whereas class 3 has comparatively more manufacturing firms (SIC = 2 and 3). Classes 2 and 4 cover a low percentage of firms in all industries, except for service firms (SIC = 7 and 8) that with both classes 16.5% are assigned to them. In general, there is no clear correspondence between the industry classification

TABLE 9–5

Estimated Mean and Variance Decomposition (in %) for Each of the Four Latent Classes

Variable	Mean (s.e.)	Components		
		Temporary	*Permanent*	*Unexplained*
		Class 1		
ROA 95	6.216 *(0.15)*	45.50	39.89	14.62
ROA 96	5.699 *(0.14)*	35.81	56.52	7.66
ROA 97	5.375 *(0.14)*	37.64	59.41	2.96
ROA 98	5.382 *(0.16)*	38.41	60.63	0.96
ROA 99	5.381 *(0.17)*	38.32	60.48	1.20
ROA 00	5.234 *(0.16)*	37.52	59.21	3.27
Average %		38.87	56.02	5.11
		Class 2		
ROA 95	3.950 *(2.53)*	0.00	53.44	46.56
ROA 96	4.865 *(2.65)*	0.00	67.62	32.38
ROA 97	5.807 *(2.87)*	0.00	61.53	38.47
ROA 98	6.835 *(3.73)*	0.00	36.64	63.36
ROA 99	7.136 *(2.92)*	0.00	45.29	54.71
ROA 00	8.915 *(3.09)*	0.00	32.34	67.66
Average %		0.00	49.48	50.52
		Class 3		
ROA 95	9.074 *(0.21)*	84.65	0.00	15.35
ROA 96	8.970 *(0.22)*	79.95	0.00	20.05
ROA 97	9.356 *(0.24)*	89.33	0.00	10.67
ROA 98	10.073 *(0.25)*	89.31	0.00	10.69
ROA 99	10.124 *(0.25)*	89.35	0.00	10.65
ROA 00	9.570 *(0.24)*	86.07	0.00	13.93
Average %		86.44	0.00	13.56
		Class 4		
ROA 95	7.025 *(1.19)*	0.00	0.00	100.00
ROA 96	7.673 *(1.11)*	0.00	0.00	100.00
ROA 97	8.926 *(1.21)*	0.00	0.00	100.00
ROA 98	6.837 *(1.39)*	0.00	0.00	100.00
ROA 99	7.176 *(1.23)*	0.00	0.00	100.00
ROA 00	9.947 *(1.12)*	0.00	0.00	100.00
Average %		0.00	0.00	100.00

TABLE 9–6

Estimated Means of Annual Sales and Total Assets for the Firms Classified in Each of the Four Classes (all annual figures are in 10^6 euros)

Year	Class 1	Class 2	Class 3	Class 4	Overall
		Total Assets			
1995	54.613	30.298	44.712	19.425	46.853
1996	59.795	34.110	50.138	22.918	52.022
1997	64.109	37.671	54.939	28.059	56.606
1998	71.003	48.276	61.689	29.213	63.228
1999	79.923	55.270	72.614	34.897	72.928
2000	90.923	58.366	87.525	42.506	85.479
Average*	70.061	43.998	61.936	29.503	62.853
Growth**	66.48	92.64	95.75	118.81	82.44
		Annual Sales			
1995	50.836	28.594	52.258	29.705	49.720
1996	54.898	30.559	57.929	30.541	54.320
1997	60.812	31.978	65.624	35.797	60.961
1998	67.268	37.011	71.478	36.625	66.761
1999	72.897	46.782	78.225	40.342	72.976
2000	82.973	54.594	89.455	51.672	83.636
Average	64.947	38.253	69.161	37.447	64.729
Growth	63.22	90.92	71.18	73.95	68.21

* Average across the six years
** Growth over six years (in %)

by first digit of SIC, [3] and the derived four-class typology based on the pattern of evolution of abnormal returns.

9.6 DISCUSSION AND CONCLUSIONS

This paper explores the patterns of evolution of abnormal returns allowing for the presence of several groups of firms that present specific dynamical behavior of ROA. Each group (or class) represents a particular case of the more general model for the persistence of abnormal returns (Bou & Satorra, in press) that decomposes the variance of abnormal returns into three components with different correlation structures over time; static, dynamic or changing, and an

---

[3] The same results are obtained when a more detailed industry classification is used (e.g., four-digit SIC code).

TABLE 9–7

For Each of the First Digit SIC Code This Table Shows the % of Firms Classified to Each of the Four Latent Classes (with last column being the number of firms)

		Class				
Digit	Sector	1	2	3	4	# firms
0,1	Agriculture Mining Construction	48.15	2.82	39.69	9.33	461
2,3	Manufacturing	34.08	2.45	59.22	4.25	2,327
4	Transportation Communication	44.62	5.38	45.38	4.62	260
5	Wholesale Retail Trade	49.11	2.56	42.68	5.65	1523
7,8	Services	31.73	8.53	51.73	8.00	375

Note. SIC code was not available for 54 firms.

unexplained firm-by-year specific component. The evolution of ROA in each group is characterized by the size of these three components.

In the most common pattern of evolution, class 3 (51% of firms), abnormal returns are modeled as an AR(1) process. In this class, abnormal returns persist some time, but disappear *progressively*. This pattern of evolution is consistent with many of the previous empirical work in the "persistence of profit" literature, such as Mueller (1986, 1990), Jacobson (1988), McGahan and Porter (1997) and Jacobson and Hansen (2001) among others. Using time-series methodology, these authors have modeled persistence of profits as an AR(1) process, and have demonstrated that profits do not vanish quickly, but persist over time. The estimated autoregressive coefficient ($\beta = 0.83$) indicates high persistence, because only 20% of abnormal returns dissipate per year. This autoregressive coefficient is in line with those obtained in previous work in other countries (see Jacobson, 1988, for the U.S.A. and Odagiri & Yamawaki, 1990, for an international comparison).

A related pattern of evolution is suggested by class 1 that comprises transient, but also permanent differences in abnormal returns. Results for Spanish firms show that in this class, roughly 40% of abnormal returns converge to the mean following an AR(1) process with $\beta = 0.67$. In comparison with class 3, the process of convergence is quicker (less persistence), as indicated by the lower level of the autoregressive coefficient. In turn, the variance of the temporary differences is almost 10 times lower than in class 3 (3.9% and 31.75%, respectively) indicating that this class is formed by very homogeneous firms. As the variance of the transient component captures the size of the nonsustainable differences, the previous results indicate that firms in class 3 have a greater ability to generate short-run or nonsustainable rents that take longer to vanish than in class 1.

Class 1 also takes account of permanent differences among firms; 56% of the total variance of abnormal returns remain constant in the 6-year period of study. The stability of abnormal returns reveals that competitive forces cannot erode the potential sources of competitive advantages, whichever they are, that generate these abnormal returns, at least during the period of study. Consequently, firms in this class exhibit different levels of profitability measured by the individual score obtained in the permanent component, and maintain the profit differential over time. Firms that are more (less) profitable at the beginning of the period remain more (less) profitable at the end, at least in the portion of variance of abnormal returns that is static.

Classes 1 and 3 also differ in their profit rates, as well as in their growth rates. Firms in class 3 have a high average of ROA (9.5%) and an upward trend, whereas class 1 is formed by less profitable firms (ROA average = 5.5%), with a slight downward trend. In turn, although assets and sales average growth in both classes, firms in class 3 have a comparatively faster growth in two magnitudes, especially in assets with a difference of almost 30 points over the 6-year period of study. Firms in class 3 are thus not only more profitable, but also have a faster growth than firms in class 1. As a consequence, the gap in sales between the two groups increases to 6.5 million euros in 2000, whereas difference in total assets decreases to 3.4 million euros.

These differences suggest that in the more profitable group of firms and with a faster growth, differences across firms in abnormal returns are transitory and based on the successive introduction of short-run rents. Although the objective of this chapter is not to directly contrast the alternative theoretical predictions about differences in abnormal returns, some preliminary insights can be advanced. Our results suggest that firm profit rates are more related to the generation of short-run rents (as in class 3), than to the sustainability of the present rents, and are more consistent with the Schumpeterian and efficiency point of view that supports that persistence is related to the ability of firms to introduce innovations continually (Roberts, 1999; 2001) in a process of creative destruction (Schumpeter, 1934).

As a whole, 90% of Spanish firms in our sample can be classified into classes 1 and 3. Both classes denote persistence in abnormal returns, but they differ in the path that their abnormal returns follow and in their level of profitability and growth. Firms in class 1 have a stable firm-specific component, whereas in class 3, all abnormal returns vanish. As different classes are formed based on their path of abnormal returns, differences in profit rates and growth across classes show that profitability depends, at least partially, on the dynamic behavior of abnormal returns.

Mixture analysis allows identifying two additional paths in abnormal returns, as classes 2 and 4 show. They are the extreme cases in the continuum of no persistence and complete persistence, and are paths that are followed by only a few firms. Class 2 is characterized by the stability of abnormal returns and by the high within-class variability, that is, large differences in profit rates across firms that do not vanish over time. Consequently, firms that persistently achieve very high or low profit rates have high probabilities to follow the path described by class 2. In our sample, only 174 firms (4%) follow this path, indicating that this is a path that departs from the classical assumptions of the economic theory and from the previous empirical studies in profit persistence.

On the other hand, class 4 (316 firms, 6% of the sample) highlights completely different dynamics of abnormal returns. This class contains firms that have highly unstable ROA across the years, thus highly unpredictable profits. Besides, the high variance means that profit rates fluctuate around zero with a high variability. In this class, firms that obtain returns above the norm are not capable to sustain it, and abnormal returns are eroded instantaneously (or over a shorter term than the time sequence of the observations). This dynamic behavior is in accordance with predictions arising from neoclassical economics and the work of Austrian School of Economics that predict that factors such as imitation, entry, or substitution prevent abnormal returns from persisting (Wiggings & Ruefli, 2002).

From a methodological point of view, it is interesting to note the importance of classes 2 and 4 in our analysis. Although these classes are not common paths (10% of firms), they group firms whose dynamics of the abnormal returns departs markedly from the regular paths of the majority of firms. Traditionally these firms are considered "outliers" that have to be excluded to avoid their influence on the results, or because they cause problems of nonnormality that impede the application of statistical analysis based on normality. Nevertheless, there are no clear criteria to determine outliers, which introduce some degree of arbitrariness in the research. In the sustainability of abnormal returns analysis, the problem of outliers has compelled some researchers to avoid the use of autoregressive models because this technique is based on measures of central tendency (Wiggings & Ruefli, 2002, p. 89) that do not allow disentangling outliers from regular firms.

Instead of excluding outliers from the analysis, or to avoid the use of autoregressive models, our mixture analysis approach encompasses the presence of "outlier" firms. We treat outliers as groups of firms with a singular pattern of behavior of abnormal returns. We thus adopt a different perspective than do Wiggings and Ruefli (2002), considering the existence of outliers and in turn using autoregressive models to model persistence as the previous literature does. That is, in our sample of Spanish firms, classes 2 and 4 are outliers, with a pattern of evolution of abnormal returns that differ from the regular paths represented by classes 1 and 3.

Mixture models are a suitable approach to longitudinal studies in which heterogeneity is present and it is assumed that a finite number of subpopulations have different associations among the time points, with the dynamic of the abnormal returns being different in each subpopulation or (latent) classes. Figure 9–3 shows the profiles of ROA for 20 firms simulated from the different classes estimated by the fitted model. In this figure, we can see how classes 1 and 3 have stable patterns of evolution, whereas classes 2 and 4—the outlier groups—have highly unstable ROA across years.

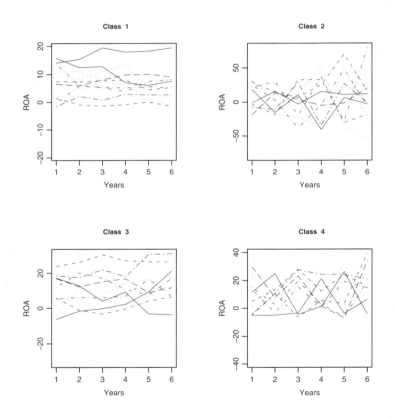

Figure 9–3. For each of the classes 1 to 4, we plot the profiles of 20 firms simulated from the fitted model.

Our approach of finite mixture models also represents an alternative to standard cluster analysis, because the posterior probability of membership of a firm in a class can be used to assign latent class membership. In addition, mixture analysis offers a clear advantage over the traditional K-MEANS cluster analysis, because we have better inference tools for assessing the appropriate number of classes. Further, our approach permits the formation of groups based on a priori defined structure of variance and covariance that, as in this case, reflect a specific pattern of evolution of abnormal returns. Our approach is more in line with recent empirical work, such as that of McGahan and Porter (2003). In our study of the emergence and sustainability of the abnormal returns, groups of firms are formed based on their dynamic behavior, instead of the more traditional group formation based on cluster analysis using data only at the beginning of the period studied (see among others, for example, Mueller, 1986; Odagiri & Yamawaki, 1986; Schohl, 1990), or the industry classification (Wiggings & Ruefli, 2002). In the case of Spanish firms, there is a lack of correspondence between the four derived classes and the first-digit SIC code. These results suggest that the identification of patterns of persistence of abnormal returns is best captured by decomposing abnormal returns into the static and dynamic components, and that the industry classification cannot capture the *unobserved dynamic heterogeneity* in the sample, because the firms in each industry follow different patterns of evolution.

This chapter can be extended in a number of ways. Explanatory variables can provide additional insights into the patterns of evolution of abnormal returns. Further research could be done on assessing the role of independent variables such as resources, capabilities, and other variables usually used in this literature, in explaining the pattern of variation of abnormal returns.The present modeling approach could also be applied to sample data from other countries, where a different mix of firms in each class can be found. Differences across countries should offer additional insights about the persistence of abnormal returns and the "efficiency" of the competitive markets.

ACKNOWLEDGMENTS

The comments by Nick T. Longford on an earlier draft of this chapter are very much appreciated. This work has been partially supported by the Spanish MCYT grant SEC2003-04476 and by the grant GV05/125 of Generalitat Valenciana (Spain).

REFERENCES

Akaike, H. (1974). A new look at statistical model identification. *IEEE Transactions on Automatic Control, 19,* 719–722.

Anderson, T., & Hsiao, C. (1982). Estimation of dynamic models using panel data. *Journal of Econometrics, 18,* 47–82.

Arrow, K., & Hahn, F. (1971). *General competitive analysis.* San Francisco, CA: Holden Day.

Bain, J. (1956). *Barriers to new competition.* Cambridge, MA: Harvard University Press.

Barney, J. B. (1991). Firm resources and sustained competitive advantage. *Journal of Management, 17,* 99–120.

Benston, G. (1985). The validity of profits-structure studies with particular reference to the FTC's line of business data. *American Economic Review, 75,* 37–67.

Bou, J. C., & Satorra, A. (in press). Persistence of abnormal returns at industry and firm levels: Evidence from Spain. *Strategic Management Journal.*

Caves, R, & Porter, M. E. (1977). From entry barriers to mobility barriers. *Quarterly Journal of Economics, 91,* 421–441.

Connolly, R. A., & Schwartz, S. (1985). The intertemporal behavior of economic profit. *International Journal of Industrial Organization 3,* 379–400.

Demsetz, H. (1979). Accounting for advertising as a barrier to entry. *Journal of Business, 59,* 345–360.

Fisher, F. M., & McGowan, J. J. (1983). On the misuse of accounting rates of return to infer monopoly profits. *American Economic Review, 73,* 82–97.

Geroski, P. A., & Jacquemin, A. (1988). The persistence of profits: A European comparison. *The Economic Journal, 98,* 375–389.

Hunt, M. (1972). *Competition in the major home appliance industry.* Unpublished doctoral dissertation, Harvard University.

Jacobson, R. (1988). The persistence of abnormal returns. *Strategic Management Journal, 9,* 415–430.

Jacobson, R. (1992). The "Austrian" school of strategy. *Academy of Management Review, 17,* 782–807.

Jacobson, R., & Hansen, G. (2001). Modeling the competitive process. *Managerial and Decision Economics, 22,* 251–263.

Kenny, D., & Zautra, A. (1985). The trait-state-error model for multiwave data. *Journal of Consulting and Clinical Psychology, 63,* 52–59.

Kenny, D., & Zautra, A. (2001). Trait-state models for longitudinal data. In L. M. Collins & A. G. Sayer (Eds.), *New methods for the analysis of change* (pp. 243–263). Washington, DC: American Psychological Association.

McGahan, A. M., & Porter, M. E. (1997). How much does industry matter, really? *Strategic Management Journal, 18,* 15–30.

McGahan, A. M., & Porter, M. E. (1999). The persistence of shocks to profitability. *Review of Economics and Statistics, 81,* 143–153.

McGahan, A. M., & Porter, M. E. (2003). The emergence and sustainability of abnormal profits. *Strategic Organization, 1,* 79–108.

McLachlan, G., & Peel, D. (2000). *Finite mixture models.* New York: Wiley.

Mueller, D. C. (1986). *Profits in the long run.* Cambridge, UK: Cambridge University Press.

Mueller, D. C. (1990). Profits and the process of competition. In D. Mueller (Ed.), *The dynamics of company profits: An international comparison* (pp. 1–14). Cambridge, UK: Cambridge University Press.

Muthén, B. O. (2002). Beyond SEM: General latent variable modeling. *Behaviormetrika, 29,* 81–117.

Muthén, B. O., & Muthén, L. K. (2004). *Mplus User's Guide.* Los Angeles, CA: Authors.

Odagiri, H., & Yamawaki, H. (1986). A study of company profit-rate time series, Japan and the United States. *International Journal of Industrial Organization, 4,* 1–23.

Odagiri, H., & Yamawaki, H. (1990). The persistence of profits: International comparison. In D. Mueller (Ed.), *The dynamics of company profits: An international comparison* (pp. 169–185). Cambridge, UK: Cambridge University Press.

Porter, M. E. (1979). The structure within industries and companies' performance. *Review of Economics and Statistics, 61,* 214–227.

Roberts, P. W. (1999). Product innovation, product-market competition and persistent profitability in the U.S. pharmaceutical industry. *Strategic Management Journal, 20,* 655–670.

Roberts, P. W. (2001). Innovation and firm-level persistent profitability: A Schumpeterian framework. *Managerial and Decision Economics, 22,* 239–250.

Rumelt, R. P. (1984). Toward a strategic theory of the firm. In M. Lamb (Ed.), *Competitive strategic management* (pp. 556–570). Englewood Cliffs, NJ: Prentice-Hall.

Schohl, F. (1990). Persistence of profits in the long run a critical extension of some recent findings. *International Journal of Industrial Organization, 8,* 385–404.

Schumpeter, J. A. (1934). *The theory of economic development.* Cambridge, MA: Harvard University Press.

Schwartz, G. (1978). Estimating the dimension of a model. *The Annals of Statistics, 6,* 461–464.

Waring, G. (1996). Industry differences in the persistence of firm-specific returns. *American Economic Review, 86,* 1253–1265.

Wernerfelt, B. (1984). A resource-based view of the firm. *Strategic Management Journal, 5,* 171–180.

Wiggings, R., & Ruefli, T. (2002). Sustained competitive advantage: temporal dynamics and the incidence and persistence of superior economic performance. *Organization Science, 13,* 82–105.

Williams, J. (1992). How sustainable is your competitive advantage? *California Management Review, 34,* 29–51.

Winter, S. (1987). Knowledge and competence as strategic assets. In D. J. Teece (Ed.), *The competitive challenge: Strategies for industrial innovation and renewal* (pp. 159–183). Cambridge, MA: Ballinger.

Chapter 10

The Development of Deviant and Delinquent Behavior of Adolescents: Applications of Latent Class Growth Curves and Growth Mixture Models

Jost Reinecke

University of Bielefeld, Germany

10.1 INTRODUCTION

Longitudinal research studies with repeated measurements are quite often used to examine processes of stability and change in individuals or groups. With panel data it is possible to investigate intraindividual development of substantive variables across time as well as interindividual differences and similarities in change patterns. Whereas the traditional analysis of variance (ANOVA) and the analysis of covariance (ANCOVA) assume homogeneity of the underlying covariance matrix across the levels of the between-subjects factors and the same covariance patterns for the repeated measurements, the structural equation methodology offers an alternative strategy, the *latent growth curve models*. These models describe not only a single individual's developmental trajectory, but also capture individual differences in the intercept and slopes of those trajectories. Based on the formative work of Rao and Tucker's basic model of growth curves (Rao, 1958; Tucker, 1958), Meredith and Tisak (1990) discussed and formalized the model within the structural equation framework. Further developments of the growth curve model were proposed by McArdle and Epstein (1987), McArdle (1988), Muthén (1991, 1997), and Muthén and Curran (1997).

The formal representation of a growth curve model can be seen either as a multilevel, random-effects model (Liang & Zeger, 1986) or as a latent variable model, where the random effects are latent variables (cf. for example Curran & Hussong, 2002, p. 69). In the latent variable model the repeated measurements are the manifest variables while the intercept and the slope are the latent variables (cf. the discussion in Hox, 2002, chap. 14). Extensive applications of different growth curve models with structural equations using the programs LISREL (Jöreskog & Sörbom, 2004) and EQS (Bentler, 2001) are discussed by Duncan, Duncan, Strycker, Li, and Alpert (1999).

Observed heterogeneity in growth curve models can be captured by covariates (e.g., gender) explaining part of the variances of the intercept and slope. But the assumption of a single population underlying the growth curves has to be relaxed in the case of unobserved heterogeneity. Instead of considering individual variation around a single growth curve, in unobserved heterogeneity, different classes of individuals vary around different mean growth curves. A very suitable framework to handle the issue of unobserved heterogeneity is *growth mixture modeling* introduced by Muthén and Shedden (1999). These mixture models differ between continuous and categorical latent variables. The categorical latent variables represent mixtures of subpopulations where the membership to those subpopulations is inferred from the data. Like the conventional growth curve models, intercept and slope variables capture the continuous part of the model. The framework of growth mixture models can also be seen as an extension of the structural modeling approach with techniques of latent class analysis. The inferred membership of each individual to a certain class is produced with the information of the estimated latent class probabilities. The growth mixture model can be applied with the program M*plus* (Muthén & Muthén, 2004). Extension and further developments of growth mixture models are discussed in several papers by Muthén (2001a, 2001b, 2003, 2004).

The simplest specification of a growth mixture model is the so-called *latent class growth analysis* where no variation across individuals is allowed within classes. This model was also discussed by Nagin and Land (1993), Nagin (1999) and Roeder, Lynch, and Nagin (1999) with normal and nonnormal outcomes especially focused on deviant and delinquent behavior. Due to the substantive similarity of the data used in our study, special attention is given to the underlying distributions of the longitudinal measurements. Our measurements represent numbers of different deviant and delinquent behaviors and can be treated as count variables. The underlying statistical model of a count variable is the Poisson distribution (see, e.g., Ross, 1993). If the count variables are biased to zero, that is, the particular behaviors seldom occur, the zero-inflated Poisson model (Lambert, 1992) should be the best statistical representation. A brief introduction of the growth mixture model including its special cases will be given in Section 10.2.

Major methodological developments in criminological longitudinal research are influenced by the debate whether distinctive groups about criminal behavior can be explored and in which way the development of a "criminal career" can be incorporated in a statistical model. The major controversy stems from fundamental disagreements about whether people with criminal activities form a distinctive group and in which way those "careers" can be explored (Nagin & Land, 1993). Several long-term studies, like the "Cambridge Study" (Farrington & West, 1990), the "Philadelphia Study" (Tracy, Wolfgang & Figlio, 1990) or the "Montreal Study" (Tremblay, Desmarais-Gervais, Gagnon, & Charlebois, 1987) were analyzed by Nagin and collaborates to find population heterogeneity in behavioral trajectories. Depending on the type of dependent variable, the nature of the sample, and the characteristics of the community, three to five trajectories reflecting different intensity and growth of delinquency were detected. These analyses can differ between nonoffenders, a time-limited delinquent behavior through adolescence, and a more or less chronic group of offenders (D'Unger, Land, McCall, & Nagin, 1998; Nagin 1999). Furthermore, background variables like household income or educational level of the parents are included via a multinomial logit model to explain differences in growth of criminal offending (Land, McCall, & Nagin, 1996; Nagin, 1999). The major statistical limitation of those analyses is the assumption that within each group, the individual developments are the same meaning that the growth parameters have no variance. This restriction can be relaxed within the growth mixture model of Muthén and collaborates.

The major aspect of this chapter is the systematic comparison of the latent class growth model and the more general growth mixture model within the framework of M*plus*. A representative panel study of adolescents' deviant and delinquent behavior served as database for the systematic study of growth mixtures. Design of the study, variables, and descriptive statistics are introduced in Section 10.3. Section 10.4 addresses the question of how many distinctive groups exists in the data under the assumption of the latent class growth model. Based on the results, Section 10.5 studies various growth mixture models allowing random intercepts and slopes. Differences from the previous results of the latent class growth analyses are emphasized. In both sections, models are extended by time-independent exogenous variables to control for observed heterogeneity. Section 10.6 summarizes the results and discusses suggestions for further research with growth mixture models.

10.2 METHOD AND MODELS

10.2.1 Growth Mixture Models

The possibility that the individual trajectories of a dependent variable can vary is one of the main advantages of the growth curve model. This variation is captured by the growth curve factors. But the model assumes that all individuals are drawn from the same population, that is, the means of the random effects have no variance. Growth mixture modeling relaxes this assumption and gives information about parameter differences across unobserved subpopulations. Instead of considering individual variation of a single mean of the intercept and slope, the growth mixture model allows different classes of individuals to vary around different intercepts and slopes (Muthén & Shedden, 1999). The classes are introduced by a latent categorical variable where the categories (classes) represent the unobserved heterogeneity of the data.

Following Muthén (2002, 2004), a growth mixture model (GMM) contains both latent growth variables η and a latent categorical variable c for $c = 1, 2, \ldots, K$. The variable c captures latent trajectory classes representing the different subpopulations. An unconditional growth mixture model can be formalized by the following equation:[1]

$$
\begin{aligned}
y_{tk} &= \lambda_{1tk}\eta_{1k} + \lambda_{2tk}\eta_{2k} + \epsilon_{tk} \\
\eta_{1k} &= \alpha_{1k} + \zeta_{1k} \\
\eta_{2k} &= \alpha_{2k} + \zeta_{2k}
\end{aligned}
\tag{1}
$$

y_{tk} is the manifest variable measured in wave t and class k, η_{1k} is the *initial level factor* whereas η_{2k} is the *linear growth factor*. Both latent variables η can be estimated specifically for class k; ϵ_{tk} is the random error term. In an unconditional model the latent variables are only described by their class specific means (α_{1k}, α_{2k}) and variances (ζ_{1k}, ζ_{2k}).

For a conditional growth mixture model, the structural equations in Equation 1 are extended by exogenous latent variables ξ_n:

$$
\eta_{mk} = A_k + \Gamma_k\xi_{nk} + \zeta_{mk}
\tag{2}
$$

Matrix A_k contains the levels and slopes within k-classes whereas matrix Γ_k refers to the regressions of ξ_n within the kth class. Figure 10–1 gives an example of a growth mixture model with one latent exogenous variable ξ_1.

The relation between the exogenous variable ξ_1 and the categorical class variable c is given by a multinomial logistic regression model:

$$
logit(\pi_k) = \alpha_c + \Gamma_c\xi_1
\tag{3}
$$

with $\pi_k = P(c_k = k|\xi_1)$ and α_c as a $(K - 1)$-dimensional parameter vector. Γ_c is a $(K - 1)\times q$-parameter matrix containing regression coefficients of K classes on predictor ξ_1. Assuming two classes, matrix Γ_c contains one parameter for the first class whereas the second parameter stands for the reference class. In M*plus*, the reference class is always the last class of the mixture

---

[1]For simplicity, person suffix i is ommited in the following equations.

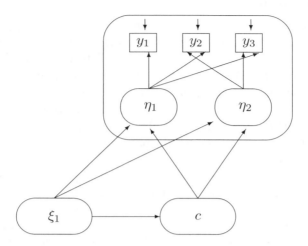

Note. A measurement model for the exogenous variable ξ_1 is omitted in the figure as well as in the description of the model.

Figure 10–1. General growth mixture model.

model. With an unordered number of categories k of the latent class variable, the probability expression $P(c_k = k|\xi_1)$ can be formalized as follows (Muthén & Muthén, 2004, p. 346):

$$P(c_k = k|\xi_1) = \frac{e^{\alpha_{ck} + \gamma'_{c_k}\xi_1}}{\sum_{k=1}^{K} e^{\alpha_{ck} + \gamma'_{c_k}\xi_1}} \qquad (4)$$

For the last class $e^{\alpha_{cK} + \gamma'_{cK}\xi_1}$ equals 1. Therefore, the probability to be in class c is simply the ratio of the exponentiated value of the logit and the sum of all exponentiated values. The categorial part of the growth mixture model in Figure 10–1 can be enlarged by adding *outcome variables* or *distal indicators* that are formally incorporated as a logistic regression with covariates c and ξ_1 (cf. Muthén, 2004, p. 349). The applications in Sections 10.4 and 10.5 do not consider this part of the mixture model.

10.2.2 Model Estimation and Evaluation

Growth mixture models can be estimated by maximizing the log likelihood function within the admissible range of parameter values given classes and data. M*plus* (Version 3.11) uses the principle of maximum likelihood estimation and employs the EM-algorithm for maximization (Dempster, Laird, & Rubin, 1977; Muthén & Shedden, 1999). A set of starting values are provided by the program before one set is used for the final estimation of the parameters. Version 3 of M*plus* includes a so-called *integration method* that tests sets of different starting values evaluating the maximum initial stage log likelihood value. The seed number corresponding to that value is used for the final estimation of the model. For reestimation of the model parameters, the *optimal seed value* of the previous run can be included in the input file (for details see Muthén & Muthén, 2004). For a given solution, each individual's probability of membership in each class is estimated. Individuals can be assigned to the classes by calculating the posterior probability that an individual i belongs to a given class k. Each individual's posterior probability estimate for each class is computed as a function of the parameter estimates and the values of the observed data (cf. Muthén & Muthén, 2001, p. 367f).

It is always an empirical question how many classes are sufficient to describe the unobserved heterogeneity of the data. By classifying each individual into the most likely class, a table with rows corresponding to individuals classified into a given class can be constructed. The columns of that table show the average conditional probabilities to be in the particular class. High diagonal and low off-diagonal probabilities indicate a good classification. The entropy measure E_k summarizes the quality of the classification (Muthén & Muthén, 2001, p. 372):

$$E_K = 1 - \frac{\sum_i \sum_k (-\hat{p}_{ik} \, ln\hat{p}_{ik})}{n \, lnK} \tag{5}$$

$\hat{p}_{ik}$ denotes the estimated conditional probability for individual i in class k. E_K ranges from zero to one, where values close to one indicate a good classification of the data.

Maximum likelihood estimates and standard errors are obtained by maximizing the log likelihood function, given the observed data and the number of classes. Standard errors of estimates are asymptotically correct if the underlying mixture model is the true model. In general, test statistics require well-defined classes in a mixture model. Muthén (2004, p. 356) pointed out that the likelihood ratio comparing a $k-1$ and a k-class model does not have the usual large-sample χ^2-distribution because the class probability parameter can be at the boundary of its admissible space, that is, a latent class probability can be zero. In addition to that, a χ^2-difference between two models is only suitable for model selection when the models are nested. In mixture models, a k class model is not nested within a $k + 1$ group model. Therefore, conventional mixture tests are the Akaike information criterion (AIC; Akaike, 1987) and the Bayesian information criterion (BIC; Schwartz, 1978) being used for model comparisons:

$$AIC = -2logL + 2p \qquad (6)$$

$$BIC = -2logL + p\,ln(n) \qquad (7)$$

L is the value of the model's maximized likelihood, p is the number of parameters, and n the sample size. The second term in both equations is the so-called *penalty term* that penalizes an increase of the likelihood with additional parameters. In addition, the BIC includes the sample size. Usually, the model with the smallest AIC or BIC is accepted within model comparisons. Furthermore, M*plus* calculates a sample size adjusted BIC with $n = (n + 2)/24$, which was found to give superior performance for model selection (Yang, 1998). If the k-class model contains a redundant class, the $k - 1$ class model with the smaller AIC or BIC value should be chosen. An expansion of the model by adding a class is desirable only if the resulting improvement in the log likelihood exceeds the penalty for more parameters. But accepting or rejecting a model on the basis of the AIC or BIC is more or less descriptive and does not imply any statistical test.

Recently, Lo, Mendell, and Rubin (2001) proposed a likelihood ratio-based method for testing $k - 1$ classes against k classes in mixture models. The Lo-Mendell-Rubin likelihood ratio test (LMR-LRT) considers the usual likelihood ratio for testing the $k - 1$ model against a k model but with the correct distribution. The p-value from the test represents the probability that H0 is true, that is, that the model is sufficient with one less class. Therefore, a low p-value indicates that the $k - 1$ class model has to be rejected and the k-class model is sufficient to represent the mixture of the data. LMR-LRT has been critized by Jeffries (2003), but importance of the critics in applications is unknown (Muthén, 2004, p. 356). BIC, adjusted BIC, and the LMR-LRT test will be used for model selection in Sections 10.4 and 10.5.

10.2.3 Special Cases of Growth Mixture Models

Latent Class Growth Analysis. A special case of the growth mixture model is the latent class growth analysis (LCGA), which has been studied by Nagin and Land (1993), Nagin (1999) and Roeder, Lynch, and Nagin (1999). Jones, Nagin, and Roeder (2001) discussed different applications of latent class growth models assuming Poisson distributed count data as well as the more general zero-inflated Poisson model discussed later. Those analyses are based on a special SAS program called PROC Traj.[2] LCGA is a submodel of Equation 1 and characterized by having zero variances and covariances of the intercept and slope variables η. In an unconditional model, the structural part of Equation 1 reduces to:

$$
\begin{aligned}
\eta_{1k} &= \alpha_{1k} \\
\eta_{2k} &= \alpha_{2k}
\end{aligned}
\tag{8}
$$

Individuals within a class are treated as homogeneous with respect to their development. As Muthén (2004, p. 350) pointed out, LCGA has two major advantages: It can be used to find cut points in the within-class variation on the growth factors. This leads to the question of which different latent classes represent substantially different trajectories and which classes exist only due to minor variations. On the other hand, the latent classes can be viewed as a nonparametric representation of the distribution of the growth factors, resulting in a semiparametric model (Nagin, 1999; Nagin & Land, 1993). LCGA serves here as a starting point for the growth mixture model (GMM) with random intercepts and/or random slopes. The random component in the GMM is represented by a mixture of k classes. The stepwise procedure from LCGA to GMM is discussed with substantive applications in Section 10.4 and 10.5.

To study development of deviant and delinquent behavior is one of the main topics in criminal sociology or criminology. Very often the longitudinal data gives information about the incidence rate of that behavior or the number of convictions. From a methodological point of view, the distribution of those variables are counts and have to be treated differently compared to continuous data. The so-called "key approach in the modeling of delinquent and criminal careers" (Land, McCall, & Nagin, 1996) is the Poisson distribution with the corresponding regression models.

Poisson Model. The Poisson model assumes count variables instead of continuous variables. Let $Y = 0, 1, 2 \ldots$ be a random variable for a given time interval and y be the number of observed occurences. The number of events in an interval of a given length is Poisson distributed with the probability density function:

$$
Pr(Y = y) = e^{-\nu} \left[\frac{\nu^y}{y!} \right]
\tag{9}
$$

---

[2]The SAS procedure called PROC Traj can be obtained free of charge from the authors (*http://lib.stat.cmu.edu/~bjones/traj.html*). The program runs only with the PC-version of SAS. Results of the analyses should be equivalent to those obtained with the program M*plus*, although differences were reported (Li, Duncan, Duncan, & Acock, 2001).

The expected value or mean of the Poisson distribution is $E(Y) = \nu$ with $Var(Y) = \nu$.[3] Usually, the parameter ν is refered as the mean rate of occurrence of events. Small values of ν yield high probability for zero occurences of the random variable Y. The higher the value of ν, the lower the skewness of the distribution. The Poisson distribution is considered most appropriate for modeling events that seldom occur (for an overview with applications to criminal careers data, cf. Land et al., 1996). If ν is indexed to each individual i in a sample, exogenous variables X can be incorporated to specify a Poisson regression model (Land et al., 1996, p. 395):

$$ln(\nu_i) = X_i\beta \qquad (10)$$

β contains the regression coefficients. The mean rate parameter ν implies a conditional expectation function ($E[Y_i|X_i]$). The expected values of the count variable Y for each individual i is conditional on the specific values of the regressor variables X for each individual i.

Instead of a simple regression model, the growth curve model can be used to explain the Poisson distributed count data:

$$ln(\nu_{it}) = \lambda_{1t}\eta_1 + \lambda_{2t}\eta_2 + \epsilon_t \qquad (11)$$

ν_{it} is the expected number of occurences of the measurement y of individual i at time t, η_1 is the intercept and η_2 is the linear slope describing the growth. Equation 11 assumes that the growth parameters do not differ between unobserved groups.

To cover the unobserved heterogeneity, a Poisson-based latent class growth model can be formulated (Nagin, 1999, p. 144; Nagin & Land, 1993, p. 335; for specification in M*plus* see Muthén & Muthén, 2004, p. 190):

$$ln(\nu_{it}^k) = \lambda_{1t}^k\eta_1^k + \lambda_{2t}^k\eta_2^k + \epsilon_t^k \qquad (12)$$

ν_{it}^k is the expected number of occurences of the measurement y of individual i at time t given the membership in class k. The conditional number of events, $P(y_{it}^k|k)$, should follow the Poisson distribution.

Zero-inflated Poisson Model. If the number of zeros in the count variable are very large, a variant of the Poisson regression model is more appropriate; the so-called *zero-inflated Poisson model* (ZIP) originally proposed by Lambert (1992). The ZIP model combines the regression model in Equation 10 with a

---

[3]Note, that in the literature the greek letter λ is often used for the expected value of a Poisson distribution. In structural equation models, λ is reserved for vectors of factor loadings. Therefore, I use the letter ν here for the expected value.

logit model to cover the zero inflation in the count variable Y with probability p that Y is zero (Lambert, 1992, p. 3):

$$logit(p) = ln(p/(1-p)) \tag{13}$$

Two parallel growth mixture models are estimated simultaneously when zero inflation of the data is assumed: The first model contains the count part of the outcomes with values of zero and above (variables y_1 to y_4 in Figure 10–2). Intercepts of the outcomes are fixed to zero as the default. The means of growth curve variables (variables i, s) are estimated for each class. The second model refers to the zero-inflation part of the outcome with only values of zero in all measurements (variables y_1^i to y_4^i). Intercepts of the outcomes are estimated and held equal as the default. The mean of the intercept variable (variable ii) are fixed to zero for all classes while the mean of the slope (variable si) is estimated and held equal for all classes (cf. Muthén & Muthén, 2004, p. 190).

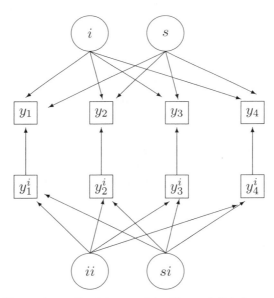

Figure 10–2. Two-part growth mixture model with zero-inflated measurements.

Those two parallel growth curve models can be combined in M*plus* to get simultaneous parameter estimates. If rare events (e.g., counts of deviant and delinquent behavior) are under study, the ZIP model should be more appropriate than the Poisson model (see the applications with PROC Traj in Jones, Nagin, & Roeder, 2001).

10.3 DESIGN OF THE STUDY AND DESCRIPTIVE STATISTICS

The empirical basis for the following analyses with mixture models is taken from the longitudinal research project *Juvenile Delinquency in Modern Towns*.[4] The main focus of the study is on the emergence and the development of deviant and delinquent behavior of juveniles and the social control surrounding it; both formal, meaning the police and the judiciary, and informal, referring to school and family.

The panel data contains self-administered interviews with pupils from the town of Münster located north of Cologne in West Germany. The initial survey was conducted in the year 2000 with pupils from 7th, 9th and 11th grade considering all relevant school types in the community. Note that the German school system differs between local communities. The highest educational level is on the *Gymnasium*, the medium one is on the *Realschule* and the lowest on the *Hauptschule*. Further on, those educational levels will be labeled as *high*, *medium*, and *low* in the analyses of the conditional models in Section 10.4 and 10.5. One cohort (7th grade) has been interviewed annually until the pupils reached the 10th grade in the year 2003. Thirty-one schools participated over the whole time period. The mean response rate was about 85%. The relatively high response rate is due to confidentiality restrictions. Almost every longitudinal study with sensitive topics avoids collecting data that can identify respondents easily (e.g., home adresses). Panel attritions can rise up to 50% depending on the time period under study. Instead of collecting pupils' home adresses, an individual encryption code was created. To generate the code, a specific code sheet was administered prior to the questionnaire in each panel wave. For example, the code sheet included questions about specific letters of respondent's eye and hair color and number of respondent's birthday. Additional information (e.g., change of class, school) was used to avoid equal codes belonging to different persons (see Pöge, 2005 for details).

Table 10–1 shows the distributions of gender and educational level for each panel wave. Compared to official statistics, the distribution of the educational level is biased. Low educated pupils are somewhat underrepresented whereas the high educated pupils are overrepresented in the data. It should also be noted that the capability to remember the answers to the code sheet questions generating the encryption code is correlated to the educational level of the schools. There is also a somewhat higher proportion of females (56%) in the four-wave panel data reflecting the greater ability to remember the answers of the code variables. Due to improvements of the encryption code sheet in

[4]This interdisciplinary research project is located at the universities of Münster (Institute of Criminology) and Bielefeld (Faculty of Sociology) and supported by the German National Science Foundation (DFG) under grant numbers Bo1234/6 and Re832/4.

TABLE 10–1

Sample of Respondents in the Four-Wave Panel Study (2000–2003)

	Wave 1	Wave 2	Wave 3	Wave 4	Wave 1-4
Gender	n (%)	n (%)	n (%)	n (%)	n (%)
male	665 (48.1)	816 (48.9)	868 (50.3)	716 (48.1)	353 (43.4)
female	717 (51.9)	852 (51.1)	857 (49.7)	774 (51.9)	460 (56.6)
	1382 (100)	1668 (100)	1725 (100)	1441 (100)	813 (100)
Level of Education	n (%)	n (%)	n (%)	n (%)	n (%)
low	282 (20.4)	402 (24.1)	423 (24.5)	341 (22.9)	129 (15.9)
medium	410 (29.7)	525 (31.5)	560 (32.5)	487 (32.7)	241 (29.6)
high	690 (49.9)	741 (44.4)	742 (43.0)	662 (44.4)	443 (54.5)
	1382 (100)	1668 (100)	1725 (100)	1441 (100)	813 (100)

the following panel waves, the bias could be reduced. In addition, a higher mobility between the schools and dropouts of 9th grade pupils after the third panel wave have to be considered. In Germany, pupils have to go to school by law until the age of 16. Pupils with low achievement and low learning abilities tend to finish their school career after the 9th grade. But the majority remain in the school system and finish either with the 10th grade (low and medium educational level) or with the 13th grade (high educational level). The last column of Table 10–1 presents the distribution of respondents that participated in all panel waves and could be detected via the encryption code (N = 813). Those respondents are used for the mixture models described in subsequent sections.

The occurrences of different types of deviant and delinquent behaviors are summarized in Table 10–2 for each panel wave. Only those delinquencies are considered that were asked in all four waves. On the average, most of them increase until the third wave (9th grade pupils) and decrease one year later. This development would give empirical evidence of an adolescent-limited group of offenders that were detected in other longitudinal studies (cf. D'Unger et al., 1998; Nagin, 1999). Using or dealing with drugs shows a somewhat different picture. The rates increase from 5% in the first wave up to 27% in the fourth wave for drug use and from nearly zero up to 4% for drug dealing in the fourth wave.

Table 10–3 shows the wave-specific overall prevalence rates as additive indexes of the particular delinquencies listed in Table 10–2. The mean rate of deviant and delinquent behavior increased from 0.46 (7th grade) to the peak of 0.86 (9th grade). One year later the mean rate decreased to 0.82 (10th grade). The percentage of zeros reflecting no particular delinquency of the pupils decreased from 77% (7th grade) to nearly 63% (10th grade).

TABLE 10–2
Prevalence Rates of Delinquency for Four Panel Waves

	Wave 1	Wave 2	Wave 3	Wave 4
Robbery	13 (1.6%)	11 (1.4%)	15 (1.8%)	11 (1.4%)
Purse snatching	0 (0.0%)	2 (0.2%)	3 (0.4%)	2 (0.2%)
Aggravated assault with a weapon	1 (0.1%)	7 (0.9%)	5 (0.6%)	4 (0.5%)
Aggravated assault without a weapon	42 (5.2%)	47 (5.8%)	55 (6.8%)	48 (5.9%)
Vandalism	56 (6.9%)	66 (8.1%)	81 (10.0%)	65 (8.0%)
Graffities	21 (2.6%)	58 (7.1%)	69 (8.5%)	40 (4.9%)
Burglary (House, App.)	8 (1.0%)	16 (2.0%)	20 (2.5%)	16 (2.0%)
Accepting stolen goods	36 (4.4%)	43 (5.3%)	40 (4.9%)	44 (5.4%)
Theft out of motor-vehicles	1 (0.1%)	4 (0.5%)	7 (0.9%)	8 (1.0%)
Motor-vehicles theft	3 (0.4%)	3 (0.4%)	7 (0.9 %)	5 (0.6%)
Theft from cash-machine	14 (1.7%)	13 (1.6%)	17 (2.1%)	11 (1.4%)
Bicycle theft	12 (1.5%)	27 (3.3%)	37 (4.6%)	51 (6.3%)
Shoplifting	107 (13.2%)	131 (16.1%)	122 (15.0%)	94 (11.6%)
Other thefts	16 (2.0%)	17 (2.1%)	22 (2.7%)	17 (2.1%)
Drug use	41 (5.0%)	100 (12.3%)	169 (20.8%)	216 (26.6%)
Drug dealing	2 (0.2%)	20 (2.5%)	30 (3.7%)	35 (4.3%)

Note. Percentages are calculated on the basis of N = 813.

Correlations within the overall prevalence rates reflect a time-dependent pattern (Table 10–4). The longer the time distance between the measurements, the lower the correlations. In accordance with our expectations, both exogenous variables correlate negatively to the prevalence rates: Females show less deviant and delinquent behavior than males, pupils in schools with a higher educational level are also less deviant and delinquent than pupils from schools with a lower educational level. The overall prevalence rates for each year will serve as the time-dependent measurement variable of the growth mixture models discussed in the following sections.

TABLE 10–3
Descriptive Statistics of the Overall Prevalence Rates (Prev) for Four Panel Waves

Index	$\bar{x}$	s	% Zeros
Prev (t_1)	0.46	1.16	76.9
Prev (t_2)	0.69	1.42	68.3
Prev (t_3)	0.86	1.65	63.5
Prev (t_4)	0.82	1.59	62.9

TABLE 10–4

Correlation Matrix of the Overall Prevalence Rates and the Exogenous Variables

	Prev (t_1)	*Prev* (t_2)	*Prev* (t_3)	*Prev* (t_4)	*Gender*	*Educ. Level*
Prev (t_1)	1.000					
Prev (t_2)	0.542	1.000				
Prev (t_3)	0.406	0.629	1.000			
Prev (t_4)	0.346	0.518	0.606	1.000		
Gender	-0.131	-0.146	-0.189	-0.171	1.000	
Educ. Level	-0.110	-0.173	-0.138	-0.171	-0.002	1.000

10.4 LATENT CLASS GROWTH ANALYSIS

To explore unobserved heterogeneity in adolescent deviant and delinquent behavior in the aforementioned panel data of Section 10.3, it is assumed that distinct classes exist, each of which follows a different developmental growth trajectory. Latent class growth analysis (LCGA) was used as a preliminary step exploring different developmental processes of the subjects under study (Muthén, 2004, p. 350): First, unconditional models with K classes using the Poisson and the zero-inflated Poisson distribution of the overall prevalence rates are calculated to detect differences in terms of model fit. In addition, the necessity to include a quadratic growth term in the models is proven (Section 10.4.1). Second, conditional models incorporating background covariates gender and educational level are tested. These analyses focused on the observed heterogeneity of the data, that is, a test of substantive relationship between the covariates and the latent classes as well as the growth variables (Section 10.4.2).

10.4.1 Unconditional Models

Latent class growth analysis of the unconditional model is performed on up to four classes as a linear and as a quadratic growth curve model as well. Assuming a Poisson distribution (abbreviated LCGA-Poisson), the BIC and the adjusted BIC favor a four-class model whereas the LMR-LRT points to a three-class model (cf. first part of Table 10–5). The LMR-LRT p-values of 0.17 (linear model) and 0.23 (quadratic model) indicate that the addition of the fourth class is not a significant improvement.

Assuming a zero-inflated Poisson distribution (abbreviated LCGA-ZIP), the BIC and the adjusted BIC favor again a four-class model. But the LMR-LRT p-values of 0.15 (linear model) and 0.19 (quadratic model) indicate that the four-class solutions contain a redundant class (cf. second part of Table 10–5). In both solutions, the fourth classes would contain less than 15 persons that do not allow substantive interpretations. The correction of the zero-inflation gives a better representation of the data in all model variants. There-fore, further analyses will focus on the ZIP-models with three classes.

TABLE 10–5

Fit of the Unconditional LCGA-Models with Different Classes

LCGA-Poisson					
Type	Test	C1	C2	C3	C4
Linear model	BIC	8994	6853	6540	6523
	Adj. BIC	8987	6837	6514	6488
	LMR-LRT		2059	317	35
	p-value		0.00	0.00	0.17
Quadratic model	BIC	8970	6835	6528	6510
	Adj. BIC	8961	6813	6493	6463
	LMR-LRT		2084	322	43
	p-value		0.00	0.00	0.23
LCGA-ZIP					
Type	Test	C1	C2	C3	C4
Linear model	BIC	7613	6724	6484	6473
	Adj. BIC	7601	6702	6452	6431
	LMR-LRT		866	248	30
	p-value		0.00	0.00	0.15
Quadratic model	BIC	7613	6734	6500	6494
	Adj. BIC	7594	6702	6456	6437
	LMR-LRT		873	251	32
	p-value		0.00	0.00	0.19

Table 10–6 shows the class distribution for the zero-inflated (ZIP) and the quadratic zero-inflated model (Quadrat-ZIP) with three classes. The criterion to be in a given class is the most likely latent class membership. For both models the distributions are nearly equal. About 32% of the respondents belong to the first, 8% to the second, and 60% to the third class. If both class member-ships are crosstabulated, only seven persons are in different classes. According to the entropy measure E_k (cf. Equation 5), the linear and the quadratic ZIP-model indicate a reasonable classification (in both models $E_k = 0.81$).

TABLE 10–6

Distributions of the Classes

Classes	ZIP		Quadrat-ZIP	
	n	(%)	n	(%)
1	262	(32.3)	265	(32.6)
2	63	(7.7)	64	(7.9)
3	488	(60.0)	484	(59.5)

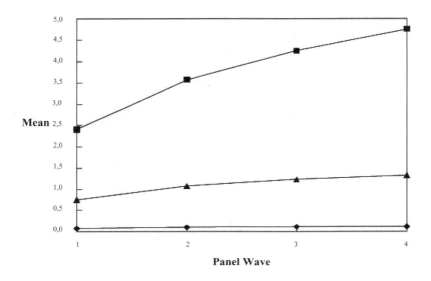

Figure 10–3. Three-class LCGA-ZIP for four panel waves.

The estimated growth trajectories of the LCGA-ZIP-model are shown in Figure 10–3. The lines next to the x-axes represents the "nonoffenders" with almost no deviant and delinquent behavior over the observed time period. This class is the largest one (Class 3 in Table 10–6). The second largest class, Class 1, shows a small development of offending starting from a low level. The estimated means range from 0.75 (t_1) to 1.33 (t_4). According to the mixture analyses of D'Unger et al. (1998), this class can be characterized as "low-rate adolescents" (intercept = 0.124; slope = 0.055). The smallest class, Class 2, reflects a somewhat stronger development of deviant and delinquent behavior starting from a high level in the first wave (intercept = 1.298; slope = 0.092). This class can be characterized as "high-rate adolescents." The estimated means range from 2.41 (t_1) to 4.75 (t_4).

Following Kreuter (2004), the intercept for the inflation part of the model is fixed to zero in all classes. The estimate of the slope is restricted to be equal across classes. In addition, intercepts of the manifest variables (y_1^i to y_4^i, cf. Figure 10–1) are set to be equal within and across classes. The estimated inflation probability decreases from 0.34 (wave 1) to less than 0.10 (wave 4). Differences between the linear and the quadratic LCGA-ZIP-model are small because nonlinearity in growth is only observed after the third wave, which is due to a slight decrease of offending in Classes 1 and 2. With more panel waves the quadratic model specification would give a better representation of the data (cf. the three-class LCGA for the Cambridge study in Muthén, 2004).

Results of the categorical part of the linear LCGA-ZIP-model are discussed as follows (cf. Equation 3). Without any exogenous variables, the exponential function of the logit parameter (intercept) is simply the odds ratio for being in the particular class versus the reference class. The class of "nonoffenders" will serve as the reference class. For the first class ("low-rate adolescents"), a logit coefficient of -0.649 is estimated. The exponentiated value is $e^{-0649} = 0.522$. For the second class ("high-rate adolescents") the estimated logit coefficient is -2.026 and the exponentiated value is 0.132. Following Equation 4, the latent class probability is 0.32 for the first, 0.08 for the second, and $1 - 0.32 - 0.08 = 0.60$ for the third (reference) class. The distribution of those probabilities is equivalent to the distribution of classes given in Table 10–6.

10.4.2 Conditional Models

The aforementioned analyses of the unconditional latent class growth curve model will be the basis for the conditional models. Therefore, gender and level of education will serve as exogenous variables for the latent class distribution and the growth curve variables. The fit of the linear and quadratic specification of the latent class growth curve model is again compared up to four classes (cf. Table 10–7). Similar to the unconditional models, the linear specification results in a better model fit than the quadratic one. The BIC, adjusted BIC, and the LMR-LRT points to a three-class solution with linear growth.

TABLE 10–7

Fit of the Conditional LCGA-ZIP-Models with Different Classes

Type	Test	C1	C2	C3	C4
Linear model	BIC	7451	6665	6444	6453
	Adj. BIC	7425	6624	6387	6380
	LMR-LRT		796	247	23
	p-value		0.00	0.00	0.49
Quadratic model	BIC	7463	6688	6474	6470
	Adj. BIC	7425	6630	6398	6375
	LMR-LRT		796	248	43
	p-value		0.00	0.00	0.05

The estimated class distribution of the conditional linear LCGA-ZIP-model is comparable to the unconditional model: 58.3% of the respondents belong to the class of "nonoffenders" (Class 3), 32.6% to the "low-rate adolescents" (Class 2), and 9.1% to the "high-rate adolescents" (Class 1). If the class membership of the three-class unconditional model is crosstabulated with the conditional one, 14 persons move from Class 3 to Class 2 and 11 persons from Class 2 to Class 1. According to the entropy measure E_k, the classification is slightly worse compared to the unconditional model, but still reasonable ($E_k = 0.72$). The estimated parameters differ only slightly from the unconditional specification. The class of "high-rate adolescents" (intercept = 1.582; slope = 0.118) indicates that the larger increase of deviant and delinquent behavior gets along with a higher initial rate compared to the class of "low-rate adolescents" (intercept = 0.409; slope = 0.053).

According to Figure 10–1 and Muthén (2004, p. 355) the regressions of the growth curve variables on the covariates should be allowed unless there are theoretical reasons not to do it. Here, those regression coefficients are restricted to be equal across classes. A substantive effect is only observed for the regression of the intercept on educational level (-0.218), which is in accordance with our hypothesis: The higher the level of education, the lower the initial rate of offending.

Table 10–8 summarizes the logit part of the conditional linear ZIP-model; the logit parameters, the exponentiated values of the logits (odds) and the latent class probabilities. Calculations are discussed for Class 1 and the first combination of values of both exogenous variables (male and low educational level) in detail.

Regarding Equation 3, the logit expression for Class 1 compared to the last (reference) class is:

$$logit(\pi_1) = \alpha_1 + \gamma_1' \cdot Gender + \gamma_2' \cdot Educ.Level \tag{14}$$

The latent class probability of Class 1 can be calculated using Equation 4:

$$P(c_k = 1 | Male, low\ educ.\ level) = \frac{e^{\alpha_1 + \gamma_{1_1}' \cdot Gender + \gamma_{2_1}' \cdot Educ.Level}}{\sum_{k=1}^{3} e^{\alpha_k + \gamma_{1_k}' \cdot Gender + \gamma_{2_k}' \cdot Educ.Level}} \tag{15}$$

The values of both exogenous variables are all zero in that particular combination (male and low educational level) so that only the intercept contributes to the logit. In the first step, the estimated intercept logit values (-0.769, 0.377, 0) are exponentiated and summed. In the second step, the first exponentiated value is divided by the sum to compute the latent class probability for Class 1 (0.159). The following latent class probabilities are calculated accordingly by using Equation 15.

The probability for males with low educational level is nearly 16% to be in Class 1 ("high-rated adolescents"), about 50% to be in Class 2 ("low-rated adolescents"), and only about 34% to be in Class 3 ("nonoffenders"). The probability to be classified in Class 3 increases with the educational level of the school. The probability for females with low educational level is only 8% to be in Class 1, nearly 43% to be in Class 2, but 54% to be in Class 3. As

TABLE 10–8

Logit, Odds (e^{logit}) and Latent Class Probabilities (Prob.) of the Conditional Linear ZIP-Model (3 Classes)

Exog. Var.	Class	Logit	e^{logit}	Prob.
Male and	1	-0.769	0.463	0.159
low educ.	2	0.377	1.458	0.499
level	3	0	1.0	0.342
Male and	1	-1.113	0.329	0.142
medium educ.	2	-0.006	0.994	0.428
level	3	0	1.0	0.430
Male and	1	-1.457	0.233	0.122
high educ.	2	-0.389	0.678	0.355
level	3	0	1.0	0.523
Female and	1	-1.902	0.149	0.080
low educ.	2	-0.345	0.708	0.381
level	3	0	1.0	0.539
Female and	1	-2.250	0.106	0.067
medium educ.	2	-0.728	0.483	0.304
level	3	0	1.0	0.629
Female and	1	-2.590	0.075	0.053
high educ.	2	-1.111	0.329	0.234
level	3	0	1.0	0.713

Note. Gender is coded 0 and 1 (male/female), educational level is coded 0, 1, and 2 (low, medium, high). Class 1 represents the "high-rated adolescents", Class 2 the "low-rated adolescents," and Class 3 the "nonoffenders".

with the males, the probability to be classified in Class 3 increases with the educational level. But this increase for the females is much stronger than for the males. The chance to be a member of the "high- or low-rate adolescents" (Classes 1 and 2) is clearly greater for males than for females within all levels of education. On the average, the effect of the latent classes on gender is stronger than the effect on educational level.

10.5 GROWTH MIXTURE MODELS

Based on the results of the latent class growth analysis, the following mixture models try to generalize the previous analyses. Results of the mixture models in Section 10.4 have shown that linear models incorporating the zero-inflated Poisson distribution have the best model fits. Therefore, only the zero-inflated Poisson distribution will be considered in the growth mixture models (abbreviated GMM-ZIP). In Section 10.5.1, the unconditional GMM-model is discussed whereas in Section 10.5.2, the model will be enlarged by the exogenous variables gender and educational level.

10.5.1 Unconditional Models

In a step-by-step procedure, the unconditional GMM-ZIP models include either the variation of the intercepts within the classes or the variation of the
slopes within the classes (with the restriction of equal intercept or slope variances across classes). Both model variants have equal degrees of freedom and
fit measures can be compared easily. Table 10–9 provides the model results
up to four classes. In general, models with random intercepts have a slightly
better model fit than models with random slopes. According to the BIC and the
LMR-LRT measures, a three-class model is sufficient for the data. All four-
class models are rejected by the LMR-LRT. Results show in detail that in each
solution, one class contains less than six persons.

If the intercept variance of the class of "nonoffenders" is set to zero (cf. a
similar specification in Muthén, 2004, p. 362), the model fit gets worse compared to the previous specification (the three-class specification is rejected with
LMR-LRT = 3 and $p = 0.65$; see first model C3a in Table 10–9).[5] Alternatively,
if the slope variance of the class of "nonoffenders" is set to zero, the model fit
is nearly equal compared to the corresponding three-class solution (the three-
class specification is confirmed with LMR-LRT = 94 and $p = 0.00$; see second
model C3a in Table 10–9). Due to the fact that this model specification is more
parsimonious than the previous one, it will be accepted for further substantive
interpretations. A random slope is estimated for the second and third class
(low- and high-rated adolescents) while the variance of the slope in the first
class (nonoffenders) is fixed to zero. It should also be noted that the entropy
measure is much better in all random slope models (average $E_K = 0.70$) compared to the random intercept models. One more general specification is the
growth mixture model with random intercept and random slope estimated simultaneously. But, even with several alternative starting values, a solution of
this model with three classes could not be obtained.

Due to the most likely latent class membership, 58% of the respondents
are classified in the first (N = 473), 33% into the second (N = 270), and 9%
into the third class (N = 70). The sequence fits into the order of the class
of "nonoffenders," the class of "low-rate adolescents," and finally, the class
of "high-rate adolescents." If the class membership is crosstabulated with the
unconditional LCGA-model discussed in Section 10.4.1, most of the cases remain in the particular classes. Only 16 persons move from the "low-rate" class
to the "high-rate" class, 9 persons move vice versa. Another 15 persons move
from the "nonoffenders" class to the "low-rate" class. All in all, the zero class
is smaller in the GMM-ZIP than in the corresponding LCGA-ZIP whereas the

---

[5]Alternatively, means and variances of the growth curve variables of the "nonoffender" class can be fixed
to zero. In the same class, the means of the manifest variables are fixed to the value -15.00 (cf. the
specification in Kreuter, 2004). Again, the model fit decreases similar to model C3a.

TABLE 10–9

Fit of the Unconditional Growth Mixture Models (GMM-ZIP) with Different Classes

Type	Test	C1	C2	C3	C3a	C4
Random intercept	BIC	6464	6450	6431	6461	6445
	Adj. BIC	6448	6424	6396	6426	6401
	LMR-LRT		33	37	3	5
	p-value		0.03	0.00	0.65	0.17
Random slope	BIC	6872	6522	6442	6444	6447
	Adj. BIC	6856	6497	6408	6409	6402
	LMR-LRT		352	95	94	15
	p-value		0.00	0.00	0.00	0.62

Note. Model C3a includes the restriction that the intercept or the slope of the class of "nonoffenders" has a variance of zero.

other classes have higher proportions in the GMM-ZIP. This result is similar to the mixture analyses of the Cambridge data in Muthén (2004).

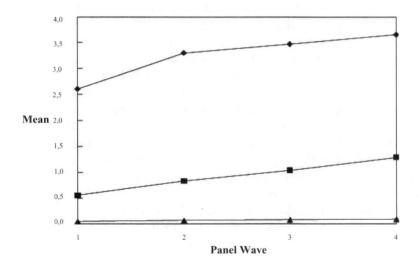

Figure 10–4. Three-class GMM-ZIP for four panel waves.

The estimated growth trajectories of the GMM-ZIP model with random slopes are shown in Figure 10–4. The line next to the x axis represents the "nonoffenders" (Class 1) with almost no deviant and delinquent behavior over the observed time period. This class is again the largest class. The second largest Class 2 shows a small development of offending starting from a low level (intercept = -0.229; slope = 0.088). The estimated means range from 0.54 (wave 1) to 1.29 (wave 4). The smallest Class 3 reflects a somewhat stronger development starting from a higher level in the first wave (intercept = 1.316; slope = 0.080). The estimated means range from 2.61 (wave 1) to 3.66 (wave 4). The three growth trajectories of the GMM-ZIP model are similar to those of the LCGA-ZIP model (Figure 10–3), the estimated slope variance restricted to be equal across classes is significant (variance = 0.049; $z = 16.27$).

Results of the categorical part of the unconditional GMM-ZIP model are also comparable to the unconditional LCGA-ZIP model. In the GMM-ZIP model, the class of "high-rate adolescents" will serve as the reference class. For the first class ("nonoffenders"), a logit coefficient of 1.656 is estimated. For the second class ("low-rate adolescents"), the estimated logit coefficient is 1.256. Following Equation 4, the latent class probability is 0.54 for the first, 0.36 for the second, and 0.10 for the third (reference) class.

10.5.2 Conditional Models

The unconditional GMM-ZIP model can now be extended by the exogenous variables gender and level of education. In a step-by-step procedure, the conditional GMM-ZIP models include either the variation of the intercepts within the classes or the variation of the slopes within the classes (with the restriction of equal intercept or slope variances across classes). Table 10–10 provides the model results up to four classes. According to the BIC and the LMR-LRT, three-class models with random intercepts or random slopes are sufficient for the data. Both four-class models are rejected by the LMR-LRT.

If the intercept variance of the class of "nonoffenders" is set to zero, the model fit gets worse according to the BIC. But different from the unconditional specification, the three-class solution is not rejected by the LMR-LRT (LMR-LRT = 41 with $p = 0.00$; see first model C3a in Table 10–10). Alternatively, if the slope variance of the class of "nonoffenders" is set to zero, the model fit is nearly equal compared to the unrestricted three-class solution (the BIC value difference between the models is only 2). The restricted model is also confirmed by the LMR-LRT (LMR-LRT = 206 with $p = 0.00$; see second model C3a in Table 10–10). So, this model specification will be accepted for further substantive interpretations. Equal to the restricted unconditional GMM-ZIP model (cf. Table 10–9), a random slope is estimated for the second and third class (low- and high-rated adolescents) while the variance of the slope in the first class (nonoffenders) is fixed to zero. According to the most likely class membership, 58.2% of the respondents belong to the class of "nonoffenders" (Class 1), 33.2% to the "low-rate adolescents" (Class 2), and 8.5% to the "high-rate adolescents" (Class 3).

The estimated class distribution of the conditional linear GMM-ZIP model can be compared to the conditional linear LCGA-ZIP model in Section 4.2 via crosstabulation of both membership files: 16 persons move from the low to the high-rated class, 9 persons vice versa and 15 persons from the nonoffender

TABLE 10–10

Fit of the Conditional GMM-ZIP-Models with Different Classes

Type	Test	C1	C2	C3	C3a	C4
Random	BIC	6402	6400	6395	6414	6421
intercept	Adj. BIC	6380	6362	6341	6361	6351
	LMR-LRT		34	32	41	8
	p-value		0.02	0.06	0.00	0.43
Random	BIC	6816	6469	6406	6408	6413
slope	Adj. BIC	6794	6431	6352	6354	6353
	LMR-LRT		369	94	206	16
	p-value		0.00	0.00	0.00	0.66

Note. Model C3a includes the restriction that the intercept or the slope of the class of "nonoffenders" has a variance of zero.

class to the low-rated class. All other "nonoffenders" of the GMM-ZIP model are also "nonoffenders" in LCGA-ZIP model. The entropy measure of this model is reasonable ($E_K = 0.71$) and nearly the same as for the conditional LCGA-ZIP model. The regression coefficients of the growth curve variables on the exogenous variables are again restricted to be equal across classes. No substantive effects are observed.

The categorical part of the conditional GMM-ZIP model is summarized in Table 10–11. The probability for males with low educational level to be in Class 3 ("high-rated adolescents") is 29%, to be in Class 2 ("low-rated adolescents") is about 46% and to be in Class 1 ("nonoffenders") is only 25%. The probability to be classified as "nonoffenders" increases with the educational level of the school. The probability for females with low educational level is about 12% to be in Class 3, nearly 42% to be in Class 2 and 46% to be in Class 3. As with the males, the probability to be classified as "nonoffenders" increases with the educational level. But, compared to the males the increase is much stronger. The chance to be a member of the "high- or low-rate adolescents" (Classes 1 and 2) is clearly greater for males than for females within all levels of education. Comparable to the conditional LCGA-ZIP model (cf. Table 10–8), the effect of gender on the latent classes is stronger than the effect on educational level. One major difference between the conditional LCGA-ZIP model and the conditional GMM-ZIP model is the distribution of the latent class probabilities within a combination of exogenous variables' categories. For example, the probability to belong to the "high-rate adolescents" is higher for males in the GMM-ZIP model than in the LCGA-ZIP model. The significant variance estimate of the slope (variance = 0.048; $z = 15.71$) leads to a more adequate classification of the respondents in the GMM-ZIP model.

TABLE 10–11

Logit, Odds (e^{logit}) and Latent Class Probabilities (Prob.) of the Conditional Linear
ZIP-Model (3 Classes)

Exog. Var.	Class	Logit	e^{logit}	Prob.
Male and	1	-0.159	0.853	0.247
low educ.	2	0.467	1.595	0.463
level	3	0	1.0	0.290
Male and	1	0.700	2.014	0.372
medium educ.	2	0.876	2.401	0.443
level	3	0	1.0	0.185
Male and	1	1.559	4.754	0.502
high educ.	2	1.285	3.615	0.386
level	3	0	1.0	0.107
Female and	1	1.360	3.896	0.464
low educ.	2	1.254	3.504	0.417
level	3	0	1.0	0.119
Female and	1	2.219	9.198	0.594
medium educ.	2	1.663	5.275	0.341
level	3	0	1.0	0.065
Female and	1	3.078	21.714	0.708
high educ.	2	2.072	7.941	0.259
level	3	0	1.0	0.033

Note. Gender is coded 0 and 1 (male/female), educational level is coded 0, 1 and 2 (low, medium, high).
Class 1 is the zero-class, Class 2 the low peaked and Class 3 the high peaked class.

10.6 DISCUSSION

The general framework of growth mixture modeling outlined by Muthén
(2002, 2004) integrates several approaches of longitudinal growth modeling,
for example, the semiparametric group-based model developed and applied by
Nagin and Land (1993), Nagin (1999), and Jones et al. (2001). This model
is equivalent to a latent class growth model that fixes the intercept and slope
variances to zero. The latent class growth analysis is useful as a first evaluation of the unobserved heterogeneity in the data. After these analyses, the
variability of the class-specific intercepts and slopes can be studied with the
more general growth mixture model. In addition, the assumption of continuously distributed variables can be replaced by the Poisson or the zero-inflated
Poisson distribution, if count data with largely skewed distributions to zero are
analyzed. M*plus* (Version 3.11) allows those tests of growth mixture models
assuming different distributions of the manifest variables under study.

Data from a four-wave panel study of adolescents are used to study unobserved heterogeneity in the development of deviant and delinquent behavior. Starting with an unconditional latent class growth model, three classes
can be obtained: "Non-offenders," "low-rate adolescents," and "high-rate ado-

lescents." The zero-inflation of the measurements results in a better model fit compared to the Poisson model only. Due to the limited number of panel waves in our data (four waves), a linear growth specification is sufficient. This result is also confirmed by a growth mixture specification allowing random slopes in the low- and high-rated classes. The conditional specifications of the mixture models include gender and educational level of the schools. These exogenous variables are related to the latent class distribution: Male adolescents with an low educational level in schools are more likely to be in the high-rated class than female adolescents on the same educational level. And female adolescents are more likely to be "nonoffenders" than male adolescents. These results confirm our hypotheses and they are similar compared to other criminological studies using mixed Poisson models with panel data of adolescents' deviant and delinquent behavior (D'Unger et al., 1998; Jones et al., 2001). These models, equivalent to LCGA, assume zero variances of the intercept and slope variable. Therefore, our analyses with the growth mixture model are more general even if it was only possible to estimate intercept and slope variances seperately. The analyses do not confirm a convex trajectory that declines from a high initial rate that was found by McDermott and Nagin (2001) using the National Youth Survey. A similar trajectory can be only obtained in a five-class solution that is rejected by several model fit criterias (BIC, adjusted BIC, and LMR-LRT). All in all, the stepwise procedure from latent growth analysis to growth mixture modeling has shown the capability of longitudinal developmental analyses where individual growth trajectories are heterogenous and belong to a finite number of unobserved populations.

The present analyses are limited due to a four-wave panel design. The mixture models were conditioned only on time-independent predictors, gender, and educational level. Note that educational level can also be analyzed as a time-dependent exogenous variable due to a certain mobility of the adolescents between different schools. But only a minor proportion of adolescents in the study have changed between the schools. In Germany, the proportion of school changes increases significantly after the 10th grade, which is beyond the period of our data collection. Several studies have considered various predictors in their studies, like socioeconomic status of the parents, parental behavior, moral beliefs, attitudes about crime, or delinquent peers (Nagin, 1999; McDermott & Nagin, 2001). Therefore, further growth mixture model explorations should also include substantively relevant time-dependent variables to test parallel developments and their interrelationships over time. These models have to cope with different assumptions about the measurement of the variables (continuous and count data), which are easy to implement in M*plus*. However, those extensions are beyond the scope of the present article.

REFERENCES

Bentler, P. M. (2001). *EQS 6: Structural equations program manual.* Encino, CA: Multivariate Software.

Curran, P. J., & Hussong, A. M. (2002). Modeling intraindividual variability with repeated measures data: Method and applications. In D. S. Moskowitz & S. L. Hershberger (Eds.), *Structural equation modeling of repeated measures data: Latent curve analysis* (pp. 59–85). Mahwah, NJ: Lawrence Erlbaum Associates.

D'Unger, A., Land, K. C., McCall, P. L., & Nagin, D. S. (1998). How many latent classes of delinquent/criminal careers? Results from mixed Poisson regression analyses of the London, Philadelphia, and Racine cohort studies. *American Journal of Sociology, 103,* 1593–1630.

Dempster, A. P., Laird, N. M., & Rubin, D. B. (1977). Maximum likelihood from incomplete data via the EM algorithm. *Journal of the Royal Statistical Society, Series B, 39,* 1–38.

Duncan, T. E., Duncan, S. C., Strycker, L. A., Li, F., & Alpert, A. (1999). *An introduction to latent variable growth curve modeling: Concepts, issues, and applications.* Mahwah, NJ: Lawrence Erlbaum Associates.

Farrington, D. P., & West, D. J. (1990). The Cambridge study in delinquent development: A long term follow-up of 411 London males. In H. J. Kerner & G. Kaiser (Eds.), *Kriminalität: Persönlichkeit, Lebensgeschichte und Verhalten* (pp. 115–138). Berlin: Springer.

Hox, J. J. (2002). *Multilevel analysis: Techniques and applications.* Mahwah, NJ: Lawrence Erlbaum Associates.

Jeffries, N. O. (2003). A note on 'testing the number of components in a normal mixture.' *Biometrika, 90,* 991–994.

Jones, B. L., Nagin, D. S., & Roeder, K. (2001). A SAS procedure based on mixture models for estimating developmental trajectories. *Sociological Methods & Research, 29,* 374–393.

Jöreskog, K. G., & Sörbom, D. (2004). *LISREL 8.7 for Windows.* Lincolnwood, IL: Scientific Software International.

Kreuter, F., (2004). *Longitudinal models with zero inflation.* Unpublished manuscript, University of California at Los Angeles, Department of Statistics.

Lambert, D. (1992). Zero-inflated Poisson regression with an application to defects in manufacturing. *Technometrics, 34,* 1–13.

Land, K. C., McCall, P. L., & Nagin, D. S. (1996). A comparison of Poisson, negative binomial, and semiparametric mixed Poisson regression models with empirical applications to criminal careers data. *Sociological Methods & Research, 24,* 387–442.

Li, F., Duncan, T. E., Duncan, S. C., & Acock, A. (2001). Latent growth modeling of longitudinal data: A finite growth mixture modeling approach. *Structural Equation Modeling, 8*, 493–530.

Liang, K.-Y., & Zeger, S. L. (1986). Longitudinal data analysis using generalized linear models. *Biometrika, 73*, 13–22.

Lo, Y., Mendell, N. R., & Rubin, D. B. (2001). Testing the number of components in a normal mixture. *Biometrika, 88*, 767–778.

McArdle, J. J. (1988). Dynamic but structural equation modeling of repeated measures data. In J. R. Nesselroade & R. B. Cattell (Eds.), *Handbook of multivariate experimental psychology* (pp. 561–614). New York: Plenum.

McArdle, J. J., & Epstein, D. (1987). Latent growth curves within developmental structural equation models. *Child Development, 58*, 110–133.

McDermott, S., & Nagin, D. S. (2001). Same or different? Comparing offender groups and covariates over time. *Sociological Methods & Research, 29*, 282–318.

Meredith, M., & Tisak, J. (1990). Latent curve analysis. *Psychometrika, 55*, 107–122.

Muthén, B. (1991). Analysis of longitudinal data using latent variable models with varying parameters. In L. Collins & J. Horn (Eds.), *Best methods for the analysis of change* (pp. 1–17). Washington, DC: American Psychological Association.

Muthén, B. (1997). Latent variable modeling with longitudinal and multilevel data. In A. Raftery (Ed.), *Sociological Methodology* (pp. 453–480). Boston: Blackwell.

Muthén, B. (2001a). Latent variable mixture modeling. In G. A. Marcoulides & R. E. Schumacker (Eds.), *New developments and techniques in structural equation modeling* (pp. 1–33). Lawrence Erlbaum Associates.

Muthén, B. (2001b). Second-generation structural equation modeling with a combination of categorical and continuous latent variables: New opportunities for latent class/latent growth modeling. In L. M. Collins & A. Sayer (Eds.), *New methods for the analysis of change* (pp. 291–322). Washington, DC: APA.

Muthén, B. O. (2002). Beyond SEM: General latent variable modeling. *Behaviormetrika, 29*, 81–117.

Muthén, B. O. (2003). Statistical and substantive checking in growth mixture modeling: Comment on Bauer and Curran (2003). *Psychological Methods, 8*, 369–377.

Muthén, B. O. (2004). Latent variable analysis: Growth mixture modeling and related techniques for longitudinal data. In D. Kaplan (Ed.), *The*

Sage handbook of quantitative methodology for the social sciences (pp. 345–368). Thousand Oaks: Sage.

Muthén, B. O., & Curran, P. J. (1997). General longitudinal modeling of individual differences in experimental designs: A latent variable framework for analysis and power estimation. *Psychological Methods, 2,* 371–402.

Muthén, L., & Muthén, B. O. (2001). *Mplus: The comprehensive modeling program for applied researchers: User's guide* (2nd ed.). Los Angeles: Muthén & Muthén.

Muthén, L., & Muthén, B. O. (2004). *Mplus user's guide* (3rd ed.). Los Angeles: Muthén & Muthén.

Muthén, B., & Shedden, K. (1999). Finite mixture modeling with mixture outcomes using the EM algorithm. *Biometrics, 55,* 463–469.

Nagin, D. S. (1999). Analyzing developmental trajectories: A semi-parametric, group-based approach. *Psychological Methods, 4,* 139–157.

Nagin, D. S., & Land, K. C. (1993). Age, criminal careers, and population heterogeneity: Specification and estimation of a nonparametric, mixed Poisson model. *Criminology, 31,* 327–362.

Pöge, A. (2005). Persönliche Codes bei Längsschnittstudien: Ein Erfahrungsbericht [Personal codes in longitudinal studies: An empirical report]. *ZA-Information, 56,* 50–69.

Rao, C. R. (1958). Some statistical methods for comparison of growth curves. *Biometrics, 14,* 1–17.

Roeder, K., Lynch, K. G., & Nagin, D. S. (1999). Modeling uncertainty in latent class membership: A case study in criminology. *Journal of the American Statistical Association, 94,* 766–776.

Ross, S. M. (1993). *Introduction to probability models* (5th ed.). New York: Academic Press.

Schwarz, G. (1978). Estimating the dimension of a model. *Annals of Statistics, 6,* 461–464.

Tracy, P. E., Wolfgang, M. E., & Figlio, R. M. (1990). *Delinquency in two birth cohorts.* New York: Plenum.

Tremblay, R. E., Desmarais-Gervais, L., Gagnon, C. & Charlebois, P. (1987). The preschool behavior questionnaire: Stability of its factor structure between cultures, sexes, ages and socioeconomic classes. *International Journal of Behavioral Development, 10,* 467–484.

Tucker, L. R. (1958). Determination of parameters of a functional relation by factor analysis. *Psychometrika, 23,* 19–23.

Yang, C. C. (1998). *Finite mixture model selection with psychometric applications.* Unpublished doctoral dissertation, University of Groningen, The Netherlands.

Chapter 11

Nonlinear Growth Mixture Models in Research on Cognitive Aging

Kevin J. Grimm and Fumiaki Hamagami

University of Virginia

John J. McArdle

University of Southern California

11.1 INTRODUCTION

The development of intelligence or cognitive ability has been a predominant focus of cognitive research since Spearman's (1904) notion of general intelligence. The divergent developmental patterns of fluid and crystallized intelligence (G_f/G_c) were an important aspect of Cattell and Horn's discovery of two broad cognitive factors (Cattell, 1963; Horn & Cattell, 1966). Horn and Cattell (1967) and Horn (1988) showed how previous thought on lifespan cognitive development was an average of the monotonically increasing development of crystallized intelligence and the rise and fall nature of fluid intelligence. Life-span cognitive developmental research has continued to evaluate the developmental patterns of multiple cognitive ability (McArdle, Ferrer-Caja, Hamagami, & Woodcock; 2002) and model the effects of demographic variables on the growth and decline of cognition. In such studies, the use of the term "development" is a group term referring to the aggregate or group change, rather than an individual term dealing with the changes occurring within a person. Other research recognizes that no two individuals follow the same exact pattern of development but many individuals may follow similar patterns of development (e.g. Horn, 1972; Wohlwill, 1973). Advances in structural equation and latent variable modeling have enabled researchers to use contemporary mathematical and statistical modeling procedures to consider such patterns of development both within and across individuals. This work was initiated with latent growth curve analysis (LGCA; McArdle, 1986; McArdle and Epstein, 1987; McArdle & Nesselroade, 2003; Meredith & Tisak, 1990; Rao, 1958; Tucker, 1958). LGCA is a combination of group and individual analyses because the growth factors (i.e., intercept, y_0 and slope, y_1) can be estimated for each individual, but the pattern of development (i.e., basis coefficients, slope loadings) is defined for the group as an aggregate and the growth factors conform to a normal distribution. Because the growth factors are constrained to a normal distribution, the estimates of the intercept and slope are restricted compared to fitting individual curves.

Latent growth curves can be used to test hypotheses regarding the shape of development (i.e., whether the development is linear, exponential, etc.) and the latent curve model has been extended to a wide variety of developmental patterns. Meredith and Tisak (1990) briefly described several different types of growth curves including the one curve model, latent basis curve, polynomial models, and a negative exponential curve. The latent basis model includes a factor with unit loadings (intercept) and a second factor with freely estimated loadings as in traditional confirmatory factor analysis. The polynomial models discussed included growth curves with linear and quadratic trends, whereas the slope loadings followed the structure of a specified mathematical function in the negative exponential. Browne and Du Toit (1991) and Browne (1993) extended the previous work on LGCA with structured curves and showed how the Exponential, Logistic, and Gompertz curves could be fit using a first order Taylor-series polynomial. Growth curves (and time-series models) were recently built upon with latent difference scores (LDS) by McArdle and Hamagami (McArdle, 2001; McArdle & Hamagami, 2001; Hamagami & McArdle, 2001). The LDS growth curves can model a series of nonlinear shapes and allow for the evaluation of time-dependent influences on the change in the variable of interest. These models are described in greater detail in the *Models* section of the chapter.

An extension of latent growth curve analysis that allows for the investigation of latent classes with differing developmental trajectories is growth mixture modeling (GMM; Muthén & Muthén, 2000; Muthén & Shedden, 1999). GMM incorporates a latent categorical variable into growth curve analysis in an attempt to locate subpopulations of people with similar relationships among the repeated measures (Nagin, 1999). This statistical technique has been employed in a variety of substantive domains (i.e., dependency, education) to uncover typical and unusual patterns of development.

The idea of using a statistical model to identify different patterns of development and to classify participants based on those patterns was originally discussed by Rao (1958) and Tucker (1958). Tucker (1966) noted that just because a group of subjects show a smooth increase in average performance on a learning task does not mean that all subjects in that group follow an individual pattern similar to the average trend (see McCall, Appelbaum, & Hogarty, 1973). Tucker's (1958, 1966) technique employed principal components analysis (PCA) to decompose the persons by occasions data matrix into component loadings, representing developmental patterns or "generalized learning curves", and component scores, representing the participants' 'saturation' on each of these curves. Tucker's method had two distinct interpretations based on the size of the component scores. When the component scores are large for a single curve and zero elsewhere, the result is the identification of participants with different growth curves. However, when there is not a dominant component score for the participants, the result is interpreted as the identification of different processes of development for all participants. McCall, Appelbaum, and Hogarty (1973) described Tucker's method using the first interpretation as their goal to cluster subjects together in such a way that there are homogenous patterns of development within a group and distinct developmental patterns between groups.

This chapter brings growth mixture models into a nonlinear framework and examines patterns of cognitive development across the lifespan. In these applications we study multiple developmental patterns for multiple cognitive abilities in the Berkeley Growth (*BGS*) and Berkeley Guidance Studies (*GS*). The previous work in nonlinear growth mixture models and cognitive development was conducted by McArdle and Nesselroade (2003). In this work, McArdle and Nesselroade fit a series of latent basis growth mixture models to cognitive data from the Bradway-McArdle Longitudinal Study (*BMLS*; $N = 111$), a longitudinal study from age 2 to 70 with six occasions of measurement. McArdle and Nesselroade concluded that there were no latent classes in the BMLS with differing developmental patterns. This chapter extends the work on nonlinear growth mixture models to include models based on structured curves (Browne, 1993; Browne & du Toit, 1991), growth models based on latent difference scores (Hamagami & McArdle, 2001; McArdle, 2001; McArdle & Hamagami, 2001) and related multivariate models. We provide a brief overview of latent growth modeling with consideration for nonlinear, multiple group, and multivariate growth models, a short introduction to growth mixture modeling, and an application of nonlinear growth mixture models to lifespan cognitive development data.

11.2 METHOD

Data
The cognitive data comes from two longitudinal studies initiated at the Institute of Human Development, University of California, Berkeley in 1928. The participants of the *Berkeley Growth Study* (N = 61) were selected from infants born in hospitals near and around Berkeley, CA. The study was initiated by Nancy Bayley to trace the normal intellectual, motor, and physical development of children through the first year. Cognitive data collection with standardized intelligence tests began in 1934 when the children were six years of age. The sample continued taking intelligence tests every year until age 16. In adulthood, the sample took an intelligence test at ages 18, 21, 25, 36, 53, and most recently at age 70.

The participants of the *Berkeley Guidance Study* (N = 206) were selected from the population of every third infant born in Berkeley between January 1928 and June 1929. Approximately half of the mothers were offered guidance by the principal investigator about general issues of childhood behavior and development (Jones & Meredith, 2000). The participants whose mother's received guidance were called the *Guidance Group* and the children whose mother's did not receive guidance were called the *Control Group*. The participants from this study took standardized intelligence tests almost every year from age 6 (1934) to age 15 and then at age 18, 40, and 53. Table 11-1 is an outline of the testing occasions for the *BGS* and the *GS*.

TABLE 11-1
The Year, Sample Size, and Type of Intelligence Tests taken by the Berkeley Growth Study (BGS) and the Guidance Study (GS)

Intelligence Test	Year	Sample	N	Max Repeats
1916 Stanford-Binet	1934- 1937	BGS	101	3
	1934- 1937	GS	410	3
Stanford-Binet Form L	1937- 1947	BGS	197	5
	1936- 1944	GS	631	6
Stanford-Binet Form M	1939- 1950	BGS	151	3

	1937- 1943	GS	375	6
Wechsler-Bellevue I	1944- 1953	BGS	141	4
	1946	GS	157	1
WAIS	1964	BGS	54	1
	1968	GS	118	1
WAIS-R	1983, 2000	BGS	74	2
	1982	GS	118	1
Woodcock-Johnson Revised	2000	BGS	33	1

Cognitive Measures

Through these longitudinal studies, the principal investigators wanted to use age-appropriate and current intelligence batteries. The intelligence tests administered to the *BGS* and *GS* participants have changed through the years to reflect this desire. The participants of the *BGS* and *GS* have taken the 1916 Stanford-Binet (Terman, 1916), Stanford-Binet Form L & M (Terman & Merrill, 1937), Wechsler-Bellevue Form I (Wechsler, 1946), Wechsler Adult Intelligence Scale (WAIS; Wechsler, 1955), Wechsler Adult Intelligence Scale – Revised (WAIS-R; Wechsler, 1981), and the Woodcock-Johnson Psycho-educational Battery Revised (Woodcock & Johnson, 1989). McArdle, Grimm, Hamagami, Bowles, and Meredith (2005) used an item analysis to equate the different measures of vocabulary and short-term memory taken by the *BGS*, *GS*, and the *BMLS*. The item linkage analysis employed common-item and common-person equating because several items were given at multiple occasions (i.e., same test at multiple occasions) and in multiple test forms (i.e., item overlap across test forms). The common scale created by the item analysis is a logit scale and an estimate of each participant's ability at each test occasion could be made regardless of which items were administered from which test. McArdle and colleagues (2005) then modeled the development of these cognitive ability estimates with growth curves.

The growth and decline of vocabulary and memory ability was evaluated using structured latent curves with PROC MIXED and NLMIXED in SAS.

The development of vocabulary matched the predicted growth of crystallized intelligence with a sharp increase through childhood and adolescence before decelerating in the twenties, reaching a peak in the late thirties, and showing a small amount of decline into the seventies. Memory ability showed a different developmental pattern, but closely matched previous work with short term memory (McArdle, Ferrer-Caja, Hamagami, & Woodcock, 2002) and fluid intelligence. Memory increased rapidly through adolescence, reaching its maxima in the early twenties before showing a marked decrease through middle and late adulthood. These vocabulary and memory ability estimates from the item analysis are used in this research project.

Age at Measurement
Latent growth curve modelling in a structural modelling framework requires a vector (person level) data file in which there is one record for each participant. In the data file the measurements are grouped into common units of time/age. To create more overlap in testing occasions, two of the measurement occasions in adulthood were grouped together. These occasions are when the participants of the *BGS* and *GS* were 36 and 40, as well as when they were 53 and 54, respectively. Figure 11-1 is a longitudinal plot of the ten occasions of measurement included in the current analysis for (a) vocabulary and (b) memory abilities.

(a)   (b)

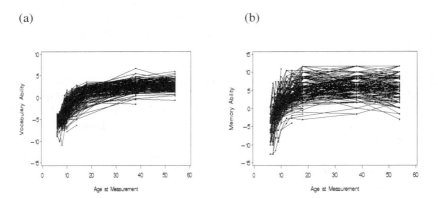

Figure 11-1. Longitudinal plot of (a) vocabulary and (b) memory data for the Berkeley Growth Study and Guidance Study.

11.3 MODELS

Latent Growth Curves

Latent growth curve analysis models the means and covariances of a set of repeated measurements ($Y[1]$ to $Y[t]$) by decomposing the observed scores into a smaller number of factors describing the changes in the measured variable(s) over time. These factors have means describing the average growth over time and variances to allow for individual differences. A latent growth curve model with two growth factors (y_0, y_1) follows the form

$$Y[t]_n = 1 \cdot y_{0n} + B[t] \cdot y_{1n} + e[t]_n \qquad (1)$$

where y_{0n}, $y_{1n} \sim MVN(\mu_0, \mu_1; \sigma_0, \sigma_{0,1}, \sigma_1)$. The uppercase letters denote observed or manifest variables, lowercase letters denote unobserved or latent variables, and the terms denoted by n indicate individual parameters. In this representation, $B[t]$ is the functional relationship of the growth model with time/age, y_0 is the intercept or predicted score when $B[t]=0$, and y_1 is the slope representing the individual's change over time. Figure 11-2 is a structural model of a latent growth curve. In this model there are four occasions of measurement ($Y1-Y4$), two growth factors (y_0, y_1), assumed to be normally distributed having means (μ_0, μ_1), deviations (σ_0, σ_1), and a covariance ($\sigma_0 \cdot \rho_{0,1} \cdot \sigma_1$). The latent variables y_0^* and y_1^* are standardized forms of the growth factors and allow the direct estimation of the correlation between the factors and factor standard deviations instead of the covariance and variances. The loadings from the intercept factor (y_0) are fixed at one, while the pattern of loadings ($B[t]$, basis coefficients) for the slope factor (y_1) determine the shape of the growth curve. The basis coefficients can be restricted to certain values (i.e., 0, 1, 2, 3) based on a theory of change or can be estimated by the data. When the basis coefficients are free to be estimated, it is a latent basis growth model (McArdle & Nesselroade, 2003; Meredith & Tisak, 1990). The latent basis model is the first nonlinear growth model discussed and is a simple nonlinear model that can fit many shapes with one dimension of change. The latent basis model is similar to a spline or segmented growth curve with a knot point at each measurement occasion.

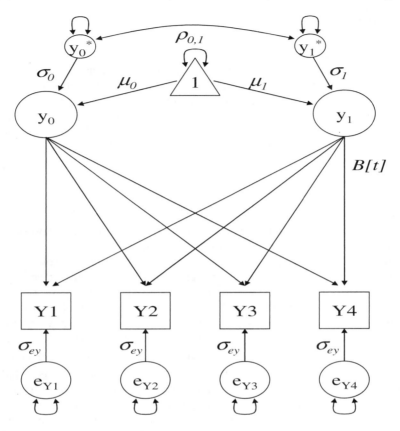

Figure 11-2. Path diagram of a latent growth curve.

There are two main drawbacks of the latent basis model. The first is the lack of structure that does not allow for projections beyond the data and the second is the relatively large increase in parameters as all but two of the slope loadings are estimated. To avoid these drawbacks, growth curves can have a structured nonlinear basis in which the basis coefficients conform to a specified nonlinear function (Browne, 1993; Browne & du Toit, 1991). In these structured curves, we assume the development follows a functional form and estimate the parameters of the function. These nonlinear models tend to be fit in a mixed-effects framework (i.e., SAS PROC NLMIXED) because of the flexibility in programming, but these structured nonlinear models can be fit with structural modeling programs that allow for nonlinear constraints. For example, a simple exponential model has the form

$$Y[t]_n = 1 \cdot y_{0n} + e^{\alpha t} \cdot y_{1n} + e[t]_n. \tag{2}$$

In this structured curve, the basis coefficients, *B[t]*, would be set equal to $e^{\alpha t}$ and α would be estimated.

Latent growth curves can also be used to model the development of multiple variables over time (McArdle, 1988; McCallum, Kim, Malarkey, & Kiecolt-Glaser, 1997). Figure 11-3 is a path diagram of a bivariate growth curve for the measured variables, *X* and *Y*. The repeated variables are decomposed into growth factors (y_0, y_1, x_0, x_1) that model the growth in each of the variables as an underlying function. The bivariate relationships between the variables are the covariances between the growth factors. The covariances among the growth factors convey a limited amount of information (i.e., a positive slope correlation indicates that participants who change more positively in the *X* variables change more positively in the *Y* variable) as these relationships are not time dependent and do not allow for the examination of relationships between the variables over time. A model that permits such investigations are based on <u>latent difference scores</u> (LDS; McArdle, 2001; Hamagami & McArdle, 2001; McArdle & Hamagami, 2001) and are described next.

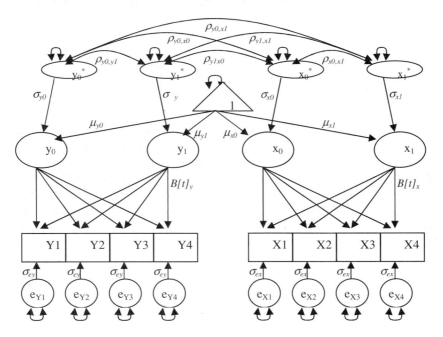

Figure 11-3. Path diagram of a bivariate latent growth curves with correlated growth factors.

Latent Difference Score Growth Modeling

Latent difference score (LDS) growth models can fit several nonlinear shapes and are linear in the parameters, so nonlinear constraints are not necessary. In the LDS model there is an initial true level of ability (y_0) from which a series of true changes occur. The equation for the measured variables, $Y[t]$, in the LDS model is

$$Y[t]_n = y_{0n} + (\sum_{t=1}^{T-1} \Delta y[t]_n) + e[t]_n, \tag{3}$$

where T is the total number of measurement occasions, y_0 is the initial level, $\Delta y[t]$ are the latent differences, and $e[t]$ is a time-dependent residual. In this framework, we also write the equation for the latent differences. In a univariate models discussed here, the latent changes can have two sources: (1) a constant amount from the slope (y_1) with weight α, and (2) an amount proportional to its previous state with weight β. When the latent changes are only predicted by the slope with a weight of 1, the model is equivalent to the linear growth model as a constant amount of change is occurring between consecutive time points. The proportional change model only includes the second source of changes (β) and the dual change model includes both sources of change. The change equation for this model is

$$\Delta y[t]_n = \alpha_y \cdot y_{1n} + \beta_y \cdot y[t-1]_n. \tag{4}$$

The dual change model approximates an exponential curve when the source of change related to its previous state (β) is non-zero. Figure 11-4 is a path diagram of the univariate dual change LDS growth model. In the path diagram, there are four observed variables ($Y1$-$Y4$) comprised of a theoretical true score ($y1$-$y4$) and an error term ($e1$-$e4$). The latent differences ($\Delta y1$-$\Delta y3$) are formed by unit autoregressions of the true scores. The latent intercept (y_0) has a unit loading to the first true score ($y1$), and the latent slope (y_1) has unit loadings to the latent changes ($\Delta y1$-$\Delta y3$).

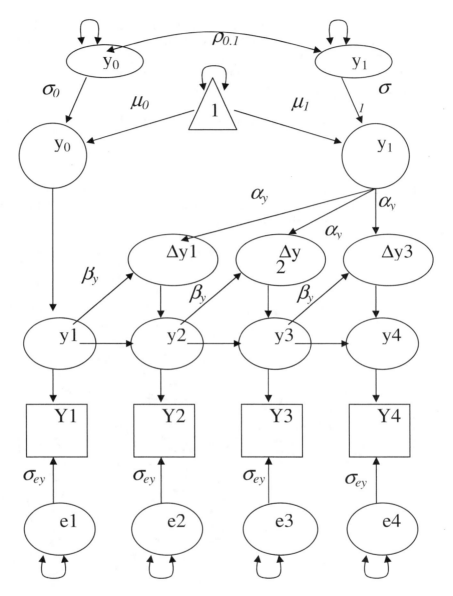

Figure 11-4. Path diagram of a univariate dual change latent difference score growth model.

One of the great benefits of the LDS models is the ability to test for leading and lagging indicators or time dependency in a set of multivariate repeated measures as the changes occurring in one variable, X, can be dependent on the previous state of another variable, Y (see McArdle, 2001 for complete write-up). For example, Figure 11-5 is a bivariate dual change LDS growth model in which the latent differences have three sources (1) a constant amount (y_1, x_1), (2) an amount proportional to the previous state of the variable (β_y, β_x), and (3) an amount proportional to the previous state of the other variable (γ_{yx}, γ_{xy}) as reflected in the change equations

$$\Delta y[t]_n = \alpha_y \cdot y_{1n} + \beta_y \cdot y[t-1]_n + \gamma_{yx} \cdot x[t-1]_n \tag{5}$$

$$\Delta x[t]_n = \alpha_x \cdot x_{1n} + \beta_x \cdot x[t-1]_n + \gamma_{xy} \cdot y[t-1]_n . \tag{6}$$

In these multivariate LDS models, we can test whether there are leading and lagging indicators by testing whether the coupling parameters (γ_{xy}, γ_{xy}) improve the fit of the model.

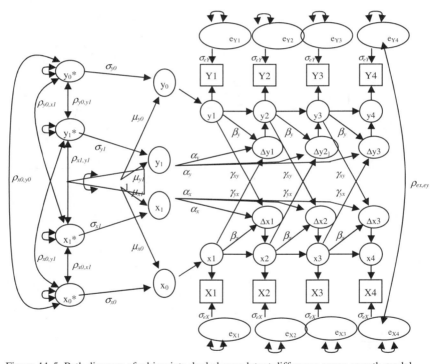

Figure 11-5. Path diagram of a bivariate dual change latent difference score growth model.

Growth Mixture Models

Growth mixture models are an extension of latent growth curve analysis, multiple group structural equation modelling (SEM), and the finite mixture model. Multiple group growth modelling (McArdle, 1989, 1994; McArdle &

Anderson, 1990; McArdle & Epstein, 1987; McArdle & Hamagami, 1996; McArdle & Nesselroade, 2003) is based on multiple group SEM (Joreskog, 1971; Sorbom, 1974) and is utilized to explore differences in estimated parameters between known groups of individuals. Multiple group growth (MGG) models differ from standard multilevel models (MLM) as the grouping variable in MLM is represented as a "fixed effects" regression on the latent growth factors, whereas in MGG models, each group, $g = 1$ to G, follows a latent growth process such that

$$Y[t]_n^{(g)} = 1 \cdot y_{0n}^{(g)} + B[t]^{(g)} \cdot y_{1n}^{(g)} + e[t]_n^{(g)}. \tag{7}$$

In multiple group models, every estimated parameter can differ over groups in a typical application. Multiple group growth models are informative for testing hypotheses about the equality of means (i.e., $\mu_0^{(1)} = \mu_0^{(2)} = \ldots = \mu_0^{(g)}$), variances, covariances, and the invariance of basis coefficients (i.e. $B[t]^{(1)} = B[t]^{(2)} = \ldots = B[t]^{(g)}$; McArdle & Bell, 2000; McArdle and Nesselroade, 2003).

Growth mixture modeling is multiple group growth modeling with one major change: The variable that defines the groupings is unknown. Growth mixture models have the same functional form as the latent growth curve (1) within each of the k ($k = 1$ to K) classes, however there is more than one class, class membership is unknown, and must be estimated. The growth mixture model estimates each participant's probability of membership ($\pi_n^{(k)}$) for each class and this probability of class membership is a multiplier of the growth model for the class. Following McArdle and Nesselroade (2003) and Equation 1, we can write the growth mixture model as

$$Y[t]_n = \sum_{k=1}^{K} \pi_n^{(k)} (1 \cdot y_{0n}^{(k)} + B[t]^{(k)} \cdot y_{1n}^{(k)} + e[t]_n^{(k)}), \tag{8}$$

given

$$\sum_{k=1}^{K} \pi_n^{(k)} = 1$$

and

$$0 \leq \pi_n^{(k)} \leq 1.$$

In linear growth mixture models, researchers tend to look for the clusters of individuals differing in the average level or slope. Other opportunities in linear growth mixture model include groups who differ in variances and covariances; however, the shape of development is the restricted to be linear.

The advantage of nonlinear GMMs is the ability to test for shape differences in development. There has been some work with higher-order polynomial models, but these models are restrictive in shape.

In nonlinear GMMs, the parameters controlling the shape of the growth function (slope loadings) can vary over the latent classes. For example, the estimated basis coefficients in the latent basis growth model, the rate parameter (α) in the exponential model, and the proportional (β) and coupling (γ) parameters in the bivariate LDS dual change model could vary across latent classes. Freeing these parameters in a mixture model allows for investigations, which would not be possible by only considering mean differences in the latent classes. Some of these possibilities in cognitive aging are subpopulations of participants with a differential decline in late adulthood or subpopulations with a stunt in growth during adolescence.

The appropriate sequential strategy for evaluating growth mixture models has not been put forward, but here we follow the principles of factorial invariance studies (i.e., McArdle & Cattell, 1994) as used by McArdle and Hamagami (2005). There are three types of growth mixture models that differ in the parameters allowed to vary across the latent classes. In the first model, the means of the growth factors are free to vary between latent classes (*Means*). The second model also allows all of the variances and covariances to vary between classes (*Means+*) and the final GMM allows the parameters that control the shape of development to vary between classes (*Curves*). This sequential strategy for fitting growth mixture models is a top-down approach. Theoretically, this approach starts with the assumption that there is a single population model (latent growth curve) and we are exploring the data for classes that differ in certain aspects of the population model. A bottom-up approach (*Curves*, *Mean+*, and then *Means*) could be employed with the same models and the same conclusions would arise (as long as the same fit criterion is used).

The three types of growth mixture models have different expectations among the latent classes and some of these models involve a large increase in the number of estimated parameters. The *Means* model is a relatively restrictive model as the variances and covariances of the growth factors and the residual variance must be equivalent between latent classes. In this model (with two growth factors) there are three additional parameters for a two class model; two means for the second class and the threshold parameter. The *Means+* model is less restrictive allowing the variance and covariance parameters to vary between latent classes. The only restriction is the invariance of the basis coefficients and this model carries seven additional parameters (two means, two factor variances, factor covariance, residual variance, and threshold) compared to the growth model. The *Curves* model is the least restrictive model as all estimated parameters in the growth model are allowed to vary between classes. This model tests for different patterns of development in the latent classes and has the greatest number of parameters. This model carries the same seven additional parameters from the *Means+* model plus additional parameters for freeing the basis coefficients. In the latent basis model, it is the number of occasions minus 2; in the exponential model there would be only one additional parameter because the rate parameter controls the basis coefficients.

In the bivariate LDS mixture models, there are interesting theoretical investigations regarding leading and lagging variables that can be evaluated. For example, there are multiple theories regarding the leading indicator of cognitive loss in adulthood. Salthouse (1996) proposed that the speed of processing is the mechanism for cognitive loss whereas Horn (1988) endorsed memory as the leading indicator of losses in fluid intelligence, which portends declines in other cognitive abilities. It could be possible that both of these theories are "partially accurate," because they apply to different groups of people. The groups of people may be different in terms of demographic variables such as gender, educational attainment, or the groups may be different in terms of level of ability. Memory may be a leading indicator of cognitive losses for people with a low level of cognitive ability (i.e., dementia) and speed of processing may be a leading indicator of cognitive loss for people with a higher level of ability. Growth mixture models with multivariate LDS growth models could investigate these differences in cognitive loss.

11.4 ANALYSIS

The analysis begins with fitting a series of linear and nonlinear latent growth curves to the vocabulary and memory data from the *BGS* and *GS*. The growth models are fit to evaluate the overall shape of development for vocabulary and memory, to obtain starting values for the growth mixture models, and to acquire baseline fit statistics for comparison. The nonlinear growth models fit to the vocabulary and memory data include the latent basis, exponential, dual exponential, logistic, logarithmic, and a series of LDS models. Table 11-2 contains the equations for the structured nonlinear growth curves.

Once the best fitting growth model is determined, the series of nonlinear growth mixture models are fit starting with the *Means* model, followed by the *Means+* and the *Curves* models. These models are fit with an increasing number of latent classes until the fit, based on the BIC, does not improve or until convergence problems surface. When the mixture models are concluded, the vocabulary and memory classes are crossed to determine the relationship between the latent classes. This step is the beginning of the bivariate analyses, but this technique does not provide information regarding the leading and lagging indicators between vocabulary and memory abilities.

TABLE 11-2
Equations of Structured Nonlinear Growth Models

Model	Equation
Exponential	$Y[t]_n = y_{0n} + y_{1n} \cdot (\exp(0 \cdot t) - \exp(-\alpha_1 \cdot t)) + e[t]_n$
Dual Exponential	$Y[t]_n = y_{0n} + y_{1n} \cdot (\exp(-\alpha_2 \cdot t) - \exp(-\alpha_1 \cdot t)) + e[t]_n$
*Logistic	$Y[t]_n = y_{1n} / (1 + \exp(-(t - y_2)/y_3)) + e[t]_n$
Logarithmic	$Y[t]_n = y_{0n} + y_{1n} \cdot \ln(t - y_2) + e[t]_n$
Michaelis-Menten	$Y[t]_n = y_{0n} + (y_{1n} \cdot t)/(y_2 + t) + e[t]_n$

*Data was transformed into a percentage score to accommodate the logistic model

The bivariate analyses with LDS models conclude the chapter. A series of bivariate LDS growth models are fit to the vocabulary and memory data to begin these analyses. The models evaluate the coupling between the two variables for the sample as a whole. The first bivariate model does not include any coupling parameters. The bivariate relationships in this model are the correlation of the growth factors and time specific covariance. The second and third model have unidirectional coupling (vocabulary to the change in memory, memory to the change in vocabulary). Finally, both of the coupling parameters are estimated in the same model.

In a next step we examine the bivariate LDS models in a mixture modelling framework and use three types of mixture models. As in the univariate analyses, the first model is the *Means* model in which the means of the growth factors are free. The second model adds free factor variances, factor covariances, residual variance, and time specific covariance. Finally, the third model allows the dynamic parameters (β, γ) to vary in the latent classes. If this third model is the best representation of the data, we may conclude that the latent classes have different developmental processes. The growth models and growth mixture models are all run using the Mplus program version 3.12 (Muthén & Muthén, 1998-2005) and the scripts are available by request.

11.5 RESULTS

Vocabulary

The series of linear and nonlinear growth curves including structured curves (Table 11-2), latent difference score growth models, and the latent basis model were fit to the repeated scores of vocabulary and memory abilities. The fit statistics for the nonlinear growth models for vocabulary ability are contained in table 11-3. The latent basis model was the best fitting model (χ^2 = 597, df = 51, RMSEA = 0.20 (0.18-0.21), BIC = 5057) based on the chi-square, RMSEA, and the BIC. The predicted growth in vocabulary is plotted in Figure 11-6a with a smoother function. There is a strong increase in ability through childhood and adolescence before a deceleration in the growth pattern in early adulthood with no decline into the fifties. However, this model shows an unusual pattern of development between ages seven and eight as there is only a slight improvement in ability. The ages surrounding these show a greater increase in ability for one year of development. The latent basis model is the best fitting model because of this stunt in growth from seven to eight years in age. The structured growth curves can not accommodate this break from a smooth increase in ability. The latent basis model is the baseline model for comparison with the growth mixture models.

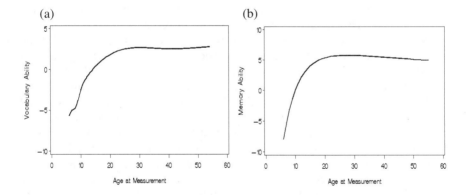

Figure 11-6. Mean predicted developmental pattern for (a) vocabulary and (b) memory.

TABLE 11-3
Fit Statistics for Nonlinear Growth Models for Vocabulary Ability

Model	χ^2/df	RMSEA	BIC
Latent Basis	597/51	0.20 (0.18-0.21)	5057
Exponential	1001/58	0.24 (0.23-0.26)	5422
Dual Exponential	970/57	0.24 (0.23-0.25)	5396
Logistic	918/60	0.23 (0.21-0.24)	5328
Logarithmic	1707/58	0.32 (0.31-0.33)	6128
Michaelis-Menten	1307/57	0.28 (0.27-0.29)	5733
Proportional Change	3193/61	0.43 (0.42-0.44)	7596
Dual Change	1001/58	0.24 (0.23-0.26)	5422

The series of growth mixture models were then fit starting with the two-class *Means* model. This model showed a slight improvement over the latent basis growth model (BIC = 5,052) and moving to three classes (BIC = 5,051) did not further improve the fit. The *Means* models did not show the promise of more classes, so the analysis continued with the *Means+* models. The two-class *Means+* model (BIC = 5,010) fit slightly better than the growth model and the three-class model (BIC = 5,024) fit worse than the two-class model so the *Means+* models were stopped. Finally, the *Curves* models were fit and the BIC had its greatest reduction. The two-class model (BIC = 4,764) reduced the BIC by 246 units over the two-class *Means+* model and the three class model (BIC = 4,741) fit slightly better than the two-class *Curves* model. The BIC is plotted by number of classes and type of growth mixture model in Figure 11-7a and based on this figure the relative increase in fit for the two-class *Curves* model is much greater than the three class model. Therefore, the classes from the two-class model are crossed with the classes from the memory analysis.

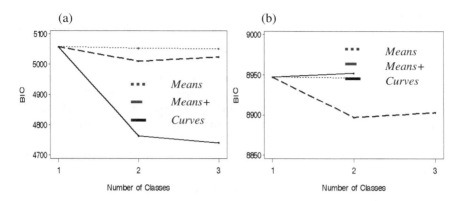

Figure 11-7. Graphical representation of the fit of the growth mixture models. The BIC is plotted against the number of classes for (a) vocabulary and (b) memory.

Because the *Curves* models fit the data the best, the two clusters of people have different patterns of development. The different patterns of development are apparent in Figure 11-8a. The two groups start at approximately the same level of ability, but the first class ($N = 179$) shows a similar stunt in growth between the ages of seven and eight as in the latent basis growth model whereas the second group ($N = 99$) shows a smooth increase in ability through childhood and adulthood. The apparent stunt in growth for the first class is probably due to the children receiving greater scores than deserved on the 1916 Stanford-Binet vocabulary test at six and seven years of age. The researchers conducting the intelligence tests in the *BGS* and *GS* did not always follow the rules for test administration and this could be the cause.

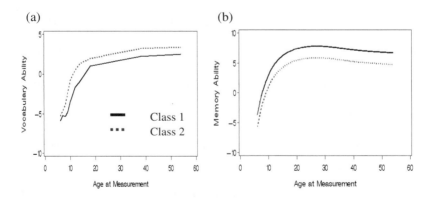

Figure 11-8. Mean predicted developmental patterns of the latent classes for (a) vocabulary and (b) memory.

Memory

As with vocabulary, the latent basis growth model was the best fitting model for the development of memory ability based on the χ^2, but the dual exponential ($\chi^2 = 246$, df = 57, RMSEA = 0.11 (0.09-0.11), BIC = 8947) fit similarly and is a more parsimonious model (Table 11-4). The dual exponential model contains two rate parameters that describe the shape of the curve: the growth and the decline rate. The estimated growth rate was 0.200 and the decline rate was 0.001. The group equation for the dual exponential model is

$$Y[t] = -33.1 + 40.2 \cdot (\exp[t \cdot (-.001)] - \exp[t \cdot (-.200)]) + e[t] \quad (9)$$

and is plotted in Figure 11-6b. The model shows a sharp increase in ability through childhood and adolescence before reaching a plateau in the mid to late twenties and showing a slow decline into the fifties. The dual exponential model is the baseline model for comparison with the growth mixture models.

TABLE 11-4
Fit Statistics for Nonlinear Growth Models for Memory Ability

Model	χ^2/df	RMSEA	BIC
Latent Basis	236/51	0.11 (0.10-0.13)	8971
Exponential	264/58	0.11 (0.10-0.12)	8959
Dual Exponential	246/57	0.11 (0.09-0.12)	8947
Logistic	495/60	0.16 (0.14-0.17)	9174
Logarithmic	881/58	0.22 (0.21-0.23)	9576
Michaelis-Menten	450/57	0.15 (0.14-0.17)	9150
Proportional Change	3510/61	0.44 (0.43-0.44)	12188
Dual Change	264/58	0.11 (0.10-0.12)	8959

The three types of growth mixture models are then fit to the data. The two-class *Means* model (BIC = 8,946) did not improve in the fit, but the two-class *Means+* model (BIC = 8,897) was a slight improvement over the growth model. The three-class *Means+* model (BIC = 8,903) did not further improve the fit. The two-class *Curves* model, in which the two rate parameters of the dual exponential would vary over the latent classes, was then fit and convergence problems were encountered. However, the investigation for different developmental curves was evaluated using the latent basis growth mixture model (two-class BIC = 8,952) and there was no improvement in fit over the two-class *Means+* model. The BIC of the growth mixture models is presented graphically by model type and number of latent classes in Figure 11-7b.

The two latent class trajectories are plotted in Figure 8b. There were 45 participants categorized into Class 1 and 251 participants in Class 2. Class 1 has a greater initial ability and a similar mean slope to Class 2 so the mean performance of the first class is always expected to be greater. However, because the *Means+* model was the best fitting model, the differences between the groups are reflected in the factor covariances and residual variance. Class 1 has greater factor variances and a greater residual variance than Class 2. Therefore Class 1 has greater spread in ability levels and is a more unstable developmental pattern.

Bivariate Analyses

The first bivariate analysis is a cross-table of the latent memory and vocabulary classes obtained from the univariate analyses. The cross-table is calculated on the 274 participants who overlapped in the vocabulary and memory analyses and a chi-square test of association was used to determine whether a relationship existed. The vocabulary classes were moderately associated with the memory classes ($\chi^2 = 7.3$, df = 1, p<.01). This association would probably have been stronger if the memory classes were more defined by differences in the means than in the covariances. The frequencies of the crossed classes are in Table 11-5.

TABLE 11-5
Cross-Table of Vocabulary and Memory Latent Classes

Memory Class	Vocabulary Class		Total
	1 – Low	2 - High	
1 – High	20	23	43
2 - Low	157	74	231
Total	177	97	274

The second set of bivariate analysis uses latent difference score models to evaluate whether memory is a leading indicator of changes in vocabulary and whether this relationship is the same for the entire sample. The series of bivariate latent difference score dual change growth models were fit to the memory and vocabulary data to obtain baseline statistics and to determine if the coupling parameters (γ_{xy}, γ_{yx}) are important for the sample (Table 11-6). The first model had correlated growth factors, zero coupling parameters, and fit the data reasonably well ($\chi^2 = 1391$, df = 211, RMSEA = 0.14 (0.13-0.14), BIC = 14210), but the fit was improved with the addition of coupling parameters. The second model with estimated coupling parameters from vocabulary to changes in memory fits better ($\chi^2 = 1345$, df = 210, RMSEA = 0.13 (0.13 - 0.14), BIC = 14,170) than the no coupling model ($\Delta\chi^2 = 46$, Δdf = 1). However, the model with memory as a leading indicator of vocabulary changes ($\chi^2 = 942$, df = 210, RMSEA = 0.11 (0.10 - 0.12), BIC = 13,767) significantly improved the fit compared to the no coupling model ($\Delta\chi^2 = 449$, Δdf = 1). Finally, the model with bidirectional coupling ($\chi^2 = 932$, df = 209, RMSEA = 0.11 (0.10 - 0.11), BIC = 13,762) fit slightly better than the model with only memory as a leading indicator of changes in vocabulary ($\Delta\chi^2 = 10$, Δdf = 1). In this final model, the changes in memory and vocabulary are based on three latent sources and the change equations for this model are

$$\Delta V[t]_n = \boldsymbol{-0.42} - \boldsymbol{0.35} \cdot V[t-1]_n + \boldsymbol{0.22} \cdot M[t-1]_n, \qquad (10)$$

$$\Delta M[t]_n = \boldsymbol{1.00} - \boldsymbol{0.15} \cdot M[t-1]_n - \boldsymbol{0.06} \cdot V[t-1]_n. \qquad (11)$$

The coupling parameter from memory to changes in vocabulary is significant and large whereas the coupling parameter from vocabulary to changes in memory is significant, but small. Based on the size of the coupling parameters and the improvement in fit, we argue that memory is a leading indicator of changes in vocabulary ability from ages 6 to 54 for the sample. Now we can perform an exploratory search for subgroups of people who have this relationship and subgroups of people who do not have this or possibly have the opposite relationship.

The two-class *Means* model (BIC = 13,783) did not improve the fit over the growth model and neither did the two-class *Means+* (BIC = 13,772) model. Finally, the two-class *Curves* model in which the proportional change (β) and the coupling (γ) parameters were free to vary between latent classes was fit and the BIC (13,763) was not reduced. Therefore, the overall relationship between the development of vocabulary and memory appears to be similar for all of the participants in this study.

TABLE 11-6
Fit Statistics for Bivariate Latent Difference Score Dual Change Growth Models

Model	χ^2/df	RMSEA	BIC
No Coupling	1391/211	0.14 (0.13-0.14)	14210
Vocabulary $\rightarrow$ ΔMemory	1345/210	0.13 (0.13-0.14)	14170
Memory $\rightarrow$ ΔVocabulary	942/210	0.11 (0.10-0.12)	13767
Bivariate Coupling	931/209	0.11 (0.10-0.11)	13762

11.6 DISCUSSION

Summary of Results

Different developmental patterns of cognitive growth and decline were evaluated using nonlinear growth mixture models. The univariate development of vocabulary and short-term memory yielded two latent classes, but were different in their patterning and participant assignment. The two vocabulary classes differed in the mean levels and in the pattern of development. The majority of participants did not show a smooth increase in ability as expected with cognitive development in childhood. For these participants, the predicted level of ability at age 8 was less than the predicted ability at age 7. This interesting developmental trajectory may be indicative of a patterned measurement error in the first two years of standardized cognitive tests (ages 6 and 7). The second vocabulary class followed a relatively smooth growth through childhood and into adulthood.

The development of short-term memory was also seen as two clusters of individuals with an invariant pattern of development and different residual variances. The first class had a slightly greater initial ability at age 6, but was relatively poorly predicted by the dual exponential model. The residual deviation for this group was almost twice that for the second class. The second and most populated class had a slightly lower level and was well predicted by the model. The crossing of latent classes showed a small relationship between the classes in the memory analysis and those in the vocabulary analysis.

Bivariate latent difference score growth and growth mixture models were then fit to the vocabulary and memory data to investigate part of Horn's theory of cognitive decline. The overall growth model showed memory to be leading the way in life-span development of vocabulary ability. Dynamic mixture models were then fit to determine whether this relationship held for all subjects. Allowing the dynamic parameters to differ across latent classes did not improve the fit and therefore it was determined that memory is a leading indicator of the vocabulary changes for the entire sample and there are no subpopulations with distinct developmental processes in this sample.

Model Fit

The fit of the latent growth curves to the vocabulary and memory data is less than ideal (i.e., RMSEA = 0.10 - 0.20) compared with conventional structural equation modeling, where an RMSEA of less than 0.05 indicates a close fit of the model to the data. The higher RMSEA values indicate room for improvement with the modeling of these data leading to two questions. The first question is whether there is another longitudinal model that would capture the observed means and covariances to a greater extent, such as a time-series model. The second question was partially answered in this chapter; whether observed or latent groupings exist in the data. If there are important groups that are not modeled, the fit of the overall model will be less than ideal. In the Berkeley data there were latent classes that improved the overall fit of the model based on the BIC. The RMSEA cannot be calculated for the mixture models as the data likelihood is not known because class membership is unknown.

Concluding Remarks

Growth mixture models are an exciting development in SEM to search for subgroups of people with different developmental patterns. Much of the previous work with GMMs has been limited to polynomial growth functions and this chapter explored a variety of nonlinear growth models that can be analyzed in a mixture framework. Nonlinear growth mixture modeling allows the researcher to investigate whether the developmental patterns conform to a single or to multiple growth functions.

This chapter also explored bivariate growth mixture models within latent difference score models (dynamic mixture models). Multivariate latent difference score models allow for the investigation of leading and lagging indicators in the study of change and incorporating the mixture component allows for different leading and lagging indicators for subgroups of people. This research becomes especially interesting when evaluating time-dependent relationships in a dyadic relationship. For example, if affect is measured in husbands and wives over many days. The growth mixture model can attempt to locate couples in which the affect of the husband drives the wife's and other couples where the affect of wife drives the husband's. Once these models are fit, explanatory variables could be used to predict which class the couple resides.

Every structural equation model can be incorporated into a mixture model giving researchers an interesting and informative exploration of the data. When evaluating these mixture models, it is important to remember the limitations (Bauer & Curran, 2003) as the models are informative for the sample at hand unless the subpopulations can be replicated across studies. Furthermore, mixture models are one way to describe data that are not normally distributed and we should consider why the data are not normal and evaluate alternative distributions (e.g., log-normal) for the data.

REFERENCES

Bauer, D. J., & Curran, P. J. (2003). Distributional assumptions of growth mixture models: Implications for overextraction of latent trajectory classes. *Psychological Methods, 8*, 338–363.

Browne, M. W. (1993). Structured latent curve analysis. In C. M. Cuadras & C. R. Rao (Eds.), *Multivariate analysis: Future directions 2* (pp. 171–197). Amsterdam: Elsevier Science.

Browne, M. W., & du Toit, S. (1991). Models for learning data. In L. M. Collins & J. L. Horn (Eds.), *Best methods for the analysis of change: Recent advances, unanswered questions, future directions* (pp. 47–68). Washington, DC: American Psychological Association.

Cattell, R. B. (1963). Theory of fluid and crystallized intelligence: A critical experiment. *Journal of Educational Psychology, 54*, 1–22.

Hamagami, F., & McArdle, J. J. (2001). Advanced studies of individual differences linear dynamic models for longitudinal data analysis. In G. A. Marcoulides & R. E. Schumacker, (Eds.), *New developments and techniques in structural equation modeling* (pp. 203–246). Mahwah, NJ: Lawrence Erlbaum Associates.

Horn, J. L. (1972). Intelligence: Why it grows, why it declines. In J. M. Hunt (Ed.), *Human intelligence* (pp. 23–31). Oxford, England: Transaction Books.

Horn, J. L. (1988). Thinking about human abilities. In J.R. Nesselroade (Ed.), *Handbook of Multivariate Psychology* (pp. 645–685). New York: Academic Press.

Horn, J. L., & Cattell, R. B. (1966). Refinement and test of the theory of fluid and crystallized general intelligences. *Journal of Educational Psychology, 57*, 253–270.

Horn, J. L., & Cattell, R. B. (1967). Age differences in fluid and crystallized intelligence. *Acta Psychologica, 26*, 107–129.

Jones, C. J. , & Meredith, W. (2000). Developmental paths of psychological health from early adolescence to later adulthood. *Psychology and Aging, 15*, 351–360.

Jöreskog, K. G. (1971). Simultaneous factor analysis in several populations. *Psychometrika, 36*, 409–426.

McArdle, J. J. (1986). Latent variable growth within behavior genetic models. *Behavior Genetics, 16*, 163–200.

McArdle, J. J. (1988). Dynamic but structural equation models of repeated measures data. In J. R. Nesselroade & R. B. Cattell (Eds.), *The handbook of multivariate experimental psychology* (Vol. 2, pp. 561–614). New York: Plenum.

McArdle, J. J. (1989). A structural modeling experiment with multiple growth functions. In R. Kanfer, P. L. Ackerman & R. Cudeck (Eds.), *Abilities, motivation, and methodology: The Minnesota Symposium on Learning and Individual Differences* (pp. 71–117). Hillsdale, NJ: Erlbaum.

McArdle, J. J. (1994). Structural factor analysis experiments with incomplete data. *Multivariate Behavioral Research, 29*, 409–454.

McArdle, J. J. (2001). A latent difference score approach to longitudinal dynamic structural analyses. In R. Cudeck, S. du Toit & D. Sorbom (Eds.), *Structural equation modeling: Present and future* (p. 342–380). Lincolnwood, IL: Scientific Software International.

McArdle, J. J., & Anderson, E. (1990). Latent variable growth models for research on aging. In J. E. Birren & K. W. Schaie (Eds.), *Handbook of the psychology of aging* (3rd ed., pp. 21–44). San Diego, CA: Academic Press.

McArdle, J. J., & Bell, R. Q. (2000). An introduction to latent growth models for developmental data analysis. In T. D. Little & K. U. Schnabel (Eds.), *Modeling longitudinal and multilevel data: Practical issues, applied approaches, and specific examples*, (pp. 69–107). Mahwah, NJ: Lawrence Erlbaum Associates.

McArdle, J. J., & Cattell, R. B. (1994). Structural equation models of factorial invariance in parallel profiles and oblique confactor problems. *Multivariate Behavioral Research, 29*, 63–113.

McArdle, J. J., & Epstein, D. (1987). Latent growth curves within developmental structural equation models. *Child Psychology, 58*, 110–133.

McArdle, J. J., Ferrer-Caja, E., Hamagami, F., & Woodcock, R. W. (2002). Comparative longitudinal structural analyses of the growth and decline of multiple intellectual abilities over the life span. *Developmental Psychology, 38*, 115 – 142.

McArdle, J. J., Grimm, K. J., Hamagami, F., Bowles, R. P., & Meredith, W. (2005). *Modeling non-repeated measures using longitudinal structural equations.* Unpublished manuscript, University of Southern California, Los Angeles, CA.

McArdle, J. J., & Hamagami, F. (1996). Multilevel models from a multiple group structural equation perspective. In G. A. Marcoulides & R. E. Schumacker (eds.), Advanced structural equation modelling: Issues and techniques (pp. 89–124). Mahwah, NJ: Lawrence Erlbaum Associates.

McArdle, J. J., & Hamagami, F. (2001). Latent difference score structural models for linear dynamic analyses with incomplete longitudinal data. In L. M. Collins & A. G. Sayer (Eds.), *New methods for the analysis of change.* (pp. 139–175). Washington, DC: APA.

McArdle, J. J., & Hamagami, F. (2005). *Multiple group modeling of linear dynamic structural equation systems applied to the Health and Retirement Study (HRS) data.* Unpublished manuscript, University of Southern California, Los Angeles, CA.

McArdle, J. J., & Nesselroade J. R. (2003). Growth curve analysis in contemporary psychological research. In J. A. Schinka & W. F. Velicer (Eds), *Handbook of psychology: Research methods in psychology* (Vol. 2, pp. 447–480). New York: Wiley.

McCall, R. B. Appelbaum, M. I., & Hogarty, P. S. (1973). Developmental changes in mental Performance. *Monographs of the Society for Research in Child Development*, 38(3), 1–85.

McCallum, R. C., Kim, C., Malarkey, W. B., & Kiecolt-Glaser, J. K. (1997). Studying multivariate change using multilevel models and latent curve models. *Multivariate Behavioral Research*, *32*, 215–253.

Meredith, W., & Tisak, J. (1990) Latent curve analysis. *Psychometrika*, *55*(1), 107–122.

Muthén, B. O., & Muthén, L. K. (2000). Integrating person-centered and variable-centered analysis: Growth mixture modeling with latent trajectory classes. *Alcoholism: Clinical and Experimental Research*, *24*, 882 – 891.

Muthén, L. K., & Muthén, B. O. (1998–2005). *Mplus user's guide* (3rd ed.). Los Angeles, CA: Muthén & Muthén.

Muthén, B., & Shedden, K. (1999). Finite mixture modeling with mixture outcomes using the EM algorithm. *Biometrics*, *55*, 463–469.

Nagin, D. S. (1999). Analyzing developmental trajectories: A semiparametric, group-based approach. *Psychological Methods, 4*, 139–157.

Rao, C. R. (1958). Some statistical methods for comparison of growth curves. *Biometrics, 14*, 1–17.

Salthouse, T. A. (1996). The processing-speed theory of adult age differences in cognition. *Psychological Review, 103*, 403–428.

Spearman, C. (1904). 'General intelligence,' objectively determined and measured. *American Journal of Psychology. 15*, 201–293.

Sörbom, D. (1974). A general method for studying differences in factor means and factor structure between groups. *British Journal of Mathematical and Statistical Psychology*, *27*, 229–239.

Terman, L. M. (1916). *The measurement of intelligence.* Boston, MA: Houghton-Mifflin.

Terman, L. M., & Merrill, M. A. (1937). *Measuring intelligence.* Boston, MA: Houghton Mifflin.

Tucker, L. R (1958). Determination of parameters of a functional relation by factor analysis. *Psychometrika*, *23*, 19–23.

Tucker, L. R (1966). Learning theory and multivariate experiment: Illustration by determination of generalized learning curves. In R. B. Cattell (Ed.), *Handbook of multivariate experimental psychology* (pp. 476–501). Chicago, IL: Rand McNally.

Wechsler, D. (1946). *The Wechsler-Bellevue Intelligence Scale.* New York: The Psychological Corporation.

Wechsler, D. (1955). *Manual for the Wechsler Adult Intelligence Scale.* New York: The Psychological Corporation.

Wechsler, D. (1981). *WAIS-R manual.* New York: The Psychological Corporation.

Wohlwill, J. F. (1973). *The study of behavioral development.* Oxford, England: Academic Press.

Woodcock, R. W., & Johnson, M. B. (1989). *Woodcock-Johnson Psycho-Educational Battery - Revised.* Allen, TX: DLM Teaching Resources.

Chapter 12

Longitudinal Multilevel Modelling: a Comparison of Growth Curve Models and Structural Equation Modelling using Panel Data from Germany

Uwe Engel, Alexander Gattig, and Julia Simonson

University of Bremen, Germany

12.1 INTRODUCTION

Panel data have become of increasing importance in the social sciences. One of their main advantages is the possibility to make causal inferences based on longitudinal data. Consequently, by now there exists a huge amount of literature on modelling techniques for panel data (e.g., Baltagi, 2001; Engel & Reinecke 1994). An early approach was to analyse growth curve models for panel data in a MANOVA repeated measures design (e.g., Potthoff & Roy, 1964; Rao, 1965). Another related option is to make use of the multi-level method to estimate growth curve models (Bryk & Raudenbusch, 1992, pp. 130; Engel, 1998, pp. 113; Hox, 2002, pp. 73; Maas & Snijders, 2003). Further authors started applying the structural equation approach for modeling latent curve models for longitudinal data (e.g., Engel & Reinecke, 1994; Hox, 2002, pp. 263; Meredith & Tisak, 1990; Reinecke, 2005).

Recently, there has been much discussion as to whether panel data is best being modelled within a multilevel approach by growth curve models, or within a structural equation approach by latent growth curve models and how these two methods are linked (e.g., Hox, 2002; Willett, 1997; Willett & Keiley 2000).

In this chapter, both approaches are used for modelling panel data with a *genuine multilevel structure*, that is in our case the structure time i < persons j < households k. We explain how the two techniques are suited to analyze panel data with a real multilevel structure, how they are related, what the respective advantages and drawbacks are, and how one can be transformed into the other.

In addition, we empirically compare both methods by using panel data from the Federal Republic of Germany (German Socio-Economic Panel - GSOEP). In substantial terms, we focus on the effects of status inconsistency at the individual level and on the effects of status incongruence at the household level.

The chapter is structured as follows: First, we explain the two different modelling approaches and how one can be transformed into the other, second, we introduce the data and elaborate on the substantial arguments and the respective index constructions to measure status inconsistency and status incongruence, and third, we report the empirical results for both modelling approaches. Finally, we draw a short conclusion about the major benefits and drawbacks of the two different modelling approaches.

12.2 MULTILEVEL ANALYSIS FOR PANEL DATA: LINEAR GROWTH CURVE MODELLING

Multilevel modelling offers important advantages over traditional analytic strategies that ignore the multilevel structure of data. By taking the hierarchical data structure into account, in contrast to conventional statistical methods, multilevel techniques do not lean on the assumption of independence of observations, which is violated if we have hierarchically structured data. Therefore standard errors for hierarchical data can be estimated correctly by using multilevel models. In addition, in multilevel models, variables measured on different levels can be analyzed simultaneously in an adequate way, and cross-level interaction effects can be estimated.

In current social research, there is ample use of multilevel modelling. These methods have been employed in a variety of settings, including research on educational performance, public health, or in the analysis of voting behaviour (see Engel & Simonson, in press) for an empirical assessment of the areas where this method is most prominent).

One option for modelling repeatedly measured data in general and panel data in particular is a special form of multilevel analysis: Linear growth curve modelling. Table 12-1 summarizes the typical data structure for panel data. The data comprise information for ten persons (*no*), three waves (t_1, t_2, t_3), one dependent variable available for all three waves ('y_1'), two independent variables available for all waves (x_1, x_2), and a time-constant variable (x_0). The first subscript indexes the variable and the second subscript indexes the wave.

TABLE 12-1
Structure of Panel Data With Additional Context Information

no.	id3	id2	t_1			t_2			t_3			$t.$
			y_{11}	x_{11}	x_{21}	y_{12}	x_{12}	x_{22}	y_{13}	x_{13}	x_{23}	$x_{0.}$
1	1	1	..	..	..	..	..					
2	1	2	..	..	..	..						
3	1	3	..	..								
4	1	4	..	..								
5	1	5	..									
6	1	6										..
7	2	1									..	..
8	2	2									..	..
9	2	3							..	..	..	..
10	2	4					..		..	..	..	..

In this table, one line represents one individual, identified by variable *id*. Variable *id3* provides information on the specific context of an individual, such as membership in a joint household. For example, in the previous table individuals 1 to 6 are members of the same household (context); the same holds for individuals 7 to 10. This context information allows the use of multilevel modelling by linking elements of level *n* with the accompanying elements of level *n + 1*.

When using the latent growth curve modelling approach described in detail later, we will use a data matrix as described in Table 12-1, however, for 'linear growth curve modelling' we will have to rearrange the data matrix as described in Table 12-2. Recoding can be done by using relatively simple routines available in standard statistical software such as SPSS or in multilevel software as MLwiN (Rasbash et al. 2000). In Table 12-2, lines have been transposed into columns, such that lines now represent time-points within persons and for each wave there exists an additional line. Hence, we added another variable *id1* to identify the particular time-point, that is, in our case the particular wave. This results in a hierarchical data structure: "time-point i < person j < context k". The time-constant variable x_0 in this structure has to be extended across the respective time-points of the individual and consequently has to be replicated accordingly.

TABLE 12-2
Rearranged Data Structure For Growth Curve Modelling

no.	id3	id2	id1 (t)	y_1	x_1	x_2	x_0
1	1	1	1	y_{11}	x_{11}	x_{21}	$x_{0.}$
2	1	1	2	y_{12}	x_{12}	x_{22}	$x_{0.}$

3	1	1	3	y_{13}	x_{13}	x_{23}	$x_{0.}$
4	1	2	1	y_{11}	x_{11}	x_{21}	$x_{0.}$
5	1	2	2	y_{12}	x_{12}	x_{22}	$x_{0.}$
6	1	2	3	y_{13}	x_{13}	x_{23}	$x_{0.}$
7	1	3	1	..	..	..	..
8	1	3	2	..	..	..	..
9	1	3	3	..	..	..	..
10	1	4	1				
11	1	4	2				
12	1	4	3				
13	1	5	1				
14	1	5	2				
15	1	5	3				
16	1	6	1				
17	1	6	2				
18	1	6	3				
19	2	1	1				
20	2	1	2				
21	2	1	3				
22	2	2	1				
23	2	2	2				
24	2	2	3				
25	2	3	1				
26	2	3	2				
27	2	3	3	..	..	..	..
28	2	4	1	..	..	..	..
29	2	4	2	..	..	..	..
30	2	4	3	..	..	..	..

In growth curve modelling level 1 usually represents the time dimension; it therefore contains the time-varying characteristics of an individual. Level 2 represents the individual and its time-constant characteristics. The third level k represents time-constant characteristics of the aggregate, time-varying characteristics of the aggregate are covariates at level 1. This approach allows for flexible modelling (see Maas & Snijders, 2003) as well as simple estimates of nonlinear time effects (by using polynoms). It also has the advantage that it does not require that for each person there has to be an identical number of repeated measures, thereby relaxing the problem of missing data caused by panel attrition (see Engel, 1998, chapters 4.1 and 6). According to Marsh and Hau (2002), however, it is vulnerable against regression toward the mean artifacts likewise other analyzing strategies.

In our examples, as described in detail later, y_1 is satisfaction with household income, x_1 is a time-varying characteristic (individual status inconsistency with respect to education/income), x_2 is a time-constant index for education, that is number of years spent in the educational system, the status incongruence variables x_3 and x_4 are variables that contain information at the context level, whether the subject lives in a single household and whether there is relational status incongruence. In addition, we could introduce x_0 as a time-constant individual characteristic.

The model is defined by the following Level 1, Level 2, and Level 3 equations,

$$y_{ijk} = b_{0jk} + b_t t_{ijk} + b_1 x_{1ijk} + b_3 x_{3ik} + b_4 x_{4ik} + e_{ijk} \tag{1}$$

$$b_{0jk} = b_{0k} + b_2 x_{2jk} + u_{0jk} \tag{2}$$

$$b_{0k} = b_0 + u_{0k} \tag{3}$$

In this model, random effects are allowed for the intercept but not for the slopes (random intercept model), inserting (3) in (2) and (2) in (1) results in (4)

$$y_{ijk} = b_0 + b_t t_{ijk} + b_1 x_{1ijk} + b_2 x_{2jk} + b_3 x_{3ik} + b_4 x_{4ik} + u_{0k} + u_{0jk} + e_{ijk} \tag{4}$$

The respective subscripts denote that the aggregate variables x_3 and x_4 vary by time i and context k but not within person j. In this model, e_{ijk} is a normally distributed random variable with zero mean and homogeneous variances across contexts.

$$e_{ijk} \approx N(0, \sigma_e^2) \tag{5}$$

In addition, it is assumed that the residuals on Level 1 are uncorrelated with the Level 2 residuals. Additional information on model assumptions and model variants can be obtained from Bryk and Raudenbush (1992), Goldstein (1995) or Snijders and Bosker (1999).

For an extension of multilevel modelling for categorical dependent variables, see also Snijders und Bosker (1999). For a discussion of the problems associated with obtaining robust parameters from different quasilikelihood procedures, see Guo and Zhao (2000). As in the text, models for the analysis of categorical data can also be applied to the analysis of latent variables, such as by using Mplus. The question of how to arrive at robust parameter estimates is a reoccurring theme in multilevel analysis. MLwiN, for example, allows for the possibility to estimate models based on the RIGLS/IGLS criterion [(Restricted) Iterative Generalized Least Squares]. Whereas the IGLS algorithm is based on a full information maximum likelihood procedure, by which regression coefficients are assumed to be known, the RIGLS algorithm is a restricted maximum likelihood method, by which regression coefficients are assumed unknown. In addition, the Bayesian Markov Chain Monte Carlo (MCMC) procedure, which can be used for the estimation of variances when the sample size is small, likewise quasi likelihood and bootstrap procedures are possible (among others, Blien, 2001, 159-163; Goldstein, 1995, 21-24 provide additional information concerning IGLS procedures). Further reading concerning the generalization of the standard IGLS estimation procedures into CIGLS (Conditioned Iterative Generalized Least Square Estimation) is provided by Blien and Wiedenbeck (2002). With the CIGLS algorithm, coefficients can be calculated even if exogenous variables and residuals are correlated (Blien & Wiedenbeck, 2002, 322).

The question of how to deal with time-varying covariates at the aggregate might pose a particular technical problem. Consider the hierarchical data structure time i < persons j < households k, a person for whom household membership has changed during the four waves (in fact this happened for 4.7% of the sample). In a data structure such as that displayed in Table 12-2 used for growth curve modelling, this is unproblematic because for each time-point, only the characteristics at the individual and the aggregate level enter the data matrix but not the context information on which these characteristics are based. This context information might change over time and thus for an individual, the contextual information might change as well. This change does not affect model estimates.

Another remarkable point is the change of level-IDs over time in multilevel modelling. For our analyses, the household number, which was registered for a person at the last panel wave, was taken as household identifier, irrespective of whether a person changed the household during the observation time or not. In the ideal case, the household affiliation at each time point should serve as household identifier. This is possible with the data of the socioeconomic panel and by the use of common multilevel software such as MLwiN, but leads to a so-called cross-classified structure of the data, whereby the complexity and the storage volume of the data are clearly increased. For that reason, we used a time constant identifier. First, comparison analyses point out that by use of a constant identifier, the explainable variance on the household level is very easily underestimated compared to the use of time changing identifiers, but estimates of effects are not.

Sometimes the program to be used for analysis expects a sorting of cases according to the level-IDs that correspond to the hierarchical data structure (in our example: "time i < persons j < households k"). If this requirement is met by sorting the data according the household-IDs of the last measurement time-point while the individual characteristics follow the exact measurement points, this is problematic: Now the aggregate characteristics of a given context might vary across its members, if these members had been associated with other contexts, such as household, at other time points.

In our experience, this will become problematic if contexts within the structural equation approach are created by use of the "cluster" variable. In this case, variables might be defined as aggregate variables that, contrary to expectations, do not display constant values. A possible remedy for this problem might be the substitution of such nonconstant values by their mean value, if this can be justified theoretically.

12.3 STRUCTURAL EQUATION MODELLING: LATENT GROWTH CURVES AND CURVES FACTORS

Latent growth curve modelling is part of the structural equation modelling approach. To understand why this approach deals with latent growth curve models consider a simple growth curve model consisting of only two levels, time-points and individuals. We therefore leave out all information of the aggregate level and obtain a model time-point $i <$ person j. This model next to b_0 contains only the linear time effect b_t. For both fixed effects, the model allows for random components such that the intercept-slope covariance between them can be estimated. In analogy to Equations 1 to 5, the data structure described in Table 12-2 results in Equations 6 to 9:

$$y_{ij} = b_{0j} + b_{tj}t_{ij} + e_{ij} \qquad (6)$$

$$b_{0j} = b_0 + u_{0j} \qquad (7)$$

$$b_{tj} = b_t + u_{tj} \qquad (8)$$

$$y_{ij} = b_0 + b_t t_{ij} + u_{0j} + u_{tj}t_{ij} + e_{ij} \qquad (9)$$

and the estimates of the fixed effects b_0 und b_t. The variance components of the associated random effects are displayed in Equation 10:

$$\text{var}(u_{0j}) = \sigma_{u0}^2 \qquad \text{var}(u_{tj}) = \sigma_{ut}^2 \qquad \text{cov}(u_{0j}, u_{tj}) = \sigma_{u0t} \qquad (10)$$

These values can also be estimated in a model where random effects are understood as latent variables. This model in turn is based on Table 12-1. For each of the involved observation points and y indicators the model looks like that depicted in Figure 12-1 (see Chou, Bentler, & Pentz, 1998, for a detailed account of how the parameters in both approaches correspond; in addition, they translate the entries in terms generally used within structural equation modelling). Intercept b_0 and slope b_t are estimated as means of the latent factors that are related to four y indicators as displayed in Figure 12-1. All paths that relate the intercept to the indicators are fixed to one. The paths that relate the indicators with the slope are fixed to the time points of the respective observations. In our example, these observations reflect time since start of the panel in years. Simultaneously the variances of the errors are considered to be time-homogeneous: $\sigma^2(e_1)=...=\sigma^2(e_4)$.

The model is specified such that it specifies mean values k of the latent factors (see Bollen, 1989, pp. 306, or Hayduk, 1987, pp. 291 for extensive descriptions of the structural equations approach with mean values of latent variables and intercepts). In Figure 12-1 these are labelled as b_0 and b_t because they are equivalent with the estimates for the growth curve model in Equation 9. We obtain the estimates for the Level 2 variance components in Equation 10 by use of the variance/covariance matrix Φ.
In both modelling strategies, one can include time-varying or time-constant covariates. One option is to estimate the influence of time-varying covariates on y_t time-dependently $(x_t \rightarrow y_t;\ t=0, 1, 2, 3)$.

Figure 12-1. Example of a latent growth curve model.

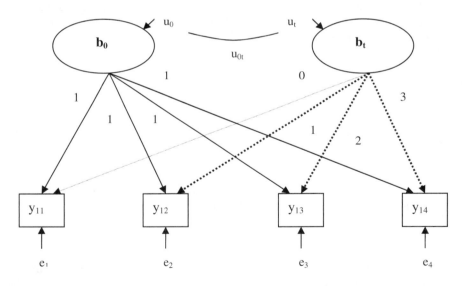

Figure 12-2 sketches a latent growth curve model with three covariates x_1, x_0, and g_1. It is assumed that the four measurement points for the individual level variable x_1 indicate a predominantly time-constant variable. Likewise, the four measurements of g_{1t} indicate a basically time-constant group-level variable. Both variables themselves represent latent constructs and we consider their possible influence on b_0 and b_t, , that is, the initially mean y value and its expected change over time. On the other hand, x_0 is an observed and completely time-constant variable. Intercept b_0 and slope b_t again are estimated as means of the latent factors that are related to four y indicators. The paths that relate the intercept to the indicators are fixed to one. The paths that relate the indicators with the slope are fixed to the time points of the respective observations.

Figure 12-2. Example of a latent growth curve model with covariates.

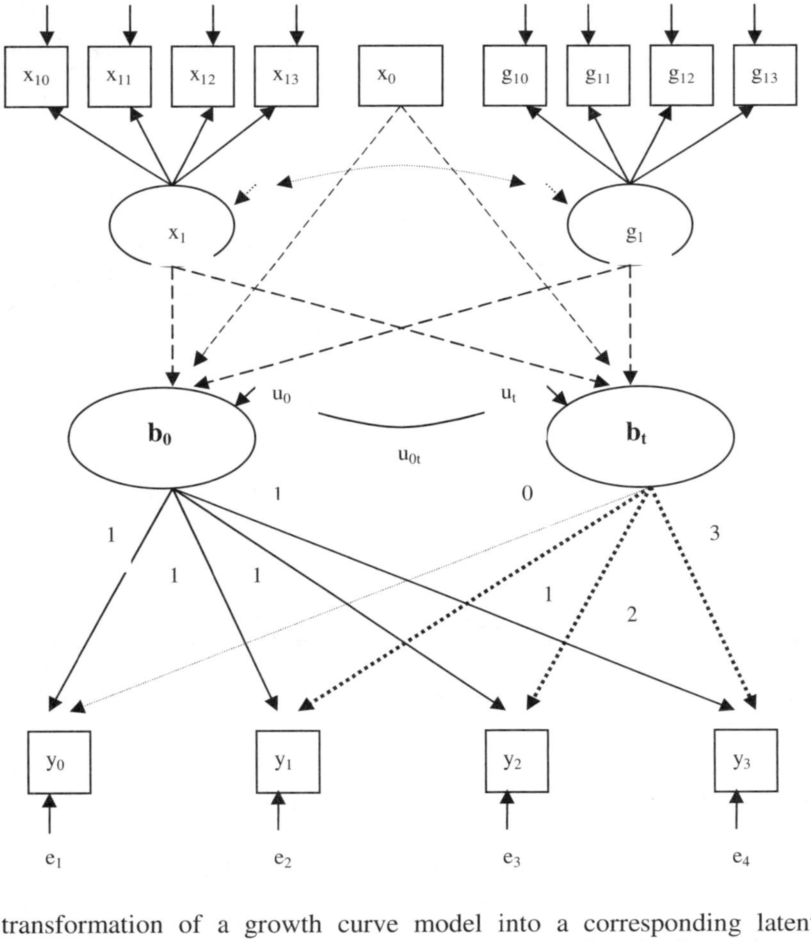

A transformation of a growth curve model into a corresponding latent growth curve model might be useful for two reasons: first, it allows the researcher to fully exploit the various possibilities in structural equation modelling for model fit assessment and second, it enables to estimate models with *multiple indicators*. This may be quite useful to control for random measurement errors.

Figure 12-3. Example of a curves of factor model.

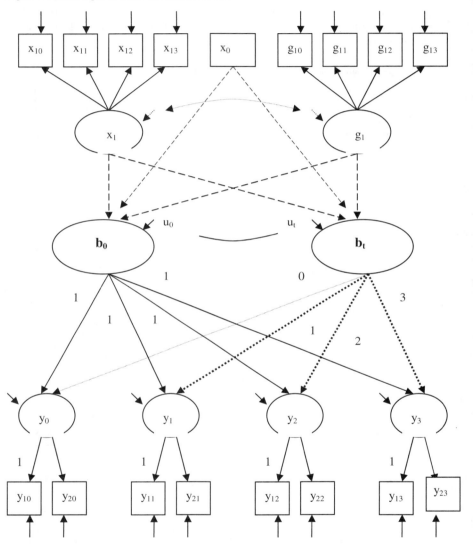

Figure 12-3 illustrates this point using a model for our four-wave panel data. We now have a so-called *curves of factor model* that measures latent factors for substantive terms on Level 1 and factors for temporal growth on Level 2 (Duncan et al., 1999; Reinecke, 2005).

The y variable is now measured by two indicators in each wave. The loadings of the first indicator are fixed to one. The loadings of the second indicator are restricted to be equal over time. The model specification does not apply to these indicators but to the latent variable y_t ($t = 0, 1, 2, 3$).

In the model displayed in Figure 12-3 likewise in Figure 12-2 it is assumed that the four measurement points for the individual level variable x_1 indicate a time-constant variable on the whole and the four measurements of g_{lt} indicate a group-level variable. Both variables themselves represent latent constructs and we consider their possible influence on b_0 and b_t. A time-constant, manifest independent variable is indexed as x_0.

12.4 DATA AND VARIABLES: STATUS INCONSISTENCY AND RELATIONAL STATUS INCONGRUENCE

We estimated both types of models with data for the Federal Republic of Germany (German Socio-Economic Panel - GSOEP). The GSOEP is a wide-ranging representative longitudinal study of private households. It provides information on all household members, consisting of Germans living in the Old and New German States, foreigners, and recent immigrants to Germany. The panel was started in 1984. In 2003, there were more than 12,000 households, and nearly 24,000 persons sampled. The data include topics such as household composition, occupational biographies, employment, earnings, and health and satisfaction indicators. In our chapter, we restrict the analysis to four waves (1998–2001), although it could easily be enlarged to include a longer timespan.

We use a balanced design, which means only persons who take part in all four waves are included in our sample. So we have a sample of 11,273 persons. Anyhow, for some persons, we do not have information about the substantive variables for all time points. Therefore, due to item-nonresponse we get a sample with varying numbers of observations at different time points. The 44,062 observations are distributed to the four measurement points as follows:

TABLE 12-3

Observations Per Year

Year	1998	1999	2000	2001	Total
Observations	10,830	10,956	11,130	11,146	44,062

In substantial terms, we focus on the effects of status inconsistency and status incongruence. Status inconsistency is defined as a difference within an individual between several aspects, which comprise status, for example income and education. People with high income and low education (or the other way round) are defined as status inconsistent, people who are either high or low on both characteristics are defined as status consistent (Blau, 1981). In our chapter status inconsistency is not, as is often done, defined in terms of deviations from equality, but as deviations from expected achievements. That is, whereas the former approach would classify someone with high educational achievements and a low income as status inconsistent, our approach does not necessarily do so. In case the composition of high educational achievements and a low income is what is usually expected for certain societal groups, for example people of a certain age, sex or nationality, this does not necessarily form a status inconsistency. Instead, we define a configuration as inconsistent if a specific status composition departs from what can be expected in a society at a given time. To determine what can be expected, we assume that what is to be expected is what typically occurs. This very well may be a state that diverges from equality.

In addition, we assume that these expectations are conditional. That is, people make comparisons with specific reference groups. These comparisons are based, among other things, on the investments that an individual has undertaken in the past. To give an example, if in a given cohort despite relatively high investments, that is educational certificates, it is not unusual to have relatively low professional achievements; this according to our definition does not constitute status inconsistency. Educational credentials will generally be the most important investments due to their influence on occupational positions and the accompanying gratifications. In the following, we measure educational achievements by the number of years an individual has spent within the educational system. To account for our argument that expectations are dependent on specific reference groups, we created 12 reference groups based on combinations of the following criteria: Nationality (German: yes/no), sex (m/f), and labor market status (working/retired/other nonworking).

We then ran regressions where we calculated the influence of education on income conditional on the specific reference groups. Status inconsistency then is defined as the difference between estimated and observed income divided by the standard deviation of residuals in the respective groups. Our index therefore becomes positive if the income is higher than what could be expected for a given group and negative if the income is lower.

Status consistency is a property of individuals. Such individuals often form groups within larger contexts, such as, households, schools, and so forth. Membership in such groups is increasingly often reflected in available data sets. For households including two or more persons, we therefore can investigate whether there is status incongruence, that is, whether both household members are status consistent or inconsistent. It should be noted that a household with two members does not exhibit status incongruence if both household members are status inconsistent in the same way. We built an index for status incongruence that takes into account the overall distance of the complete set of the respective status inconsistencies. The index is based on its numerical value because it is irrelevant which household member is defined as Individual 1 and who is defined as Individual 2.

To classify households according to their degree of incongruence, we took household size and number of classified people within the household into account. These two quantities are only identical in the absence of missing values. To calculate the degree of incongruence within a household, we calculated all $k*(k-1)/2$ distances between the k household members, which could be classified. We then took the average of these distances for each household.

We estimate effects of status incongruence on two dependent variables: satisfaction with the respective household income and satisfaction with the own socio-economic position.

12.5 RESULTS

We now report the results of different models. We begin with a two-level model with the data structure time point i within person j and a corresponding latent growth model that is exactly the same type of model as displayed in Figure 12-1. Dependent variable is satisfaction with household income. We use four waves (1998–2001) from the GSOEP data. Estimating a growth curve model with MLwiN based on Equation 9 after rearranging the data according to the structure displayed in Table 12-2 [n_1 = 44.062] resulted in the estimates displayed in the left hand side of Table 12-4.[1] The corresponding latent growth curve model [n = 10.527] based on a data structure as displayed in Table 12-1, estimated with LISREL 8.54 (see Jöreskog et al., 2001) and the specifications given in the previous text resulted in nearly the same parameters presented in the right hand sight of Table 12-4. The value for constant b_0 (= 6,125 resp. 6,126), gives the estimated y value in case t is zero. The time index t starts with zero for t_1 (t = 0, 1, 2, 3). This is done in order to get an initial value while expected change per unit time is expressed by b_t. For both models, satisfaction with household income rises slightly over time. Obviously both modelling strategies lead to nearly the same results. Subsequently, in case of modelling growth curves without taking covariates into account, both approaches are equally good. Nevertheless both methods offer different options to extend this basic model.

---

[1] As the estimation procedure in this model like in all other models estimated by MLwiN, we used the IGLS (Iterative Generalized Least Squares) criterion.

TABLE 12-4

Results of a Growth Curve Model and a Corresponding Latent Growth Curve Model

	Satisfaction with household income			
	growth curve model		*latent growth curve model*	
	b	*s.e*	*b*	*s.e*
Constant b_0	6,125	0,020	6,126	0,021
Time b_t	0,098	0,007	0,098	0,007
	Variance components			
$\Sigma^2(u_0)$	3,322	0,063	3,350	0,064
$\sigma^2(u_t)$	0,118	0,007	0,122	0,007
$\sigma(u_{0t})$	-0,238	0,017	-0,248	0,017
$\sigma^2(e)$	1,800	0,017	1,74	0,017

In the following table we present the results of a latent growth curve model with covariates, estimated with LISREL 8.54 and a corresponding 3-Level linear growth curve model, estimated by use of the multilevel software MLwiN. As we expected the two modelling approaches again lead to almost the same results.

TABLE 12-5

Results of a 3-Level Growth Curve Model and a Corresponding Latent Growth Curve Model With Covariates

	Satisfaction with household income			
	3-Level-growth curve model* [n_1=44.062]		*latent growth curve model** [n=10.527]*	
	b	s.e	b	s.e
Constant b_0	5,666	0,075	5,667	0,075
Time b_t	0,108	0,006	0,108	0,006
Individual SI (x_1)	0,047	0,009	0,047	0,009
HH-status-incongruence (g_1)	0,102	0,014	0,102	0,014
Single–HH/no comp. possible (g_2)	-0,302	0,040	-0,302	0,040
Education in years (x_0)	0,037	0,006	0,037	0,006
	Variance components			
$\Sigma^2(v_0)$ [household level]	2,491	0,054	2,491	0,054
$\sigma^2(u_0)$ [individual level]	0,289	0,017	0,289	0,017
$\sigma^2(e)$ [occasion level]	1,999	0,016	1,999	0,016

* estimated using MLwiN 2.0; ** estimated using LISREL 8.54

For each of the panel waves we created measures described in detail for individual status inconsistency with respect to education and income and relational status incongruence at the household level. The value for constant, b_0 (= 5,667), gives the estimated y value in case all t and x variables are restricted to zero. Because in this interpretation the covariates have to be taken into account, b_0 gives the initial y value for people who are status consistent ($x_1 = 0$) within status congruent households ($x_3 = 0$, $x_4 = 0$) and zero years of education ($x_2 = 0$). Contrary to the former values, zero years spent in the educational system are empirically impossible, therefore $b_0 = 5,667$ has to be altered by $7 \times 0,037 = 0,259$ to 5,926 to get the initial estimate for people with only 7 years of education. An alternative often applied in empirical research is to introduce education as a centred variable into the model. In this case "zero" expresses the average educational achievements of the sample.

To include time-dependent covariates at the individual and the aggregate level is meaningful if concurrent variation of proposed cause and effect serves as a criterion to estimate the degree to which a relationship can be considered as causal. Because our model estimates y_t as a function of such x_t variables we obtain the respective information via the respective b's. It should be noted, however, that these b-values do not provide information whether or to what extent changes did occur.

In substantial terms for both models we find a positive effect of education on the satisfaction with household income. Likewise satisfaction with household income rises over time and if there is positive status inconsistency, that is, if income is higher than what would be expected for a certain reference group. Finally, members of congruent households show higher satisfaction with their household income than members of incongruent households. As to the variance decomposition provided by growth curve modelling, by far the most variance is on the household and time level, much less on the individual level.

In Table 12-6 the results of different models for multiple indicators are presented. As displayed in Figure 12-3 y is now measured by two indicators for each time point ("satisfaction with household income" and "satisfaction with standard of living"). In all models the loadings of the first indicator are fixed to one and the loadings of the second indicator are restricted to be equal over time.

Model B corresponds to model A except that now due to the inclusion of another level, individuals are again analyzed as members of households. Thus, in this model a "within" as well as a "between" component had to be specified. Model C extends model A by the two concepts x_1 and g_1, both of them measured by four indicators, and g_2. We present our results mainly with respect to b_0 and b_t and the influence x_0, x_1, and g_1 exert on them. As explained in Figure 12-3 the model assumes effects of these variables on both the initial average value of y, b_0, and the expected change per unit time

b_t (in our case, years). The same holds for the index of educational achievements, x_0. In model C we present these effects on both b_0 and b_t.

TABLE 12- 6

Results of Different Latent Growth Curve Models

	\multicolumn{8}{c}{*Satisfaction with own socio-economic position**}
	b	s.e	b	s.e	b	s.e	b	s.e
	\multicolumn{2}{c}{A}	\multicolumn{2}{c}{B}	\multicolumn{4}{c}{C}
Latent Mean: Intercept b_0	6,245	0,017	6,203	0,024	6,246			
Latent Mean: Slope b_t	0,052	0,005	0,062	0,006	0,053			
					\multicolumn{2}{c}{effect on b_0}	\multicolumn{2}{c}{effect on b_t}
Individual SI (x_1)					0,192	0,023	0,005	0,007
HH-status-incongruence (g_1)					0,348	0,028	-0,013	0,009
Single-HH/no comp. possible (g_2)					-0,002	0,056	0,022	0,018
Education in years (x_0)					0,036	0,007	0,004	0,002
	\multicolumn{8}{c}{Variance components}
$\sigma^2(u0)$	1,874	0,038	1,856	0,050	1,749	0,036		
$\sigma(u0t)$	-0,102	0,010	-0,135	0,012	-0,100	0,010		
$\sigma^2(ut)$	0,063	0,005	0,075	0,005	0,061	0,005		
$\sigma^2(v0)$			0,241	0,026				
$\sigma(v0t)$			0,008	0,009				
$\sigma^2(vt)$			0,000	0,005				

		I1(ek)	I2(ls)	I1(ek)	I2(ls)	I1(ek)	I2(ls)	
$\sigma^2(e)$	t_0	2,058	0,578	1,402	0,415	2,044	0,596	
	t_1	1,970	0,642	1,349	0,417	1,958	0,657	
	t_2	1,782	0,600	1,177	0,368	1,772	0,612	
	t_3	1,732	0,543	1,121	0,356	1,720	0,556	

*2-Indicators model: Satisfaction with a) Household income [„I1(ek)"] and b) Standard of living [„I2(ls)"]; all models were estimated using Mplus 3.01

In all models, the estimates of intercepts and slopes are very similar, whereby the slopes, which give us the effect of time, are relatively low. What can be reported in regard to the variance components is that in terms of variance decomposition, we can notice most of the variance being positioned on Level 1. Furthermore, variances of indicator one are much higher than the variances of indicator two.

In model C effects of status inconsistency, status incongruence, and education are included. Despite that there are no significant effects on b_t, we can observe different significant effects on b_0. All effects are positive. So if there is positive status inconsistency, that means, if income is higher than expected, satisfaction with the own socio-economic position rises.

12.6 DISCUSSION

In this paper we discussed two modelling strategies for panel data: The multilevel approach by growth curve models, and the structural equation approach by latent growth curve models. We explain how these two techniques are suited to analyze panel data, and how they are related.

Both approaches were applied on modelling panel data from the Federal Republic of Germany (German Socio-Economic Panel - GSOEP), which has the multilevel structure time-point i < person j < household k. In substantial terms, we focused on the effects of status inconsistency at the individual level and on the effects of status incongruence at the household level. As we expected, and as it has been already mentioned by other authors, the two modelling approaches produced more or less equivalent outcomes.

In our view, both approaches are useful for analyzing panel data. Nevertheless, both methods have their assets and drawbacks. Some noteworthy advantages argue for the structural equation approach: It allows the researcher to make use of the various possibilities in structural equation modelling for model fit assessment and recommends model changes to improve the fit. It affords a flexible handling of error terms, that is, it is simple to allow for different or correlated errors over time, which is possible in multi-level models as well, but more difficult to handle. Finally, it enables estimating more sophisticated models, that is, models with multiple indicators or complex path models.

However, the multilevel approach as well has its advantages: First, the estimation of multilevel growth curve models is much easier and straightforward than the specification of equivalent latent growth curve models; and second, the multilevel approach is predominant if one wants to model data with a higher hierarchical structure, because in multilevel modelling it is possible to include as many levels as the data facilitate and theoretical considerations require. Multilevel regressions also allow varying relationships at different levels, and modelling this variation by cross-level interactions such as they enable the unpretentious coping of incomplete data.

Thus, the decision about which approach to prefer for analyzing panel data is a function of researchers' objectives. If one wants to take a highly nested data structure into account and is not interested in measuring latent factors by multiple indicators, the multilevel approach should be the appropriate method. The other way around, if one aim of research is to make use of the structural equation facilities as mentioned earlier, the latent growth curve method should be the suiting one.

REFERENCES

Baltagi, B. H. (2001). *Econometric analysis of panel data* (2nd ed.). Chichester, UK: Wiley.

Blau, P. M. (1981). Diverse views of social structure and their common denominator. In P. M. Blau & Robert K. Merton (Eds.), *Continuities in structural inquiry* (1–23), London: Sage.

Blien, U. (2001). *Arbeitslosigkeit und Entlohnung auf regionalen Arbeitsmärkten.* Heidelberg: Physica.

Blien, U., & Wiedenbeck, M. (2002). Mehrebenenanalyse. In G. Kleinhenz (Ed.), *IAB Kompendium Arbeitsmarkt- und Berufsforschung. Beiträge zur Arbeitsmarkt- und Berufsforschung 250* (309–324), Nürnberg.

Bollen, K. A. (1989). *Structural equations with latent variables.* New York: Wiley.

Bryk, A. S., & Raudenbush, S. W. (1992). *Hierarchical linear models: applications and data analysis methods.* Newbury Park: Sage.

Chou, C.-P., Bentler, P. M., & Pentz, M. A. (1998). Comparisons of two statistical approaches to study growth curves: the multilevel model and the latent curve analysis. *Structural Equation Modeling*, 247–266.

Duncan, T. E., Duncan, S. C., Strycker, L. A., Li, F., & Anthony, A. (1999). *An introduction to latent variable growth curve modeling: Concepts, issues, and applications.* Mahwah, NJ: Lawrence Erlbaum Associates.

Engel, U. (1998). *Einführung in die Mehrebenenanalyse. Grundlagen, Auswertungsverfahren und praktische Beispiele.* Opladen/Wiesbaden: Westdeutscher Verlag.

Engel, U., & Reinecke, J. (1994). *Panelanalyse. Grundlagen, Techniken, Beispiele.* Berlin: DeGruyter.

Engel, U., & Simonson, J. (in press). Sozialer Kontext in der Mehrebenenanalyse. In Andreas Diekmann (Ed.), *Methoden der Sozialforschung* (303–329), Sonderheft 44 der Kölner Zeitschrift für Soziologie und Sozialpsychologie. Wiesbaden: VS Verlag für Sozialwissenschaften.

Goldstein, H. (1995). *Multilevel statistical models.* London: Edward Arnold.

Guo, G., & Zhao, H. (2000). Multilevel modeling for binary data. *Annual Review of Sociology, 26,* 441–462.

Hayduk, L. A. (1987). *Structural equation modeling with LISREL.* Baltimore, Johns Hopkins University Press.

Hox, J. J. (2002). *Multilevel analysis, Techniques and applications.* Mahwah, NJ: Lawrence Erlbaum Associates.

Jöreskog, K., Sörbom, D., Du Toit, S., & Du Toit, M. (2000-2001). *LISREL 8: New statistical features.* Chicago: Lincolnwood, Scientific Software International.

Maas, C. J. M., & Snijders, T. A. B. (2003). The Multilevel approach to repeated measures for complete and incomplete data. *Quality and Quantity, 37,* 71–89.

Marsh, H. W., & Hau, K.-T. (2002). Multilevel modeling of longitudinal growth and change: Substantive effects or regression toward the mean artifacts? *Multivariate Behavioral Research, 37,* 245–282.

Meredith, W. & Tisak, J. (1990) Latent curve analysis. *Psychometrika, 55,* 107- 122.

Muthén, L. K., & Muthén, B.O. (1998-2004). *Mplus user's guide* (3rd Ed.), Los Angeles, CA: Muthén & Muthén.

Potthoff, R. F., & Roy, S. N. (1964). A generalized multivariate analysis of variance model useful especially for growth curve problems. *Biometrika, 51,* 313–326.

Rao, C. R. (1965). The theory of least squares when the parameters are stochastic and its application to the analysis of growth curves. *Biometrika, 52,* 447–458.

Rasbash, J., Browne, W., Goldstein, H., Yang, M., Healy, M., Woodhouse, G., Draper, D., Longford, I., Lewis, T. (2000). *A user's guide to MLwiN. Multilevel models Project.* London: Institute of Education, University of London.

Raudenbush, S., Bryk, A., Cheong, Y. F., & Congdon, R. (2001). *HLM 5.* Lincolnwood: Scientific Software International.

Reinecke, J. (2005). *Strukturgleichungsmodelle in den Sozialwissenschaften.* München, Oldenbourg.

Snijders, T. A. B., & Bosker, R. J. (1999). *Multilevel Analysis. An introduction to basic and advanced multilevel modeling.* London: Sage.

Willett, J. B. (1997). Measuring Change: What individual growth modeling buys you. In E. Amsel & K. A. Renninger (Eds.), *Change and development: Issues of theory, method, and application* (pp. 213–243), Mahwah, NJ: Lawrence Erlbaum Associates.

Willett, J. B., & Keiley, K. K. (2000). Using covariance structure analysis to model change over time. In H. E. A. Tinsley & S. D. Brown (Eds.), *Handbook of Applied Multivariate Statistics and Mathematic Modeling* (pp. 665–694), San Diego, CA: Academic Press.

Chapter 13

Applying Autoregressive Cross-Lagged and Latent Growth Curve Models to a Three-Wave Panel Study

Elmar Schlueter

University of Marburg, Germany

Eldad Davidov and Peter Schmidt

University of Giessen, Germany

13.1. INTRODUCTION

Recent theoretical and empirical research shows a renewed interest in authoritarianism and anomia (Herrmann 2001; Herrmann & Schmidt 1995; Kühnel & Schmidt 2002). This interest is the most recent variant of a long-standing literature that dates back to the classic contributions of Adorno and colleagues (1950) and Srole (1956). However, systematic attempts to investigate the measurement models underlying these constructs and their suggested causal relationships are still largely missing.

In this contribution, we address these issues drawing on data from a representative three-wave panel study of the German general population. In our model, we measure the latent constructs via multiple indicators. Using latent autoregressive cross-lagged (AR-CL) and latent growth curve (LGC) models, the purpose of this chapter is to apply two methods for longitudinal analysis that can be used to test different types of propositions and to gain new insights for substantive research. Whereas for some areas of research autoregressive cross-lagged or latent growth curve models appear to be commonly used, other areas of research seem just to begin to realize the potentials of such methods (Halaby, 2004; Christ, Schmidt, Schlueter, & Wagner 2006). Thus, with the present chapter we intend to contribute to the reader's interest and understanding of AR-CL and LGC for further applications.

This chapter is structured as follows. In the following second section, we introduce the specifications of authoritarianism and anomia and explicate two alternative causal models for these constructs. In the third section, we present the key characteristics of AR-CL and LGC. In the fourth section, we present our research questions and discuss how autoregressive cross-lagged and latent growth curve models can be used to investigate these questions. In the fifth section, we describe the sample and indicators of the latent constructs. Subsequently, in the sixth part, we present the empirical findings from the AR-CL including latent means and intercepts and LGC. In the seventh and last section, this contribution concludes with a summary of the substantial findings, a comparative evaluation of the different contribution of the two methods and an outlook on recent developments on the integration of complementary methods for the analysis of panel data.

13.2 THEORETICAL BACKGROUND OF THE STUDY

Ever since their invention in the 1950s, authoritarianism and anomia have played an important role in many studies on prejudice and intolerance. Regarding authoritarianism, most researchers agree that this construct reflects in equal measures (a) an individual preference for submission under authorities (authoritarian submission), (b) a strict orientation along the perceived conventions of the in-group (authoritarian conventionalism), and (c) aggressive stances towards out-groups (authoritarian aggression; Altemeyer, 1996; Stenner, 1997). However, notwithstanding the consensus on the manifestation of the construct, the question "what authoritarianism really is" is still open (Stenner, 1997). Particularly, two key approaches on the concept specification of authoritarianism need to be distinguished. A first perspective dates back to Adorno et al.'s (1950) seminal work on "The Authoritarian Personality". According to this view, authoritarianism is conceptualized as a relatively stable intrapersonal characteristic that results from enduring intrapersonal conflicts rooted in childhood experiences of harsh education. A second perspective derives from the social learning approach as introduced by Altemeyer (Altemeyer, 1996). Neglecting the idea of authoritarianism as an intrapersonal characteristic, Altemeyer conceptualizes authoritarianism as a set of coherent attitudes that are learned from peer groups and similar socializing agents (Altemeyer, 1988, 1996).

Anomia was considered by Srole (1956) to be a subjective "feeling" responding to acute societal dysfunctions (Scheepers, Felling, & Peters 1992; Srole 1956). More specifically, Srole (1956) defined anomia as consisting of five subdimensions labelled (a) political powerlessness, (b) social powerlessness, (c) generalized socioeconomic retrogression, (d) normlessness and meaninglessness, and (e) social isolation (Srole, 1956). Usually, these aspects are measured on an attitudinal level.

To explain the causal order of authoritarianism and anomia, previous research has focused on two opposing theoretical models. According to a first model, the expectation is that anomia leads to authoritarianism (Scheepers et al., 1992; Srole, 1956). This line of argumentation suggests that individuals who feel normless and meaningless adopt authoritarian attitudes in order to regain orientation in an environment perceived as increasingly complex and irritating. Thus, according to this perspective, authoritarianism serves as a coping mechanism for individuals who are anomic.

This view is challenged by an alternative model proposed by McClosky and Schaar (1965), suggesting that it is in fact authoritarianism that causes anomia. According to these authors, certain personality characteristics as reflected by authoritarianism lead to anomia as the narrow-mindedness of authoritarian people confines their opportunities for social interactions with others. Consequently, authoritarian people are assumed to possess fewer opportunities for receiving social support by which they could prevent or reduce social isolation. Therefore, authoritarian people are thought to be particularly vulnerable to anomia (McClosky & Schaar 1965).

To date, empirical evidence for these causal assumptions is largely missing. To the best of our knowledge, only Scheepers et al. (1992) have set out for an explicit test of the causal order of authoritarianism and anomia. Based on a cross-sectional representative Dutch survey dated 1987, they estimated a nonrecursive regression model and found a significant positive path with a substantial effect size leading from anomia to authoritarianism (Scheepers, et al. 1992). Although this finding supports the assumption that anomia leads to authoritarianism, the methodological assumptions underlying the nonrecursive model used by Scheepers et al. (1992) are by no means always given (see Kaplan, Harik, & Hotchkiss 2001). As a consequence, the conclusion that anomia causes authoritarianism can easily be called into question. Clearly, for investigating the dynamic relationships of authoritarianism and anomia panel data are much more desirable. Specifically, there are three reasons why panel data appear particulary adequate for such an investigation. First, regarding the construct specifications of authoritarianism and anomia, panel data offer the opportunity to test the invariance of the measurement models of these constructs by comparing individual responses to the indicator variables across different measurement points. Second, panel data are particularly appropriate for testing causal assumptions (Finkel, 1995) such as for the relations of authoritarianism and anomia as the observations are collected over two or more points in time. As Reinecke, Schmidt, and Weick (2005) point out, because panel data are not collected retrospectively, the observations remain unaffected by possibly distorting memory or reevaluation-effects. Third, panel data offer explorative insights into the dynamics of the theoretical constructs over time using different methods for longitudinal data analysis.

13.3 METHODS

Autoregressive Cross-Lagged Models.

A major approach for the analysis of panel data is the autoregressive model (Finkel, 1995; Hertzog & Nesselroade, 2003; Jöreskog, 1979). Dating back to the Markov simplex model (Guttman, 1954) which used observed variables only, subsequent developments soon allowed for the incorporation of latent variables into the autoregressive framework (Jöreskog, 1979). Such autoregressive models are based on the assumption that each latent construct η_i measured at time t is a function of its former value at time t-1 plus random error. In addition, a measurement model is needed to relate the latent variables to their respective indicators and the random measurement errors. The autoregressive process is described by stability coefficients that reflect the amount of change in the relative rank order of individuals between two or more points in time (Finkel, 1995; Jagodzinski, Kühnel, & Schmidt, 1987). Importantly, the stability coefficients do not bear information about individual change in absolute scores across different points in time. For instance, although individuals may maintain their relative standing among group members, their individual scores might indeed be subject to an increase or decrease in the period under study (Conroy, Metzler, & Hofer, 2003). Using the notation of the generalized structural equation model (Bollen & Curran, 2006; Graff & Schmidt, 1982), the equation for the latent autoregressive model in the univariate case for two measuring points is as follows:

$$\eta_{it} = \alpha_i + \beta_{t,t-1}\eta_{it-1} + \zeta_{it} \qquad (1)$$

α_i represents the intercept for the estimate of time point t and $\beta_{t,t-1}$ indicates prior influences of η_{it-1} on $\eta_{it.}$ Index i denotes the individual unit and t the point in time. Further, this model assumes that the random errors are not correlated with the explanatory variables and have an expected mean of zero. For causal analyses of panel data, structural relationships between two or more latent constructs as an extension of the autoregressive model are often of special interest. Consider for the bivariate case two latent constructs η_i measured at two or more points at time t and time t-1. Within the framework of the bivariate autoregressive cross-lagged model, each of the two latent constructs is regressed at time t on its lagged score plus the lagged score of the other latent construct at time t-1 (Finkel, 1995; Hertzog & Nesselroade, 2003). The resulting cross-lagged coefficients inform about the structural relationships between both constructs. Specifically, the magnitude of the cross-lagged coefficients indicates how much variation in η_{it-1} predicts aggregate change in $\eta_{it.}$ Due to the control of autoregression for each latent construct via the stability coefficients, the cross-lagged effects indicate the "pure" influence of each construct of interest. The equations for the latent autoregressive cross-lagged model in the bivariate case for two measuring points are:

$$\eta_{i3} = \alpha_{i3} + \beta_{31}\eta_{i1} + \beta_{32}\eta_{i2} + \zeta_{i3} \qquad (2)$$
$$\eta_{i4} = \alpha_{i4} + \beta_{41}\eta_{i1} + \beta_{42}\eta_{i2} + \zeta_{i4} \qquad (3)$$

α_{i3} and α_{i4} represent the intercepts for the estimates at each time point t. β_{31} and β_{42} are autoregressive parameters, whereas β_{32} and β_{41} represent the cross-lagged coefficients. Random errors are represented by ζ_{i3} and ζ_{i4}, while the prior assumptions of uncorrelated random errors and explanatory variables with expected value of zero for the random errors are retained. The measurement model can be expressed as follows:

$$y_{ikt} = \mu_{ikt} + \lambda_{kt}\eta_{ikt} + \varepsilon_{ikt} \qquad (4)$$

y_{ikt} is the observed value for a specific $(j = 1,2...,N)$ indicator y for each individual i at time t. μ_{ikt} denotes the intercept term and λ_{kt} the factor loadings that relate a specific $(j = 1,2...,N)$ indicator to a latent factor η_{ikt}. ε_{ikj} indicates the random error.

AR-CL models can be extended in several ways. For instance, the bivariate AR-CL model can be extended toward larger SEM's with more than two latent constructs (Burkholder & Harlow, 2003).

Likewise, additional observed or latent exogenous variables can be introduced to the model to predict the constructs of interest. Also, researchers can investigate possible moderating effects by referring to multigroup comparison using categorial grouping variables. Notwithstanding this flexibility, the statistical assumptions underlying the AR-CL have also been subject to criticism (Rogosa, 1995; Rogosa & Willett, 1985; see also Stoolmiller & Bank, 1995). Specifically, the fixed effects approach of the autoregressive model by assuming its coefficients to be the same for all individual units under study has been criticized to reflect group changes only. Also, the previously discussed aspect that the autoregressive model does not account for absolute changes in individual scores for a construct of interest has been mentioned. Alternatively, to account for such individual differences in processes of change scholars suggest the use of latent growth curve models for the analysis of panel data.

Latent Growth Curve Models.
Latent growth curve models (LGC) are another useful statistical procedure for the analysis of panel data. LGC inform about individual growth in a given construct over time by estimating a single underlying trajectory for each individual unit. Expanding on the seminal work of Tucker (1958) and

Rao (1958), LGC was firstly proposed by McArdle and Epstein (1987) and
Meredith and Tisak (1990). The idea underlying LGC is that individual
growth for a given construct is a function of a latent intercept and a latent
slope plus random error. Whereas the latent intercept indicates the average
initial starting values of the longitudinal change process, the latent slope reflects the average individual change rate over time. A univariate LGC with
observed indicators can be described as follows (see Bollen & Curran, 2006:
27):

$$y_{it} = \alpha_i + \lambda_t \beta_i + \varepsilon_{it} \tag{5}$$

y_{it} are the observed values for each person i at time t in an indicator variable
y. α_i denotes the latent intercept and β_i the latent slope factor. As indicated by
subscript i, these factors are assumed to vary across individuals. To assess
the individual's initial values of the growth process, the factor loadings of
the latent intercept term α_i are commonly constrained to 1. Because this
value is constant for all t, the equation does not contain a specific coefficient
for the factor loadings of the latent intercept. λ_t indicates the factor loadings
for the latent slope factor β_i; for instance, for a minimum of three time points
fixing these loadings to values of 0, 1, and 2 specifies a linear growth process. ε_{it} is the random error assumed to have a mean of zero and to be uncorrelated with the exogenous variables. The individual latent intercept and
slope factors are each constituted by a group mean and a disturbance term
capturing the deviations from this group mean. In an unconditional LGC
with no further explanatory variables, these deviations indicate the amount
of individual variability for the estimated latent intercepts and slopes. This is
described by Equations 6 and 7:

$$\alpha_i = \mu_\alpha + \zeta_{ai} \tag{6}$$
$$\beta_i = \mu_\beta + \zeta_{\beta i} \tag{7}$$

With α_i and β_i representing the latent intercept and the latent slope factor, μ_α
and μ_β denote the means for these latent factors whereas ζ_{ai} and $\zeta_{\beta i}$ denote the
variability for these means. These disturbances are assumed to have means
of zero and to be uncorrelated with the random error. When combining
Equations 5, 6 and 7, the following Equation 8 results:

$$y_{it} = [\mu_\alpha + \lambda_t \mu_\beta] + [\zeta_{ai} + \lambda_t \zeta_{\beta i} + \varepsilon_{it}] \tag{8}$$

LGC can also be applied to latent constructs with multiple indicators and
higher order factors. For instance, detailed applications of such a so-called
second order growth curve model are given by Hancock, Kuo, and Lawrence

(2001) and Bollen and Curran (2006). Following Bollen and Curran (2006), the second order LGC can be expressed as follows:

$$\eta_{it} = \alpha_i + \lambda_t \beta_i + \zeta_{it} \tag{9}$$

η_{it} is the repeated latent variable for individual i and time t. As for the LGC with observed indicators, α_i and β_i denote the latent intercept and slope factor, with λ_t indicating the factor loading for the latent slope. ζ_{it} is the random error assumed to have a mean of zero and to be uncorrelated with the exogenous variables. The latent intercept (α_i) and latent slope factors (β_i) in such an unconditional model are defined as before:

$$\alpha_i = \mu_\alpha + \zeta_{\alpha i} \tag{10}$$
$$\beta_i = \mu_\beta + \zeta_{\beta i} \tag{11}$$

Again, the disturbance terms $\zeta_{\alpha i}$ and $\zeta_{\beta i}$ are assumed to have means of zero and to be uncorrelated with ζ_{it} and λ_t. The measurement model for the second order LGC is expressed by the following equation:

$$y_{jit} = \nu_{jt} + \Lambda_{jt}\eta_{it} + \varepsilon_{jit} \tag{12}$$

y_{jit} denotes the observed value for a specific ($j = 1,2...,N$) indicator y for each individual i at time t.

ν_{jt} is the intercept for indicator j at time t. Λ_{jt} is the factor loading for indicator j at time t on a latent factor η_{it}. ε_{jit} is the random error.

Univariate LGC as described earlier are often extended toward bi- or multivariate LGC. Such LGC are capable to simultaneously estimate individual change in two or more observed or latent constructs of interest. In the context of such models, researchers can also investigate possible correlations between the latent intercept and latent slope factors of different constructs. Likewise, unconditional LGC are often extended to include further observed or latent exogenous variables. Such variables can then be used to explain the variance in the latent intercept or slope factors. Another opportunity in the context of LGC is to conduct multigroup analyses based on a categorical grouping variable of interest. By doing so, research can possibly examine variant growth processes between subgroups (e.g., gender, ethnicity). Further, it should be noted that LGC offer considerable flexibility in modelling individual change as it is not limited to linear growth processes, but also capable of modelling nonlinear (e.g., quadratic) forms of individual change (Hancock et al., 2001).

13.4 RESEARCH QUESTIONS

By investigating the subsequent four research questions on the dynamics of authoritarianism and anomia, we compare the use of latent autoregressive cross-lagged and latent growth curve models. Specifically, to examine research questions one and two, we use autoregressive cross-lagged models:

1. Which amount of aggregate change do we find for authoritarianism and anomia over the three measurement points?

Examining aggregate change of authoritarianism and anomia provides important information about the concept specifications of these constructs. Regarding authoritarianism, on the one hand high stability coefficients together with constant mean values would support the idea of authoritarianism as a stable intrapersonal characteristic. On the other hand, low stability coefficients would speak in favor of authoritarianism as a more flexible attitude cluster. Likewise, for anomia conceptualized as a more situation-specific construct, we expect lower stability coefficients for the period under study. To investigate these issues, we refer to the stability coefficients of authoritarianism and anomia as provided by the autoregressive model plus the latent means of these constructs.

2. Which evidence do we find for cross-lagged effects (a) from authoritarianism on anomia and (b) from anomia on authoritarianism over the three measurement points?

Current knowledge on the causal relations between authoritarianism and anomia will be advanced by investigating the cross-lagged effects between these constructs. Specifically, positive cross-lagged effects from authoritarianism on anomia would support the view of authoritarianism as antecedent of anomia. In turn, positive cross-lagged effects from anomia on authoritarianism would be consistent with the idea of anomia as antecedent of authoritarianism.

To investigate research questions three and four, we will refer to latent growth curve models:

3. Which evidence do we find for individual (a) growth and (b) variability in growth for authoritarianism or anomia over the three measurement points?

An alternative approach for investigating the conceptual underpinnings of authoritarianism and anomia using panel data is to explore possible growth processes in these constructs. According to the idea of authoritarianism as a stable intrapersonal characteristic, we would expect short-time growth processes to be rather unlikely to occur. In turn, evidence for such growth processes as indicated by a significant mean of the latent slope factor would support the view of authoritarianism as a coherent attitude cluster affected by situational circumstances. Likewise, empirical evidence for growth processes in anomia would support the idea of anomia as an individual response to specific situations.

4.   Which evidence do we find for structural relations between the latent intercept and latent slope factors of authoritarianism and anomia over the three measurement points?

Examining possible growth processes in authoritarianism and anomia offers additional opportunities to explore the dynamic relations of these constructs. Specifically, such an analysis could reveal if and how the possible latent intercepts and latent slopes of authoritarianism and anomia are statistically interrelated. For instance, it seems interesting to explore whether the initial values of one construct as measured by the latent intercept factors affects growth processes in another construct as measured by the latent slope factors.

13.5 DATA AND INDICATORS

Data for the subsequent analyses were drawn from a representative panel study of the German general population aged sixteen years and over (Heitmeyer, 2004). Data collection was done by computer-assisted telephone interviews, conducted at three measuring points each one year apart. Starting in 2002, the initial sample of the panel consisted of $N = 2,722$ German respondents. One year later at Time 2, of those $N = 2,364$ respondents who agreed at Time 1 to participate in the panel $N = 2,029$ respondents could be recontacted. From this sample, $N = 1,175$ interviews were successfully completed. Again one year later at Time 3, of those $N = 1,142$ respondents who gave their consent at time 2 to be reinterviewed, $N = 875$ respondents could be recontacted. Here, $N = 875$ interviews were successfully completed. Using the realized sample of Time 1 as baseline, response rates were 49% for the second time point and 37% for the third time point.

For measuring authoritarianism, two items were selected from an authoritarianism short-scale shown to be a valid measure of authoritarianism in previous studies in the German context (Schmidt, Stephan, & Herrmann, 1995). Respondents were asked to rate on a four-point Likert-type scale the following statements: "The most important qualities someone can have are obedience and respect to superiors." (SUBMIS1) and "We should be grateful for leaders who can tell us what to do and exactly how to do it." (SUBMIS2). These indicators reflect the partial aspect authoritarian submission. Response options ranged from "absolutely agree" (1) to "absolutely disagree" (4). These values were recoded so that higher values indicate greater authoritarianism. For measuring anomia, respondents were asked to rate on a four point Likert-type scale the following two statements: "Things have become so difficult today that you do not know what's up." (NORMLES1) and "In former times people were better off because one knew what to do" (NORMLES2). These items reflect the subdimension of anomic normlessness. Response options ranged from "absolutely agree" (1) to "absolutely disagree" (4). Again, the original responses recoded so that higher values indicate greater anomia. Regarding unit nonresponse (Engel and Reinecke 1994), separate analyses not shown here confirmed that neither those participants who gave their consent at Time 1 for reinterviewing, but were not interviewed at Time 2, nor those participants who gave their consent at Time 2 for reinterviewing but were not interviewed at Time 3, differed substantially from the respondents used in the initial panel sample with regard to sex, education, and place of living. Item nonresponse was on a very low level with a maximum of 1.5%.

13.6 RESULTS

Descriptive Results

Table 13-1 displays means and standard deviations for the observed indicators of the latent constructs. For the first indicator measuring authoritarianism, the data reveal above-average scores at each measurement point, whereas the scores for the second indicator remain slightly below the midpoint of the scale across the period under study. Further, the mean values for the indicators of authoritarianism remain essentially constant for all measurement points. Regarding anomia, the results indicate above-average scores for both indicator variables. Further, the increasing mean values indicate a clear trend across the three measurement points.

Measurement Models

Next, to test for the appropriate operationalization of the latent constructs by the observed indicators, measurement models were estimated (Anderson & Gerbing, 1988). Using the AMOS 5.0 software (Arbuckle, 2003), all analyses reported are based on FIML-estimates including means and intercepts (Enders & Bandalos, 2002; Raykov, 2005). Given the crucial importance of measurement invariance for making inferences about changes in constructs over time (Pitts,West, & Tein 1996), we subsequently tested measurement models for configural and weak factorial invariance (Meredith & Tisak, 1990).

TABLE 13-1

Means (M) and Standard Deviations (SD) for the Observed Indicators of Authoritarianism and Anomia Across the Three Measurement Points.

	t1 (2002)			t2 (2003)			t3 (2004)		
Authoritarianism	N	M	(SD)	N	M	(SD)	N	M	(SD)
SUBMIS1..........	2706	2.68	(.93)	1166	2.70	(.91)	817	2.69	(.91)
SUBMIS2..........	2698	2.13	(.85)	1168	2.21	(.83)	821	2.2	(.84)
Anomia									
NORMLESS1......	2705	2.57	(.91)	1166	2.78	(.9)	825	2.9	(.88)
NORMLESS2......	2705	2.53	(.89)	1173	2.73	(.9)	824	2.87	(.87)

Note. All values are based on raw data. N = sample size.

The initial measurement model (1) allowed the latent constructs to correlate and included autocorrelations for the measurement errors. Visual inspection of model (1) indicated that all factor loadings for the latent constructs of authoritarianism and anomia were of sufficient size and approximately equal for each measurement point as shown in Table 13-2.

According to the fit statistics, model (1) matched well to the data (χ^2 = 64.73; df = 33; χ^2/df = 1.96; CFI = .996; RMSEA = .019; *p*-value of close fit = 1.0). Thus, configural factorial invariance was given (Meredith & Tisak, 1990).

In the subsequent measurement model (2), factor loadings for authoritarianism and anomia were constrained to be equal across the three measurement points. Following the insignificant χ^2-difference test, these constraints did not significantly reduce the fit of model (2) ($\Delta\chi^2$ = 4.98; *ns*). Thereby, weak factorial invariance of the measures was established (Meredith & Tisak, 1990). For all subsequent AR-CL and LGC, these constraints for weak factorial invariance as well as autocorrelated measurement errors were retained. Further, model (2) also provides the implied latent means for authoritarianism and anomia that are discussed in the context of our first research question.

TABLE 13-2

Standardized Factor Loadings of the Latent Factors for Authoritarianism and Anomia

	t1 (2002)	t2 (2003)	t3 (2004)
Authoritarianism			
SUBMIS1.....................	.79	.79	.80
SUBMIS2.....................	.68	.66	.67
Anomia			
NORMLESS1.................	.83	.88	.89
NORMLESS2.................	.83	.88	.88

Note. Coefficients are based on FIML-estimates.

Structural Models

Next, we turn to the findings from the structural models. We start with model (3) depicted in Figure 13-1.

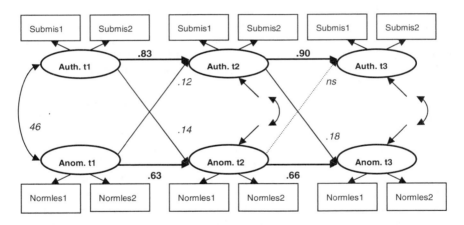

Figure 13-1. Path diagram of a latent autoregressive cross-lagged model for authoritarianism and anomia.

Note. Bold parameters represent standardized stability coefficients. Cursive parameters represent standardized cross-lagged coefficients (Pearson correlation coefficient for Auth. t1 and Anom. t1). Factor loadings of the latent constructs and measurement errors are not shown (for factor loadings, see Table 13-2).

This model comprises the stability coefficients for authoritarianism and anomia and the mutual cross-lagged coefficients from authoritarianism to anomia as well as from anomia to authoritarianism. Accordingly, this model showed a good fit to the data ($\chi^2 = 127.19$; df = 43; $\chi^2/\text{df} = 2.95$; CFI = .99;

RMSEA = .027; *p*-value of close fit = 1.0). In our first research question we hypothesized that low levels of change in authoritarianism would support the idea of authoritarianism as a relatively stable intrapersonal characteristic. In turn, considerable amounts of change would point to the alternative conception of authoritarianism as a situational adaptive attitude cluster. For evaluating the amount of change in authoritarianism, we consider the stability coefficients in conjunction with the latent means. The data reveal considerably high stability coefficients (i.e., standardized regression coefficients) between the two time intervals (β = .83, *p* < .001; β = .90, *p* < .001). Although the differences in the stabilities appear rather small, a χ^2-difference test reveals that this difference is significant ($\Delta\chi^2$ = 5.31; *p* < .05). These findings suggest that only very little change in authoritarianism took place over the period under study. Consistent with this conclusion, the latent means for authoritarianism as shown in Table 13-3 revealed basically constant values for the three measurement points (μ_{t1} = 2.67; μ_{t2} = 2.71; μ_{t3} = 2.71).

TABLE 13-3

Implied Latent Means for Authoritarianism and Anomia

	t1 (2002)	*t2 (2003)*	*t3 (2004)*
Authoritarianism............	2.67	2.71	2.72
Anomia......................	2.56	2.77	2.91

Note. Coefficients are provided by measurement model (1) based on FIML-estimates.

Taken together, we conclude that these findings support the conceptualization of authoritarianism as a stable intrapersonal characteristic.

For anomia, we hypothesized that considerable amounts of aggregate change would support its conceptualization as individual reaction contingent on situational conditions. In fact, the lower stability coefficients (β = .63, *p* < .001; β = .66, *p* < .001) for anomia point to substantial amounts of change in the period under study. When these stabilities were constrained to be equal, the nonsignificant χ^2-difference test shows that model fit was not altered ($\Delta\chi^2$ = .13; *ns*). The finding of substantial amounts of aggregate change for anomia is also supported by the latent means for this construct as given in Table 13-3. The latent means for anomia denote an increase in anomia over the three measurement points (μ_{t1} = 2.56; μ_{t2} = 2.76; μ_{t3} = 2.91). For a further test of the apparent differential longitudinal developments of authoritarianism and anomia, we constrained the stabilities between both constructs to be equal for each time interval. Doing so resulted in a significanlty altered model fit ($\Delta\chi^2_{t1-t2}$ = 6.14, *p* <.05; $\Delta\chi^2_{t2-t3}$ = 25.47, *p* < .001). Thus, we conclude that the stabilities of anomia are indeed substantially lower than the stabilities for authoritarianism. Stated differently, for anomia there is considerably greater amount of change than for authoritarianism. In sum, we reason that this result supports the conceptualization of anomia as an individual reaction to situational circumstances.

Next, following our second research question we examined the alternative causal models for authoritarianism and anomia. According to the suggestions of Srole (1958), the expectation was that heightened levels of anomia would lead to heightened levels of authoritarianism. Contrary to this view, McClosky and Schaar (1965) suggested that heightened levels of authoritarianism would lead to heightened levels of anomia. To get evidence on the empirical adequacy of these opposing predictions, we consider the cross-lagged effects (i.e., standardized regression coefficients) as incorporated in the present model (3). As suggested by McClosky and Schaar (1965), the results show that authoritarianism exerts significant and positive effects on anomia for Time 1 to Time 2 ($\beta = .14$, $p < .001$) as well as from Time 2 to Time 3 ($\beta = .18$, $p < .001$). However, consistent with the assumptions of Srole (1958), the data also reveal a significant and positive cross-lagged effect from anomia at Time 1 to authoritarianism at Time 2 ($\beta = .12$, $p < .001$), whereas no significant cross-lagged effect was found for anomia at Time 2 to authoritarianism at Time 3. To conduct an even stricter test of these findings, we compared the fit of the present model (3) that was comprised of cross-lagged effects for both authoritarianism and anomia to two alternative models: In model (3a), only cross-lagged effects from authoritarianism to anomia were estimated while the reverse effects leading from anomia to authoritarianism were constrained to zero. In turn, in model (3b) only cross-lagged effects from anomia to authoritarianism were incorporated, with the reverse effects leading from authoritarianism to anomia set to zero. Both model (3a) ($\Delta\chi^2 = 47.83$, $p < .001$) and model (3b) ($\Delta\chi^2 = 16.64$, $p < .001$) adjusted significantly worse to the sample than did the initial model (3). Thus, we conclude that in this study McClosky and Schaar's suggestion (1965) that it is authoritarianism that causes anomia gains most support, albeit the data revealed some evidence for a reverse effect of anomia.

Keeping these findings from the autoregressive cross-lagged analyses in mind, we turn to our third research question. Here, our aim was to utilize latent growth curve models for an improved understanding of the conceptual nature of authoritarianism and anomia. For this purpose, we first estimated separate LGC models for authoritarianism and anomia, which were comprised of both a latent intercept and a latent slope factor. Under the assumption of linear growth, factor loadings for the latent slope factor were set to 0, 1, and 2 (Bollen & Curran, 2004; Bollen & Curran, 2004, 2006; Duncan et al., 1999). For authoritarianism, the initial latent growth curve model (4) showed a very good fit to the data ($\chi^2 = 2.67$; df = 5; χ^2/df = .535; CFI = 1.0; RMSEA = .000; p-value of close fit = 1.0). Substantially, in this model the significant latent intercept factor ($\mu = 2.69$, $p < .001$) indicates that the respondents displayed on average a significant group mean of authoritarian attitudes of 2.7 at the initial time point. In addition, the significant variance found for the intercept (φ = .453, p < .001) denotes substantial individual variability around the group mean of authoritarianism at the initial time point.

However, as might have been expected from the basically invariant latent means, the latent slope factor for authoritarianism turned out not to be significantly different from zero (μ = .005, *ns*). Also the variance of the slope was not significantly different from zero (φ = .003, *ns*). Hence, the subsequent LGC model (5) was estimated with a latent intercept factor for authoritarianism only. Even this model matched the data very well (χ^2 = 2.87; df = 7; χ^2/df = .411; CFI = 1.0; RMSEA = .000; *p*-value of close fit = 1.0), hence it was retained for further analyses.

Regarding anomia, the initial LGC labelled model (6) showed a good fit to the data (χ^2 = 29.68; df = 11; χ^2/df = 2.67.; CFI = .996; RMSEA = .025; *p*-value of close fit = 1.0). Both the latent intercept and the latent slope of anomia turned out to be significantly different from zero. Specifically, for anomia the mean of the latent intercept factor was estimated as μ = 2.56 (*p* < .001), while the mean of the latent slope factor reached μ = .204 (*p* < .001). These findings suggest that on average, the respondents displayed a significant group mean of 2.56 for anomia plus a linear increase in anomia of .204 for each time point, a finding consistent with the increasing latent means for each time-point discussed earlier. Further, the significant amounts of variance for both the latent intercept (φ = .41, *p* < .001) as well as for the latent slope (φ = .025, *p* < .001) indicate substantial interindividual differences in the growth process of anomia. In a final step, we estimated a dual LGC labelled model (7) that integrates the prior LGC-analyses shown for authoritarianism and anomia. This model is depicted by Figure 13-2.

According to the fit measures, model (7) matched well to the data (χ^2 = 94.88; df = 53; χ^2/df = 1.79; CFI = .995; RMSEA = .017; *p*-value of close fit = 1.0).

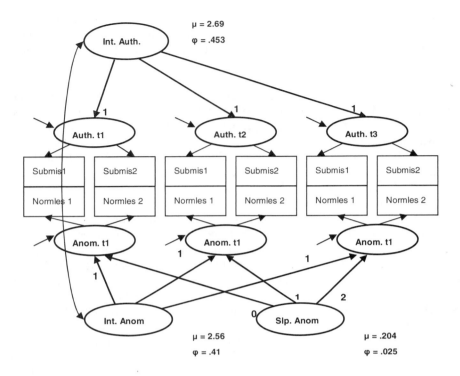

Figure 13-2. Path diagram of a latent growth curve model for authoritarianism and anomia.
Note. μ represent the means, φ represent the variances of the latent intercept and latent slope factors. Bold parameters represent fixed factor loadings for the latent intercept and latent slope factors. Cursive parameters represent Pearson correlation coefficients. Factor loadings of the latent constructs and measurement errors are not shown (see Table 13-2).

In addition to the means and variances of the latent intercept and slope factors as obtained from the prior models, this dual model also provided the necessary information for investigating our fourth research question, that is to examine possible statistical relations between the latent intercept factor of authoritarianism and the latent intercept and slope factors of anomia. The model reveals a significant and substantial positive correlation among the intercepts of authoritarianism and anomia ($r = .54$, $p < .001$). This indicates that respondents with a higher initial level of authoritarianism also exhibit a higher initial value of anomia and vice versa. However, no significant co-variance was found between the intercept of authoritarianism and the slope of anomia, implying that there was no relation between the initial level of authoritarianism and the change process over time of anomia. Finally, the covariance between the intercept and slope of anomia was not significantly different from zero, suggesting that the initial level of anomia and its changing process are not related.

13.7 DISCUSSION

In this chapter, we examined the dynamics of authoritarianism and anomia using data from a nationally representative three-wave panel survey in Germany. By investigating the measurement models and causal relationships of these constructs, we sought to demonstrate the complimentary application of latent autoregressive cross-lagged and second-order latent growth curve models to substantial research problems. Below, we summarize the findings and methodological aspects of these analyses.

Following our first research question, we aimed to shed new empirical light on the concept specifications of authoritarianism and anomia. For this task, we capitalized on the statistical assumptions of the latent autoregressive model by examining the stabilities and latent means of the constructs. With regard to authoritarianism, the data revealed considerably high stabilities plus latent means with essentially constant values. Taken together, these findings indicate that the German adult populations' authoritarianism did not change significantly between 2002, 2003, and 2004. Thereby, the conceptualization of authoritarianism as a relatively invariant intraindividual characteristic was supported. Contrary to the results for authoritarianism, the findings from the autoregressive models for anomia showed significantly lower stabilities. In line with this outcome, the data also revealed increasing latent means for anomia in the course of time. Thus, consistent with the ongoing process of rapid social change in the period under study (Heitmeyer, 2004), we consider these results to support the idea of anomia as an individual reaction to certain situational circumstances.

According to our second research question, we examined the causal order of authoritarianism and anomia. Based on two alternative theoretical models, we investigated whether authoritarianism leads to anomia or anomia leads to authoritarianism. For this analysis, the cross-lagged effects as provided by the latent autoregressive model were of central importance. In short, the findings provided mixed support for the competing causal models. On the one hand, consistent with the idea that authoritarianism causes, anomia significant and positive cross-lagged effects from authoritarianism on anomia were found for each time interval. On the other hand, we also found a significant cross-lagged effect from anomia at Time 1 to authoritarianism at Time 2, as suggested by the alternative view that it is anomia which causes authoritarianism. However, the cross-lagged path from anomia at Time 2 to authoritarianism at Time 3 turned not out to be significant. From these findings, we concluded that McClosky and Schaar's (1965) suggestion that it is authoritarianism which leads to anomia gains most support from the present data, albeit somewhat weaker evidence points to the possibility that authoritarianism is also affected by anomia.

In our third research question, we focused on possible growth processes in authoritarianism and anomia for a further understanding of the concept specifications of these constructs. For authoritarianism the analyses showed that no growth process took part for the period under study, a finding consistent with the prior result of high stabilities and essentially constant latent means of the authoritarianism-construct. However, evidence for a growth process was found for anomia. More specifically, the data revealed a linear increase in anomia for the period under study, coupled with a significant amount of population variance. Again, these outcomes complement the insights provided by the autoregressive model in that they are consistent with the lower stabilities and increasing latent means discussed earlier.

Continuing the use of latent growth models for exploring the dynamics of authoritarianism and anomia, in our fourth and last research question we set out to examine if the respondent's initial values for these constructs as measured by a latent intercept would affect possible growth processes as measured by a latent slope. The positive and significant correlation found for the latent intercepts of authoritarianism and anomia indicates that higher initial values in authoritarianism correspond with higher initial values in anomia and vice versa. However, no further significant correlations were detected for the latent intercept of authoritarianism and the latent slope and intercept of anomia.

Although not crucial for the purpose of this chapter, for future research it would seem promising to introduce further exogenous variables such as education, class, or general economic conditions into the models. Likewise, a longitudinal analysis of the effects of authoritarianism and anomia on prejudice could contribute to an improved understanding of the dynamics of intolerance. In line with such substantial advancements, various methodological extensions seem advisable, too. In addition to the discussed extensions for autoregressive cross-lagged and latent growth curve models, subsequent research could expand on our present methodological strategy by exploring the autoregressive latent trajectory (ALT) model proposed by Curran and Bollen (2001; Bollen & Curran 2006). By integrating the statistical assumptions underlying autoregressive cross-lagged and latent growth curve models, the ALT-model allows researchers to analyze autoregressive cross-lagged and growth curve relations simultaneously. However, for three waves of data as in our present example, identification of the ALT requires nonlinear constraints. Hamaker (2005) showed that under the assumption of time-invariant autoregressive parameters, the ALT-model is equivalent to a latent growth curve model with autoregressive disturbances whereby nonlinear constraints are not required. However, currently testing for cross-lagged relations between constructs in this model remains problematic because it has not yet been clarified which coefficients would correspond to the cross-lagged coefficients in the autoregressive cross-lagged model. Finally, particularly Oud's (in press) finding of several paradoxes for cross-lagged models because of different discrete time observation intervals within and between studies seems to bear major implications for cross-lagged models with SEM. As an alternative, he proposes the application of continuous time modelling. Consistent with this argument, we agree that future research in this direction is a necessary and promising task.

ACKNOWLEDGMENTS

Work on this chapter was supported by the German Israeli Foundation (GIF), project number 627001160. We thank Oliver Christ for help and valuable comments on earlier drafts of this study.

REFERENCES

Adorno, T., Frenkel-Brunswik, E., Levinson, D. J., & Sanford, R. N. in collaboration with B. Aron, M. H. Levinson and W. Morrow (1950). *The authoritarian personality*. New York: Harper & Row.

Altemeyer, B. (1988). *Enemies of freedom: understanding right-wing authoritarianism*. San Francisco, CA: Jossey-Bass.

Altemeyer, B. (1996). *The authoritarian specter*. Cambridge, MA: Harvard Univ. Press.

Anderson, J. C., & Gerbing, D. W. (1988). Structural equation modeling in practice: A review and recommended two step approach. *Psychological Bulletin, 103*, 411–423.

Arbuckle, J. L. (2003). *Amos 5.0, update to the Amos user's guide*. Chicago, IL: SmallWaters.

Bast, J., & Reitsma, P. (1997). Matthew effects in reading: A comparison of latent growth curve models and simplex models with structured means. *Multivariate Behavioral Research, 10*, 135–168.

Bollen, K. A., & Curran, P. J. (2004). Autoregressive latent trajectory (ALT) models: A synthesis of two traditions. *Sociological Methods and Research, 32*, 336–383.

Bollen, K. A., & Curran, P .J. (2006). *Latent curve models: A structural equation perspective*. New York: Wiley.

Burkholder, G. J., & Harlow, L .L. (2003). An illustration of a longitudinal cross-lagged design for larger structural equation models. *Structural Equation Modeling, 10*, 411–423.

Christ, O., Schmidt, P., Schlueter, E., & Wagner, U. (2006). Analyse von Prozessen und Veränderungen: Zur Anwendung autoregressiver latenter Wachstumskurvenmodelle. *Zeitschrift für Sozialpsychologie*, in print.

Conroy, D. E., Metzler, J. N., & Hofer, S. M. (2003). Factorial invariance and latent mean stability of performance failure appraisals. *Structural Equation Modeling, 10*, 401–422.

Curran, P.J., & Bollen, K. A. (2001). The best of both worlds. Combining autoregressive and latent curve models. In L. Collins & A. Sayer (Eds.), *New methods for the analysis of change* (pp. 107–135). Washington DC: American Psychological Association.

Duncan, T. E., Duncan, S. C., Strycker, L. A., Li, F., & Alpert, A. (1999). *An introduction to latent variable growth curve modeling. Concepts, issues and applications.* Mahwah, NJ: Lawrence Erlbaum Associates.

Enders, C. K., & Bandalos, D L. (2001). The relative performance of full information maximum likelihood estimation for missing data in structural equation models. *Structural Equation Modelling, 8*, 430–457.

Finkel, S. (1995). *Causal analysis with panel data.* Thousand Oaks, CA: Sage.

Graff, J. , & Schmidt, P. (1982). A General Model for the Decomposition of Effects. In K. G. Jöreskog & H. Wold (Eds.), *Systems under indirect observation: Causality, structure, prediction* (pp. 131–148). Amsterdam, The Netherlands: North Holland.

Guttman, L. A. (1954). A new approach to factor analysis, the radix. In P. F. Lazarsfeld (Ed.), *Mathematical thinking in the social sciences* (pp. 258–348). New York: Columbia University Press.

Halaby, C. (2004). Panel models in sociological research: Theory into practice. *Annual Review of Sociology, 30*, 507-544.

Hamaker, E. L. (2005). Conditions for the equivalence of the autoregressive latent trajectory model and a latent growth curve model with autoregressive disturbances. *Sociological Methods and Research, 33*, 319–348.

Hancock G. R., Kuo,W. L., & Lawrence F. R. (2001). An illustration of second order latent growth models. *Structural Equation Modeling, 8*, 470–489.

Heitmeyer, W. (Ed.) (2004). *Deutsche Zustände. Folge 3.* Frankfurt a. M.: Suhrkamp.

Herrmann, A., & Schmidt, P. (1995): Autoritarismus, Anomie und Ethnozentrismus. In G. Lederer & P. Schmidt (Eds.), *Autoritarismus und Gesellschaft. Trendanalysen und vergleichende Jugenduntersuchungen 1945-1993* (pp. 287–319*).* Opladen, Germany: Leske & Budrich.

Herrmann, A. (2001). *Ethnozentrismus in Deutschland.* (287–319). Opladen, Germany: Leske & Budrich.

Hertzog, C., & Nesselroade, J. R. (2003). Assessing psychological change in adulthood: an overview of methodological issues. *Psychology and Aging, 8,* 639–657.

Jagodzinski, W., Kühnel, S., & Schmidt, P. (1987). Is there a 'Socratic Effect' in non-experimental panel studies? Consistency of an attitude toward guestworkers. *Sociological Methods and Research, 15,* 259–302.

Jöreskog, K. G. (1979). Statistical estimation of structural models in longitudinal development investigations. In J. R. Nesselroade & P. B. Baltes (Eds.), *Longitudinal research in the study of behavior and development* (pp. 303–352). New York: Academic Press.

Kaplan, D., Harik, P., & Hotchkiss, L. (2001). Cross-sectional estimation of dynamic structural equation models in disequilibrium. In R. Cudeck, S. du Toit, & S. Sörbom (Eds.), *Structural equation modeling: present and future* (pp. 315–340). A Festschrift in honor of Karl Jöreskog. Lincolnwood, IL: SSCI.

Kühnel, S., & Schmidt, P. (2002). Orientierungslosigkeit. Ungünstige Effekt für schwache Gruppen. In Heitmeyer , W. (Ed.), *Deutsche Zustände. Folge 2* (pp. 83–95). Frankfurt a.M.: Suhrkamp.

McClosky, H., & Schaar, J. H. (1965): Psychological dimensions of anomy. *American Sociological Review, 30,* 14–40.

Meredith, W., & Tisak, J. (1990). Latent curve analysis. *Psychometrika, 55,* 107–122.

Oud, J. H. L. (2006). Continuous time modelling of reciprocal relationships in the cross-lagged panel design. In S. M Boker & M. J. Wenger (Eds.), *Data analytic techniques for dynamical systems in the social and behavioral sciences.* Mahwah, NJ: Lawrence Erlbaum Associates.

Pitts, S. C., West, S. G., & Tein, J.-Y. (1996). Longitudinal measurement models in evaluation research: Examining stability and change. *Evaluation and Program Planning, 19,* 333–350.

Rao, C. R. (1958). Some statistical methods for the comparison of growth curves. *Biometrics, 14,* 1–17.

Raykov, T. (2005). Analysis of longitudinal studies with missing data using covariance structure modeling with full-information maximum likelihood. *Structural Equation Modeling, 12,* 493–505.

Reinecke, J., Schmidt, P., & Weick, S. (2005). Dynamic modeling with structural equations and stochastic differential equations: Applications with the German socio-economic panel. *Quality and Quantity, 39,* 483–506.

Rogosa, D. R. (1995). Myths and methods: Myths about longitudinal research. In J. M. Gottman (Ed.), *The analysis of change* (pp. 3–66), Mahwah, NJ: Lawrence Erlbaum Associates.

Rogosa, D. , & Willett, J. B. (1985). Satisfying a simplex structure is simpler than it should be. *Journal of Educational Statistics, 10*, 99–107.

Scheepers, P., Felling, A., & Peters, J. (1992). Anomie, authoritarianism and ethnocentrism: Update of a classic theme and an empirical test. *Politics and the Individual, 2*, 43–60.

Schmidt, P., Stephan, K., & Herrmann, A. (1995). Entwicklung einer Kurzskala zur Messung von Autoritarismus. In G. Lederer & P. Schmidt (Eds.), *Autoritarismus und Gesellschaft. Trendanalysen und vergleichende Jugenduntersuchungen 1945-1993* (pp. 221–227). Opladen: Leske & Budrich.

Srole, L. (1956). Social integration and certain corollaries: an exploratory study. *American Sociological Revue, 21*, 709–716.

Stenner, K. (1997). *Societal threat and authoritarianism: Racism, intolerance and punitiveness in America, 1960-1994*. Ann Arbor, MI: University of Michigan.

Stoolmiller, M., & Bank, L. (1995). Autoregressive effects in structural equation models: We see some problems. In J.M. Gottman (Ed.), *The analysis of change* (pp. 261-278). Mahwah. NJ: Lawrence Erlbaum Associates.

Tucker, L. R. (1958). Determination of parameters of a functional relation by factor analysis. *Psychometrika, 23*, 19–23.

Chapter 14

Markov Process Models for Discrimination Learning

Ingmar Visser, Verena D. Schmittmann, and Maartje E. J. Raijmakers

University of Amsterdam, The Netherlands

14.1 INTRODUCTION

The focus of this chapter is on models with discrete states. The system of states evolves according to transition dynamics with Markov assumptions. Discrete state models have proven useful in such diverse areas as sociology, psychology, and economics. In particular, whenever discrete underlying constructs are plausible, and the data are longitudinal, Markov models are a good option to start modeling such data. They are usually applied when the data to be modeled are categorical, but Markov models are not limited to such data.

Because Markov models are extremely flexible for the purpose of modeling change, their use is widespread. For example, in operational research, so-called Markov decision models have been applied to problems in water resource management, epidemics, and sales promotion. See White (1993) for a survey of applications in operational research. In epidemics, for example, equilibrium states of predator-prey relationships can be modeled as states in Markov models. In economic science, Markov models are applied in predicting successive stages of economical development, periods of regression and expansion of the economy, and to pursue the holy grail; predicting the stock markets. The different stages of development, and regression or expansion form the discrete states in the Markov models applied in these areas. See for an application Ghysels (1994), and for a rather more theoretical treatment of Markov-switching dynamics Kim (1994).

In psychology, Markov models have a long history, going back at least to Miller (1952) and Miller and Chomsky (1963). Applications range from the analysis of social interactions in a situation where people are negotiating (Weingart, Prietula, Hyder, & Genovese, 1999), to the analysis of EEG measurements in the prefrontal cortex (Rainer & Miller, 2000). See Wickens (1982) for an overview of applications of Markov models in psychology. In most applications in psychology, the discrete states of Markov models are used to model knowledge or other states or characteristics of individuals, and possibly their interactions. A recent example is Böckenholt (1999) who applies Markov models to emotional states and their relationship to personality factors. In this chapter, an application is presented of Markov models in a learning experiment in which children of different ages and adults are compared as to the learning strategies they bring to bear on the task.

The organization of the rest of this chapter is as follows. In the next section, the conceptual background of discrete state models and the transition dynamics that are used to model processes of change is described. At the end of that section some pointers to the existing literature on those models are provided. In the next section, a formal treatment of the Markov model and extensions is presented. That section also includes the basics of computing likelihoods for such models and how to estimate and optimize parameters of Markov models. Then, in the following two sections, a discrimination learning experiment is presented that is used to illustrate a number of possibilities in applying Markov models to longitudinal data. In the final section, the results, possible extensions, and suggestions for further research are discussed.

14.2 THE MARKOV MODEL: STATE SPACE AND TRANSITION DYNAMICS

Markov models are characterized by two main features: a state-space and the transition dynamics. The state-space consists of a denumerable number of possible states that a system can be in, usually a finite number. Each state is characterized by a particular set of measurement results. The time-dependence of different measurement occasions is, in the Markov model, governed by a transition dynamical system. The transition dynamics can be both in discrete or in continuous time, however, in this chapter only data with measurements at regular discrete time intervals are considered. In the case of discrete time measurement occasions and a finite state-space, transitions between states can be described by a transition matrix containing the probability of remaining in a given state and the probabilities of moving to another state. An important assumption in Markov modeling is that the distribution of states at a certain time only depends on the distribution of states at the previous measurement occasion, but not on earlier occasions. This assumption, the Markov assumption, is detailed below.

Note that in log-linear models, which are frequently applied with discrete, longitudinal data, the time-dependence of the variables is not explicitly modeled in the same way as in Markov models. That is, in Markov models the transition dynamics is an explicit part of the model in the form of transition parameters. In log-linear models however, transition parameters may be estimated using a three-way table where one of the variables represents time (see Bijleveld & van der Kamp, 1998, for discussion).

The transition dynamics are the main point of interest in Markov models. That is, the transition dynamics provide us with the changes occurring over time in data, which is generally the focus of longitudinal research. Even so, a few words need to be said about the relationship between the states and the measured variables that are being modeled. There are a number of different options for this relationship. In the following, measured variables are referred to as indicators. States in a Markov model are levels of a possibly latent, nominal variable. In the case of simple Markov models, there is a one-to-one relationship between indicators and states. When someone votes democrat, we count her in the democrat camp. The focus of research when elections are near is how many people change their voting intention, due to a debate, say. In many social science situations unfortunately, things are not that easy. There are two ways in which the relationship between states and indicators may be different from a one-to-one relationship. First, there may be measurement error, as frequently occurs in social science testing and measuring. Subjects may get answers right by a lucky guess or they may make a mistake and erroneously get an answer wrong to a question they would otherwise answer correctly. When we wish to accommodate the possibility of measurement error, we need to use so-called *latent* Markov models. In latent Markov models, the relationship between indicator and state is not one-to-one, but rather modeled by a probability density. Note however that the relationship would be one-to-one in the absence of measurement error, that is, in an ideal world. The second way in which the relationship between indicator and states in the model can be different from a one-to-one relationship is usually based on theoretical arguments. For example, in models of learning, as elaborated in later sections, it is customary to include a so-called guessing state. At the start of some learning task, subjects have not gained any knowledge yet, and consequently their best strategy is guessing for the correct answer. In such a situation, the relationship between a latent state of the Markov model and the indicators is some probability function over the different alternatives, usually the multinomial distribution. Concluding, it may be said that the main distinction between simple Markov models and latent Markov models is in the relationship between the states of the model and the indicators. This part of the model is the *measurement* part of the model, that is, it relates the measurements with the structural variables in the model, the (latent) states. Extending this vocabulary, the transition matrix, containing the probabilities of switching between (latent) states, constitutes the *dynamic* part of the model.

Three other extensions of Markov models are important to mention; they deal with (1) multiple indicators, or multiple variables measured at each occasion of measurement, (2) heterogeneity in the population, and (3) heterogeneity in time. Until now it was assumed that at each occasion, a single variable was measured, a single indicator, such as correct/incorrect or Democrat/Republican. More often than not, however, in the social sciences we measure more than one variable or indicator. These indicators are all supposed to be indicative of some latent state. Hence, extending Markov models to include the possibility of multiple indicators is certainly useful. In the formal description of Markov models in the next section, we not only deal with multiple indicators of the same type, for example, two binary indicators for the latent state, but also with the case of mixed indicators. That is, in the model described fully below, it is also possible to have for example, one continuous and one binary response at each measurement occasion such that we have one continuous and one binary indicator. This is particularly useful in the analysis of psychological data, where we often have a categorical response, but also a reaction time corresponding with that response. Modeling those reaction times may prove useful in testing substantial hypotheses about the data at hand.

The second extension of Markov models deals with heterogeneity, which occurs when subgroups of the population have different transition dynamics or different response distributions (measurement part of the model). In this case, a multiple group (latent) Markov model is the appropriate model. Population heterogeneity is frequently encountered in the social sciences. For example, one can assume that elderly people are more conservative in their voting behavior. As a consequence, the transition dynamics, that is, changing preference from Republicans to Democrats or vice versa, of elderly people would be different from the dynamics of younger people. These assumptions could be tested using a multiple group model.

Another important form of population heterogeneity is latent heterogeneity. In the previous example, the population subgroups are known a priorily. However, this may not always be the case. As an example, that is treated extensively later in our illustration, consider learning strategies. For example, in discrimination learning, two types of learning strategy are used. These strategies can be expressed in terms of different latent Markov models. Because it is unknown how many and which subjects use which strategy, the models need to be combined into a mixture of latent Markov models. Langeheine and Van de Pol (1990) use the term mixed Markov model and a mixture of Markov models interchangeably. However, in this chapter we also use Markov models with mixed indicators, discrete and continuous indicators for the latent states, which are denoted here as mixed Markov models. Note also that Böckenholt

(1999) use the term mixed Markov model to refer to a single latent Markov model with a combination of fixed and random effects on the parameters, in line with the use of the term "mixed" in the general linear models literature.

In the above example, there are two qualitatively different learning strategies. However, it is also possible to assume that there is a single learning strategy that is applied more efficiently as one grows older. This would result in population heterogeneity, but of a different form. In such a situation, a Markov model with a covariate would be appropriate. In this case, some of the parameters of the model could be made to depend on age as a covariate.

Finally, the third extension of the simple and latent Markov models considered so far, deals with time heterogeneity. There are two ways to deal with time heterogeneity. The first possibility is to allow the model to have the transition dynamics depend on t, the measurement occasion, such that transition parameters are estimated for each t separately. For long time series and a limited number of subjects, as in our example, this is not feasible. Therefore, we consider the second possibility that is to include time-dependent covariates in the model. Covariates may be included in a model such that the dynamics of the model changes over time, or, as is the case in our application, such that the response distributions are different at different occasions. For example, in economical regime change models, the interest rate may be a covariate that can influence the probability of changing from stable markets to unstable markets. Adding all these extensions to the base models results in a very general model, the mixture of latent mixed Markov models with time-dependent covariates.

The most comprehensive introduction to Markov models, their relationship with latent class models, and their extensions, with references to applications, is Langeheine and Van de Pol (1990). For more specific examples of dealing with population heterogeneity through mixtures of Markov models or mixed Markov models, see Böckenholt (1999) and Rost (2002). For an educational application of time-dependent covariates in latent Markov models, see Vermunt, Langeheine, and Böckenholt (1999). The best overview of applications of (latent) Markov models in the psychology of learning is Wickens (1982). For more recent developments in that area, Katsikopulos and Fisher (2001) is a good choice. Schmittmann, Dolan, van der Maas, and Neale (2005) discuss latent Markov models with continuous valued indicators in the context of structural equations models, that is, each state is characterized by its own factor structure.

14.3 THE MARKOV MODEL: PARAMETERS, LIKELIHOOD, AND ESTIMATION

Before providing the full model that is considered later, first a simple example of a model for three-wave data of two binary items O_1 and O_2 is presented.

The responses are assumed to result from an underlying (knowledge) state S. The model is depicted in Figure 14–1. Using these notations, the likelihood of the complete data, that is, when the states S are assumed to have known values, is:

$$L(O_{11}, O_{21}, O_{12}, O_{22}, O_{13}, O_{23}) =$$
$$p(S_1)p(O_{11}, O_{21}|S_1)p(S_2|S_1)p(O_{12}, O_{22}|S_2)p(S_3|S_2)p(O_{13}, O_{23}|S_3). \quad (1)$$

Here S_i denotes the latent state variable at time i, which has a discrete distribution; in general, S_i is distributed multinomially with n the number of possible values of the state variable; $p(S_1)$ is the probability distribution of the state variable at time $t = 1$; $p(O|S_i)$ is the conditional distribution of the responses O given the current state, and $p(S_2|S_1)$, and $p(S_3|S_2)$ denote transition probabilities. More generally, of course, it could be the case that the distribution S_3 depends not only on S_2, but also on S_1. In Equation 1, the core assumption of Markov models is silently applied. The assumption states that the current state S_t of the system to be modeled only depends on the previous state S_{t-1}, and not on earlier states. Formally this (first-order) Markov assumption is expressed as:

$$p(S_t|S_1, S_2, \ldots, S_{t-1}) = p(S_t|S_{t-1}), \quad (2)$$

and hence the conditional distribution of S_3 only depends on S_2, and not on S_1. This assumption is customarily made in many applications in the psychology of learning. If the assumption is not met, it is usually possible to increase the number of latent states in such a way that the assumption is met. This amounts to fitting so-called higher order latent Markov models (see Langeheine & Van de Pol, 2000, for discussion).

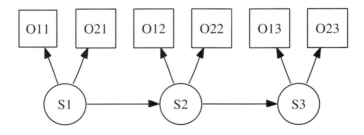

Figure 14–1. Markov model for three-wave data of two binary items.

Parameters

Throughout the rest of this chapter we use the following notations:

$$\pi_i \;\; := \;\; p(S_1 = i), i = 1, \ldots, n \tag{3}$$

$$b_i(O) \;\; := \;\; p(O|S_t = i), i = 1, \ldots, n \tag{4}$$

$$a_{ij} \;\; := \;\; p(S_t = j|S_{t-1} = i), i, j = 1, \ldots, n, \tag{5}$$

with n the number of states of the model, that is, the number of possible values the state variable S_t can assume. Here n is assumed to be finite. In words, π denotes the initial state distribution at $t = 1$, which is a probability vector with $\sum_i \pi_i = 1$. Next, $b_i(.)$ is the distribution of the responses or observations O conditional on the current state $S_t = i$, which may be written as a probability matrix when the observations are categorical. For example, for a binary item O we have $b_i(O = 1) + b_i(O = 2) = 1$, for each i. Finally, a_{ij} is the transition probability of moving from state $S_t = i$ to state $S_{t+1} = j$, which is written as a probability matrix $\mathbf{A}$. That is, for each state S_i the transition probabilities sum to one, $\sum_j a_{ij} = 1$. Heterogeneity in time can be accommodated by specifying separate distribution functions for each measurement occasion. In this general case, the distributions depend on t and we write $a_{ij} = a_{ij}(t)$. As a result, the number of parameters depends on the number of measurement occasions, which quickly becomes complicated when analyzing long time series. In particular, in the application that we consider, we have a large number of measurement occasions, and a limited number of cases. Therefore, none of the distributions depends on t in this general way. Instead, we deal with heterogeneity in time in a more parsimonious way by specifying parameters of distributions to be functions of time-dependent covariates z_t. When that is the case, we write e.g. $b_i(O|z_t) = P(O|S_t = i, z_t)$.

Using previous parameters of the latent Markov model, the likelihood of the example in Equation 1 is expressed as follows:

$$L(O_{11}, O_{21}, O_{12}, O_{22}, O_{13}, O_{23}|\lambda) =$$
$$\sum_{i,j,k} \pi_i b_i(O_{11}, O_{21}) a_{ij} b_j(O_{12}, O_{22}) a_{jk} b_k(O_{13}, O_{23}), \tag{6}$$

where the indices i, j, k run over possible sequences of states. The likelihood has to be summed over possible sequences of states, because these are unknown. Hence, when S can take n possible values, and when there are three measurement occasions, there are n^3 summands in the likelihood expression.

Likelihood

The data that we consider in this chapter consist of responses of subjects in a typical learning experiment. At each trial, a subjects' accuracy and his/her response time is measured, that is, the data consists of a bivariate time series with one binary variable and one continuous variable. The lengths of the time series vary from 10 to a maximum of 48 trials. The notation $\mathbf{O}_T^k = \mathbf{O}_1, \ldots, \mathbf{O}_T$ is used to denote a k-variate time series of length T, where $\mathbf{O}_t = O_t^1, \ldots, O_t^k$ are the responses observed at time t. Using the previous defined parameters, the likelihood for such a time series can be expressed as follows:

$$L(\mathbf{O}_T^k|\boldsymbol{\lambda}) = \sum_{S_1, \ldots, S_T} \pi_1 \, b_{S_1=i}(\mathbf{O}_1) \prod_{t=2}^{T} a_{S_{t-1}=i, \, S_t=j} b_{S_t=j}(\mathbf{O}_t). \quad (7)$$

In words, the sum runs over all possible realizations $S_1, \ldots, S_T$, which amounts to n^T summands when S_t can assume n possible values. Henceforth, as a shorthand, we write $S_i := S_t = i$.

When local independence is assumed among the items, the distribution functions $b_i(\mathbf{O}_t)$ can be simplified to:

$$b_i(\mathbf{O}_t) := b_i(O_t^1, \ldots, O_t^k) = \prod_{j=1, \ldots, k} b_i(O_t^j). \quad (8)$$

The assumption of local independence is very common in so-called latent variable models. Some even claim that local independence is *the* defining feature of latent variable models (see Bollen, 2002, for discussion). In many applications, local independence is indeed a reasonable assumption. A particular state, such as a knowledge state, an economical state, or an attitude, is supposedly the common cause of the observed variables. This assumption means that the underlying variable that we are interested in, the states in the case of Markov models, causes the observed variables to have the values that they have. As a consequence, when conditioning on that underlying variable, the observed variables are independent, which is expressed in the local independence assumption. Throughout the rest of the chapter, local independence is assumed for models that are fitted.

Note that so far we have not mentioned any particular assumptions about the distributions $b_i(.)$. The state variable S is distributed multinomially, and so are the transition probabilities, but for the observation distributions $b_i(.)$, there is no compelling reason to make any assumptions. As a consequence, they can be any estimable density function, including the multinomial distribution for categorical responses, but also the Gaussian distribution if, for example, reaction times are included. In such a case, when there is a categorical response and a continuous response, the local independence assumption proves very valuable, because there is no need to deal with the possible correlation structures among these different variables.

Mixtures of Markov Models

To deal with heterogeneity between subjects, in this chapter mixtures of latent Markov models are considered. Discrimination learning is provided here as an example to illustrate the need for mixture models. In discrimination learning, the assumption is that children of increasing age and adults apply a different learning strategy in solving the task than do younger children. Which strategy each person uses is not immediately clear, but has to be inferred from the responses that a subject generates. This is in contrast with population heterogeneity between, say boys and girls, in which case the researchers know a priorily to which group the subjects belong. In the case of discrimination learning, the goal is to infer the learning strategy a particular subject has applied from his/her response pattern. Two strategies are considered here that are proposed by theoretical considerations. Each of these can be translated into a latent Markov model. The resulting mixture of latent Markov models consists of two components, one for each strategy. Before discussing the interpretation of each of the proposed components in the next section, first, the equations for efficiently computing the log-likelihood of a mixture of Markov models is presented. Suppose the first component of the mixture has two states and the following parameters:

$$\mathbf{A} = \begin{pmatrix} a_{11} & a_{12} \\ a_{21} & a_{22} \end{pmatrix} = \begin{pmatrix} 1 & 0 \\ \alpha & 1-\alpha \end{pmatrix} \quad \text{and} \quad \boldsymbol{\pi} = \begin{pmatrix} \pi_1 \\ \pi_2 \end{pmatrix}. \tag{9}$$

The response parameters b are all freely estimated. The second component of the mixture has three states and the following parameters:

$$\mathbf{A} = \begin{pmatrix} a_{11} & a_{12} & a_{13} \\ a_{21} & a_{22} & a_{23} \\ a_{31} & a_{32} & a_{33} \end{pmatrix} = \begin{pmatrix} 1 & 0 & 0 \\ 0 & g & 1-g \\ \alpha & \beta & \gamma \end{pmatrix} \quad \text{and} \quad \boldsymbol{\pi} = \begin{pmatrix} \pi_1 \\ \pi_2 \\ \pi_3 \end{pmatrix}, \tag{10}$$

where $\gamma = 1 - \alpha - \beta$. When combining these transition matrices and initial state distributions in Equations 9 and 10, it can be easily seen that a mixture of latent Markov models is itself a latent Markov model:

$$\mathbf{A} = \begin{pmatrix} 1 & 0 & 0 & 0 & 0 \\ \alpha & 1-\alpha & 0 & 0 & 0 \\ 0 & 0 & 1 & 0 & 0 \\ 0 & 0 & 0 & g & 1-g \\ 0 & 0 & \alpha & \beta & \gamma \end{pmatrix} \quad \text{and} \quad \boldsymbol{\pi} = \begin{pmatrix} \pi_1^1 \\ \pi_2^1 \\ \pi_1^2 \\ \pi_2^2 \\ \pi_3^2 \end{pmatrix},$$

with the constraint that the π's sum to unity. It can easily be seen that computing the likelihood of such a model leads to many unneccessary computations because the transition matrix $\mathbf{A}$ contains blocks of zeroes that have to be multiplied T times for each time series under consideration. Therefore, the likelihood is computed as a mixture of the previous components with mixture proportion parameters p_k. The likelihood of a K-component mixture is written as follows:

$$L_T(\mathbf{O}|\boldsymbol{\lambda}) = \sum_{k=1}^{K} p_k L_T(\mathbf{O}|\boldsymbol{\lambda}_k), \tag{11}$$

where $\boldsymbol{\lambda}$ denotes $\boldsymbol{\lambda}_1, \ldots, \boldsymbol{\lambda}_K$, the parameter vectors for the different components of the mixture, and $L_T(\mathbf{O}|\boldsymbol{\lambda}_k)$ denotes the likelihood of each component model. The mixture proportions sum to unity, $\sum_k p_k = 1$. Details of the likelihood computation are provided next.

Likelihood and Parameter Estimation

It should be clear from Equation 7 that computing the likelihood for even moderately long time series leads to serious problems. For example, when the number of states of the model is two, and there are two binary variables measured at each occasion, i.e., we have $n = m = k = 2$, and T is 20, the contingency table to be analyzed has $4^{20} = 1099511627776 \approx 10^{13}$ cells. Moreover, the number of summands to compute the likelihood equals $2^{20} = 1048576 \approx 10^6$, for each case. Last but not least, the number of terms in the products for computing the likelihood is $2 \times T$ multiplied by the number of items. When this product becomes too high, it will cause underflow problems on every computer, that is, the numbers get too small to compute and/or the round-off errors increase exponentially. For this reason, common programs to do Markov analysis have limits on T. Panmark (Van de Pol, Langeheine, & Jong, 1996) limits T to 20 with a single observed variable at each occasion, whereas in the following illustration, T goes up to 48 with two observed variables at each t. To avoid these problems, we use a common estimation procedure from the hidden Markov model literature (Lystig & Hughes, 2002; Rabiner, 1989). This estimation procedure differs in three ways from the standard latent Markov estimation procedures. First, scaling is used to prevent underflow problems. Second, the raw data likelihood is computed instead of a sufficient statistic, a contingency table based likelihood. An added advantage of this is that missing data can be easily dealt with in a similar vein as is done in for example the Mx-program (Neale, Boker, Xie, & Maes, 2003). Third, a recursive scheme is used to compute the likelihood that is known as the forward algorithm such that the number of computations is limited.

Scaling. To deal with underflow problems, the joint probability of the data is first written as a product of conditional probabilities as follows (Lystig &

Hughes, 2002):

$$L_T = p(\mathbf{O}_1, \dots, \mathbf{O}_T) = \prod_{t=1}^{T} p(\mathbf{O}_t | \mathbf{O}_1, \dots, \mathbf{O}_{t-1}), \tag{12}$$

where $p(\mathbf{O}_1 | \mathbf{O}_0) := p(\mathbf{O}_1)$. Note that rewriting the joint likelihood in this way does not depend on any particular assumption of (latent) Markov models. Therefore, the dependence on the model parameters is dropped in the above equation. The log-likelihood can now be expressed as:

$$l_T = \sum_{t=1}^{T} \log[p(\mathbf{O}_t | \mathbf{O}_1, \dots, \mathbf{O}_{t-1})]. \tag{13}$$

This formulation of the likelihood prevents underflow to occur for long time series because the conditional probabilities $p(\mathbf{O}_t | \mathbf{O}_1, \dots, \mathbf{O}_{t-1})$ are computed, rather than the usual probabilities $p(\mathbf{O}_1, \dots, \mathbf{O}_T)$. Next we need to compute these conditional probabilities using the model parameters.

Forward Algorithm. Define the forward recursion variables as follows:

$$\phi_1(j_k) = p(\mathbf{O}_1, S_1 = j_k) = p_k \pi_{j_k} b_{j_k}(\mathbf{O}_1), \tag{14}$$

$$\phi_t(j_k) = p(\mathbf{O}_t, S_t = j_k | \mathbf{O}_1, \dots, \mathbf{O}_{t-1})$$
$$= \left[\sum_{k=1}^{K} \sum_{i=1}^{n_k} \phi_{t-1}(i_k) a_{ij_k} b_{j_k}(\mathbf{O}_t) \right] \times (\Phi_{t-1})^{-1}, \tag{15}$$

where $\Phi_t = \sum_{k=1}^{K} \sum_{i=1}^{n_k} \phi_t(i_k)$. Note first that the double sum over k and n_k in equation (15) is simply an enumeration of all the states of the model. Because $a_{ij_k} = 0$ whenever S_i is not part of component k, the sum over k can be dropped from the equation. These equations for computing the likelihood are a generalization of the work of Lystig and Hughes (2002) with the inclusion of mixtures of latent Markov models. Here $\phi_t(j_k)$ is the probability of observing $\mathbf{O}_t$ in state S_{j_k} conditional on having observed $\mathbf{O}_1, \dots, \mathbf{O}_{t-1}$. Hence, $\Phi_t = \sum_{k=1}^{K} \sum_{i=1}^{n_k} \phi_t(i_k)$ is the probability of observing $\mathbf{O}_t$ conditional on having observed $\mathbf{O}_1, \dots, \mathbf{O}_{t-1}$. The recursion includes an efficient enumeration of all possible latent state sequences. Note that computing the Φ_t takes in the order of S^2 computations, and hence computing the likelihood takes $S^2 \times T$ computations. Writing out Φ_t for $t = 3$ makes explicit its relationship with equation (7):

$$\Phi_3 =$$
$$\left\{ \sum_{i_3} \left[\sum_{i_2} \left(\sum_{i_1} \pi_{i_1} b_{i_1}(O_1) a_{i_1 i_2} \right) b_{i_2}(O_2) \right] a_{i_2 i_3} b_{i_3}(O_3) \right\} \times (\Phi_1 \times \Phi_2)^{-1}. \tag{16}$$

Note that the triple summation between braces is identical to Equation 7 for the case that $t = 3$. The multiplication of this term by $(\Phi_1 \times \Phi_2)^{-1}$ takes care of the scaling at each time point to prevent underflow.

Combining $\Phi_t = p(\mathbf{O}_t | \mathbf{O}_1, \ldots, \mathbf{O}_{t-1})$, and Equation 13 gives the following expression for the log-likelihood:

$$l_T = \sum_{t=1}^{T} \log \Phi_t. \tag{17}$$

Lystig and Hughes (2002) also provide gradients of the parameters for the log-likelihood. Existing programs for latent Markov models such as Panmark (Van de Pol et al., 1996) and Latent Gold (Vermunt & Magidson, 2003), cannot handle arbitrarily long time series and do not use raw data likelihoods, such that missing data can be problematic. The algorithm for computing the log-likelihood and the gradients are implemented as a package called depmix in the R-language for statistical computing (R Development Core Team, 2004). Depmix uses direct optimization of the log-likelihood with a Newton type algorithm using the gradients whenever they are available (Visser, 2005). Box constraints on parameters and general linear constraints between parameters (such as the sum constraints between the mixture proportions and the transition parameters) are handled by the optimization routines using either penalized log-likelihood or Lagrange multipliers.

14.4 DISCRIMINATION LEARNING AND CONCEPT IDENTIFICATION

As an illustration of the possibilities of mixtures of latent Markov models, they are applied in analyzing a discrimination learning experiment. Discrimination learning is typically assessed in a two-choice learning task. After a choice is made, feedback is given as to the correctness of the choice. From a series of such trials, subjects have to learn to discriminate which stimuli are correct and which are false. The data analyzed here are from a study by Raijmakers, Dolan, and Molenaar (2001). The study is described in some detail before presenting the analyses.

Experiment

Subjects.   The sample consisted of 249 children from a primary school in The Netherlands in the age range of 4 to 12 years old and 26 adults, who were first year psychology students.

Materials and Procedure.   Discrimination learning was assessed on a two-choice learning task. Stimuli differed on two dimensions; shape (triangle/

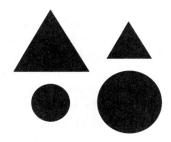

Figure 14–2. Stimuli used in the experiment.

square) and color (black/white). Stimuli were presented in pairs on a computer screen. The stimuli that were used in this study are shown in Figure 14–2. The stimulus pairs were randomized in groups of four. The subjects responded by choosing either the left or the right stimulus by pressing a marked key on the left or the right of a keyboard. Feedback consisted of either a cross or a smiley for incorrect and correct responses respectively. The task of learning to discriminate was continued until the criterion, that 9 of the last 10 trials were correct, was reached. The task comprised a maximum of 48 trials after which the test was interrupted. Each subject was tested once. Subjects' responses, including their reaction times, were recorded on each trial.

Sample. Eighty-four subjects did not satisfy the learning criterion of 9 correct trials in 10 successive trials within the maximum of 48 trials. They were not included in the analysis because subjects probably did not fully understand the task. Furthermore, 8 subjects were excluded who made a response in less than 150 ms more than twice. Such selection is done regularly in reaction time experiments: when subjects respond faster than 150 ms, it is considered unlikely that they have perceived and processed the stimulus. The remaining reaction times below 150 ms were coded as missing data. However, the accuracy data were kept on these trials, because during feedback the correct and incorrect choices were indicated below the stimuli, such that subjects still had the possibility to learn from such a trial. This resulted in a total of 185 subjects (82 males and 103 females) who were included in the analyses.

14.5 MIXTURE MODELS

There has been considerable debate about the nature of discrimination learning in the psychological literature. One aspect of the debate focuses on the question whether there are two distinct modes of learning rather than a single mode. The two proposed modes of learning are rational learning and slow learning (cf. Kendler, 1979). These modes of learning correspond to two latent Markov models which are compared here; the all-or-none model, which has two states, and the concept identification model, which has three states. Both models have a learned state, in which subjects are when they have mastered the task (Wickens, 1982). In this state, the probability of producing a correct answer is one or close to one. The all-or-none model proposes that learning is an all-or-none process: Either subjects have mastered the concept or they have not. If they have not, the probability of producing a correct answer is hypothesized to be 0.5, because there are two possible alternatives. This is the guessing probability and the knowledge state that underlies this is called the guessing state. In Figure 14(a) this model is represented graphically. Once subjects enter the learned state they cannot leave it, and hence the transition probability a_{ll} of remaining in the learned state is one. The probability of learning α, that is, the probability of moving from the guessing state to the learned state, is estimated. In Markov models of discrimination learning, this parameter is usually called the learning rate (Wickens, 1982).

In the concept identification model (ci-model henceforth), an extra assumption is introduced into the model. This assumption is that learning is an hypothesis-testing process and that learning only occurs after an error has been made (Wickens, 1982). Just as the all-or-none model, the ci-model has a learned state, which represents the knowledge state of subjects who have mastered the concept. In this state the probability of an error is zero or close to zero. In addition there are two other states, a correct state and an error state. Subjects are in the correct state as long as they produce correct answers, but fail to identify the concept. Similarly, they are in the error state, when they make an error. By definition, the probability of an error in the error state is 1, and similarly, the probability of answering correctly is 1 in the correct state. When in the error state, subjects choose a new hypothesis about the concept to be learned that is informed by their last error. The ci-model is depicted in Figure 14–3(b).

Based on this theory, Raijmakers et al. (2001) investigated the existence of two learning modes. They did this by deriving from each model its predicted distribution of errors in the first 16 trials, and fitting a finite mixture distribution model on the observed numbers of errors. In this chapter, we extend their work by fitting mixtures of latent Markov models to the full sequences of responses, instead of the derived distribution of the number of errors in the first

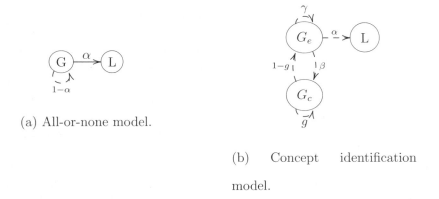

(a) All-or-none model.

(b) Concept identification

model.

Figure 14–3. Models for discrimination learning.

16 trials. The most important addition to the Raijmakers et al. analysis is that in our approach, *all* the parameters of the models can be estimated, whereas for example the error rates in the learned states were not estimated by Raijmakers et al. These error rates may in turn influence estimates of other parameters in the model, which in our approach are estimated simultaneously.

We fitted a number of models to the data. Note that the data consist of a series of correct/incorrect responses of a maximum of 48 trials. So, we have series of responses of different lengths, in fact varying from 9 to 48 trials for 185 subjects. In the next two sections, the reaction times were not included in the analyses.

All-or-None Models

A number of one component all-or-none models were fitted to the data. The full all-or-none model has four freely estimated parameters. First, the learning parameter α, which is the transition probability of moving from the guessing state to the learned state. Second, it has an error parameter in the learned state, denoted e_l, which is the probability of making an error even though the task has been mastered. This occurs sometimes, especially so in young children, due to lack of attention or due to inaccuracy. The third parameter is the guessing parameter, the probability of a correct answer in the guessing state; it is denoted c_g. The parameter estimates are in the first line of Table 14–1, Model 2. The fourth parameter (not in the table), is the initial state parameter π_l: It is the probability of starting in the learned state at the first trial. It is estimated at 0.085 with a standard error of .049. In Model 2a, this parameter is fixed at zero.

In Models 2b–2d this parameter is also fixed at zero. In the third model (2b), the guessing parameter c_g is fixed to 0.5, its theoretical value. This restricted model is nested within the first model and hence the constraint can be tested by means of a log-likelihood ratio test. The statistic $lr = -2 \times (l_c - l_u)$, where l_c is the log-likelihood of the constrained model, and l_u is the log-likelihood of the unconstrained model (2a), is χ^2-distributed with the difference in number of estimated parameters as df. In this case, $lr = 2.64$ with $df = 1$, which has $p = .104$. Hence, the constraint does not significantly worsen the goodness of fit of the model, and the constraint can be retained. The fourth model (2c) constrains the error parameter e_l to zero, and the fifth model (2d) constrains both parameters e_l and c_g. These models are not nested under the other models and so cannot be tested by the lr-statistic. Therefore, in Table 14–1, the AIC and BIC criteria (Akaike, 1979; Bozdogan, 2000; Golden, 2000) are included as well. As can be seen from those criteria, both Models 2c and 2d fit the data worse than do Models 2a and 2b. According to the AIC, Model 2 is the best fitting model, and according the BIC, Model 2b is the best fitting model. We discuss this point further in the section on mixture models.

TABLE 14–1

All-or-None Model Fits and Parameter Estimates

model	α (se)	c_g (se)	e_l (se)	logl	AIC	BIC	free
2	.116 (.010)	.511 (.019)	.050 (.010)	−1532.2	3072.4	3096.3	4
2a	.120 (.010)	.527 (.017)	.044 (.009)	−1534.05	3074.1	3092.1	3
2b	.125 (.010)	0.5 (fixed)	.048 (.009)	−1535.37	3074.7	3086.7	2
2c	.087 (.007)	.589 (.013)	0 (fixed)	−1556.64	3117.3	3129.3	2
2d	.095 (.007)	0.5 (fixed)	0 (fixed)	−1578.89	3159.8	3165.8	1

Note. These models have 3 parameters: α is the learning parameter, i.e. the probability of a transition from the guessing state to the learned state, c_g is the probability of a correct answer in the guessing state, and e_l denotes the probability of making an error in the learned state.

Concept Identification Models

The ci-model is depicted in Figure14–3(b), it has 3 states. The learned state, denoted L, is identical to the learned state in the all-or-none model: it represents the knowledge state when subjects have mastered the task. The other two states follow from the assumption that learning by hypothesis testing can only proceed after an error has been made. The states are labeled G_e and G_c respectively denoting the state in which errors are made and a state in which correct responses are produced. Hence, for those states, the observation function b_i is fixed such that in G_e the probability of a correct response is zero, whereas in state G_c the probability of a correct response is fixed to one. Learning can only occur after an error has been committed and as a consequence, there is a nonzero probability of moving from state G_e to state L, whereas the transition probability between G_c and L is zero. The probability of moving to state L from state G_e is called the learning rate α. The other parameters of the model are denoted β, γ, g, e_l, and the initial state probabilities $\boldsymbol{\pi}$, as they are called in the example in (10). The parameter g is the probability of staying in state G_c, hence it is the probability of getting a correct answer provided that the subject has not yet learned the task. Similarly, parameter $1 - g$ is the probability of moving to state G_c, and hence can be interpreted as the probability of making an error when the subject has not yet mastered the task. Parameters β and γ are related to the error state. The assumption in the CI-model is that subjects can only learn after an error, and they do this by selecting a new hypothesis after making an error. Consequently, α is interpreted as the probability of generating the correct hypothesis, β is interpreted as the probability of generating a wrong hypothesis leading to an incorrect answer, and γ is the probability of generating a wrong hypothesis leading to a correct answer on the next trial. The goodness-of-fit measures for this and other ci-models are in Table 14–2.

Assuming that subjects indeed respond according to their current hypothesis, the probability of committing an error in the presolution states should equal 0.5. This assumption translates into two constraints on the transition matrix parameters: Parameter g should be fixed at 0.5 and parameters β and γ should be equal to each other. These constraints about the parameters are tested both separately and together and the resulting log-likelihood ratio statistics with the full ci-model are reported in Table 14–2 as Models 3b, 3c, and 3d. Table 14–2 also provides log-likelihood ratio statistics that are all with respect to Model 3a. From those, it can be seen that both constraints, and the combined constraint are tenable, that is, they do not lead to worse models.

In the ci-models, the learning parameter α has a very specific interpretation: It is the probability of selecting the correct hypothesis after committing an error, in such a way that the new hypothesis is consistent with the last error made. Its magnitude depends on the hypothesis space that subjects consider. Subjects can also of course select the correct hypothesis immediately at the first trial. At the first trial, subjects have not made an error yet, and as a consequence, the probability of selecting the correct hypothesis should be equal to half the learning rate α (Kendler, 1979). This is the case if it is assumed that an error eliminates half of the possible hypotheses, which is plausible due to the symmetry of the given hypothesis space. This assumption translates into a constraint on parameters α and π_1 such that $\alpha = 2 \times \pi_1$. When at the first trial an incorrect hypothesis is selected, the probability of a correct answer is equal to the probability of an incorrect answer. Consequently, similar to the earlier fitted constraints about the equality of β and γ, the initial state probabilities π_2 and π_3 should be equal as well. The resulting models and their goodness-of-fit statistics are reported in Table 14–2 as Models 3e, 3f, and 3g for the two constraints combined. Table 14–2 also provides log-likelihood ratio statistics with respect to Model 3a. From the likelihood ratio statistics, it is clear that the constraints, both singularly and combined lead to models with poorer goodness-of-fit.

TABLE 14–2

Concept Identification Models for Discrimination Learning

model	logl	AIC	BIC	free	llr	df	p(llr)	constraint
3a	−1532.0	3076.0	3111.9	6	-	-	-	
3b	−1533.3	3076.6	3106.5	5	2.6	1	.107	$g = 0.5$
3c	−1533.7	3077.5	3107.4	5	3.4	1	.058	$\beta = \gamma$
3d	−1534.6	3077.1	3101.1	4	5.2	2	.074	$g = 0.5$ & $\beta = \gamma$
3e	−1536.7	3079.3	3097.3	3	9.4	3	.024	$\alpha = 2 \times \pi_1$
3f	−1536.4	3078.7	3096.7	3	8.8	3	.032	$\pi_2 = \pi_3$
3g	−1537.4	3078.7	3090.7	2	10.8	4	.029	$\alpha = 2 \times \pi_1$ & $\pi_2 = \pi_3$

Mixture Models

There are three important reasons that the single component models are not adequate descriptions of the data. First, as can be seen in Table 14–1 of the results of the all-or-none models, Model 2 turned out to be the best model according to the AIC criterion. For theoretical reasons however, having an initial state parameter different from zero for the learned state is very undesirable. That is, the all-or-none model is supposed to describe an incremental learning process, much like in conditioning. In such a learning process, it is highly unlikely that the stimulus-response connection already exists before any conditioning has taken place, i.e., before the presentation of the first trial. Consequently, this model is not very attractive. Second, in the ci-models, the constraints on the learning parameter turned out to be not tenable according to the log-likelihood ratio statistic. Again, from a theoretical point of view, this is undesirable, because it contradicts the basic assumption of the model, which is that subjects are using hypothesis testing to induce the relationships between stimuli and responses. Third, and finally, theory predicts that during development people shift from an all-or-none learning strategy to an hypothesis testing strategy. Because subjects from different ages took part in the experiment, it is natural to expect that the data reflect different learning strategies. Therefore, in this section, we discuss a number of mixture models, consisting of all-or-none and ci-model components.

We started with fitting a mixture model consisting of component Models 2 and 3a, an all-or-none and CI component respectively. Note that in this model all the parameters in each component are freely estimated. The fit statistics of this baseline model are in Table 14–3, Model 5a. In the following, this baseline model is constrained in three ways. The first parameter that we are interested in constraining is the nonzero initial probability of the all-or-none component, π_l. Remember that the interpretation of the all-or-none model is that subjects master the task slowly. This assumption is hard to reconcile with a nonzero probability of starting in the learned state, that is, mastering the task at the first trial. Hence, in Model 5b parameter π_l in the all-or-none model is constrained to zero. This constraint is on the boundary of the parameter space, and as a result the log-likelihood ratio test cannot be applied. Using the information criteria AIC and BIC, however, it may be concluded that Model 5b is more adequate in describing the data than Model 5a: it is more parsimonious than Model 5a, and has a better BIC value (AIC values are equal).

TABLE 14–3

Goodnes-of-Fit Measures for Mixture Models

model	logl	AIC	BIC	free	llr	df	p(llr)	add'l constr.
5a	−1519.6	3061.2	3127.1	11	-	-	-	
5b	−1520.6	3061.2	3121.1	10	-	-	-	$\pi_l(AN) = 0$
5c	−1521.1	3060.1	3114.0	9	1.0	1	.317	$c_g = 0.5$
5d	−1522.0	3054.0	3084.0	5	2.8	4	.592	$g = 0.5 \ \& \ \beta = \gamma \ \& $
								$\alpha = 2 \times \pi_1 \ \& \ \pi_2 = \pi_3$

The second constraint that we entered into the mixture model concerns the guessing parameter c_g of the all-or-none model. Model 5c implements the constraint in which c_g equals 0.5, the same constraint that was fitted in Model 2b. The first state of the all-or-none model is the so-called guessing state, and hence it is interesting to test whether indeed the behavior in that state has a probability correct of 0.5. The so-constrained model is nested under Model 5b, and hence the constraint can be tested with the likelihood ratio test, which is also reported in Table 14–3. The associated p-value is $p = 0.317$, and it can be concluded that constraining the guessing parameter does not result in worse model fit.

The third constraint, or rather set of constraints, relates to the ci-component of the model. It contains the four constraints that were also fitted in the ci-Models 3b and 3c, and 3e and 3f. First, the guessing parameter g is fixed at a value of 0.5, corresponding to the idea that having a wrong hypothesis leads to a wrong answer in 50% of the trials. Second, β and γ are constrained to be equal. The interpretation of this constraint is as follows: When subjects make an error, they choose a new hypothesis consistent with their last error.

They choose the correct hypothesis with probability α, and hence they choose the wrong hypothesis with probability $1 - \alpha$. Assuming that the hypothesis space they choose from is symmetrical, the probability of getting the next trial correct equals the probability of getting an incorrect answer at the next trial. As a result, these transition probabilities β and γ should be equal. The third and fourth constraints in the ci-component of the mixture model concern the initial state probability vector $\boldsymbol{\pi}$. The parameters π_e and π_c of the correct and error presolution states, are estimated to be equal for similar reasons as that β and γ should be equal. The initial probability of the learned state π_L is constrained as: $\pi_L = 1/2 \times \alpha$, that is, guessing the correct hypothesis by chance on the first trial can be done with half the probability of getting the correct hypothesis after an error because an error deletes half of the possible hypotheses. Model 5d in Table 14–3 implements these constraints.

The log-likelihood ratio statistic for Model 5d compared with Model 5c equals 1.8 with 4 degrees of freedom, which corresponds to a p-value of .592. Consequently, it can be concluded that the constraints are tenable. Also, the information criteria AIC and BIC assume their lowest values for this model compared with the other two-component models, and the single component models. Hence, it can be concluded that this mixture model is the best model among the models that we have fitted to these data.

The parameter values for this model are as follows (standard errors between parentheses). The mixture proportions are .483 (.109) and .517 (.109) for the all-or-none and ci-model components, respectively. In the all-or-none component, there are two free parameters, the learning rate α and the probability of an error in the learned state e_l. The values for these parameters are $\alpha = .078 \,(.013)$ and $e_l = .063 \,(.021)$, respectively. For the ci-model component, there is one free parameter in the learned state, the probability of committing an error in the learned state $e_l = .037 \,(.014)$. The other parameters are the transition matrix and the initial state parameter:

$$
\mathbf{A} = \begin{pmatrix} 1\ (\text{fixed}) & 0\ (\text{fixed}) & 0\ (\text{fixed}) \\ 0\ (\text{fixed}) & 0.5\ (\text{fixed}) & 0.5\ (\text{fixed}) \\ 0.530\,(.100) & 0.235\,(.050) & 0.235\,(.050) \end{pmatrix} \text{ and } \boldsymbol{\pi} = \begin{pmatrix} .265\,(.050) \\ .367\,(.025) \\ .367\,(.025) \end{pmatrix}.
$$
$$(18)$$

The comparison of the fitted models clearly shows that there are two modes in discrimination learning; one component with subjects who are comparatively slow learners, with a learning rate of .078, and a component with subjects who learn by hypothesis testing, which is a much more efficient learning strategy, with a learning rate of .530. In the sample that we tested, about half of the subjects (.483) belonged to the slow learners, and the other half to the hypothesis testers. In the following section, we have a closer look at each of these subgroups. Moreover, so far, we have only looked at relative measures of goodness-of-fit whereas it is interesting to know whether the proposed mixture model is adequate in terms of absolute goodness-of-fit.

A Posteriori Distributions

From the fitted models, Model 5d best describes the data, providing evidence for the existence of two distinct learning modes. However, we do not know whether it is an adequate model in absolute terms. The usual goodness-of-fit test for Markov models (and latent class models as well), is the χ^2-statistic, which is defined over the complete contingency table of the data. Three characteristics of the data and the model under consideration prevent the use of this goodness-of-fit statistic. First, because of the different lengths of the observed time series, the cells in the contingency table would have different reliabilities, thereby compromising the trustworthiness of the χ^2-statistic. Second, and more importantly, because of the length of the time series involved, the complete contingency table would have $2^{48} \approx 10^{15}$ and as a result the table would be very sparse. Third, even if the observed contingency table were available, computation of the expected contingency table is problematic in the models that we fitted. The reason for this is that the Markov models have so-called absorbing states and as a consequence the time series produced by them are not stationary. This means that the distribution of the possible states changes at each time point. In particular, the switching process between states ends in the learned state. For example, what would be the observed proportion of correct responses at trial 15? The answer to that question depends not only on the model parameters but also on the number of subjects that have not yet learned until criterion at that trial. There are two ways around this problem.

First, the contingency table could be made to depend on the criterion that was used to cut off the time series produced by the human subjects. This could be done by a bootstrapping procedure; generating series of responses from the model, and cutting them off using the discrimination learning criterion described earlier. The second possible solution to this problem is getting rid of the learned states in the model: The trials leading up to the learned state do form a stationary time series. Later we use this second approach to compute the expected number of trials until the learned state is reached.

From the parameters of the model, the distribution of the number of trials n before entering the learned state can be derived as follows. For the ci-model, the distribution $d(n)$ is the following:

$$d_{ci}(0) = \alpha/2, \tag{19}$$

$$d_{ci}(n) = (g(1 - \alpha/2))\alpha(1 - g\alpha)^{(n-1)}, n > 0, \tag{20}$$

where α and g are the estimated parameters of the model. For the all-or-none model the distribution is as follows:

$$d_{an}(n) = \alpha(1-\alpha)^{(n-1)}, n > 0, \tag{21}$$

where α is the learning parameter of the model. Note that the error parameter e_l, that is, the probability of making an error in the learned state, does not enter into these computations. The distribution d for the mixture model (5d) can simply be written as:

$$d_{mix} = p_{an}d_{an}(n) + p_{ci}d_{ci}(n), \tag{22}$$

where p_{an} and p_{ci} are the mixture proportions of the respective component models, and $d_{an}(0) = 0$, because in the all-or-none model one cannot have correct knowledge before the first trial.

In Figure 14–4, the expected frequencies are plotted as a line. From the observed sequence of trials, it is not clear when someone has mastered the task, and therefore we need another criterion. The criterion for learning in the experimental task was to have 9 out of the last 10 trials correct. Hence, as a criterion for the trial at which subjects master the task, we used the trial of the last error that subjects made before they started their run of trials that fulfilled the criterion. This run of trials that fulfills the criterion can be either 9 or 10 trials long. When it is 10 trials long, it contains one error at an arbitrary position, except the first trial. Using this criterion, we computed the lengths of the series of trials before mastering the task; this number is denoted t_m. The resulting observed frequencies t_m are plotted in Figure 14–4.

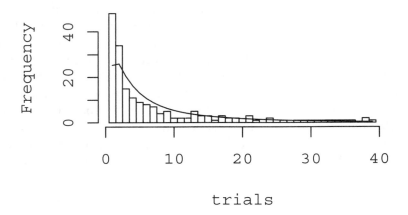

Figure 10–4. Trials until criterion.

With the model derived frequencies and the observed frequencies, we can now compute goodness-of-fit measures for the model. In particular, the χ^2 statistic and the L^2 statistic. For these frequencies, these are $\chi^2 = 54.29$ and $L^2 = 53.52$. These statistics both follow a theoretical χ^2-distribution. The degrees of freedom for the statistics are computed as the number cells minus one minus the number of parameters in the model. In this case, there are 39 observed frequencies, and three parameters (α_{ci}, α_{an} and one of the mixing proportions p_{an} or p_{ci}), resulting in $df = 35$. The corresponding p-values are $p(\chi^2 = 54.29, df = 35) = .012$, and $p(\chi^2 = 53.52, df = 35) = .023$, respectively. Consequently, the model fails to be completely adequate.

There are a number of possible reasons for this lack of fit. First, the observed frequencies in the tail of the distribution are very low and hence unreliable. As can be seen in Figure 14–4, the observed frequencies of t_m trials upwards of 25 are mostly one or zero, except where trials equal 38, where the frequency is two. The contribution of this cell to the χ^2-statistic is 6.7. This contribution is disproportionate in comparison to those of the other cells, which have a mean contribution of .37 to the χ^2. Leaving this cell out of the computation leads to $p(\chi^2 = 47.62, df = 34) = .061$, which is evidence of a reasonable model fit. Another, probably more important, reason for the lack of fit of the model is the criterion for determining when subjects have mastered the task from the observed sequence of responses. This is especially problematic for subjects who apply hypothesis testing.

Suppose that a subject produces the following series of trials: 1 0 1 1 1 1 1 1 1 1, that is, one correct response, followed by an error, followed by 8 correct trials. According to the criterion used earlier, this subject is scored as having mastered the task at trial 1, and hence a 0 is entered into the observed frequency table in Figure 14–4. However, it is quite likely that this subject has in fact used the feedback at trial 2 to figure out the correct hypothesis. Note that the criterion was introduced for errors that were made due to lack of attention, or other non-task related errors. This proved especially useful for young children who frequently commit such errors. As a consequence, a typical final run of trials would look something like: 1 1 1 1 0 1 1 1 1 1, that is, 4 correct answers followed by an error, and again followed by 5 correct answers. As a result of our criterion, we may have overestimated the number of subjects who master the task at trial 1, and underestimated the number of subjects who master the task at trials 2 or 3 instead. This suspicion is confirmed by looking at the contributions to the χ^2 at early trials. In particular, the individual cell contributions are 20.3, 2.5, 1.4 and 1.7 respectively in the first four cells. In the first two cells, the model underestimates the number of subjects, whereas in cells 3 and 4, the model overestimates the number of subjects. For these reasons, we believe the model actually captures the data quite adequately, and that the deviations that we find between observed and expected frequencies are an artifact of the criterion that we used to determine the observed frequencies. Bootstrapping could possibly resolve these issues (Langeheine, Pannekoek, & Van de Pol, 1996).

14.6 MODELS: INTERPRETING THE MIXTURE COMPONENTS

The logical next step is to find out what the subgroups corresponding to the mixture components look like. Based on the parameter values of the fitted model, we computed a posteriori probabilities for subjects to belong to either one of the components of the model. Next, to categorize subjects in one of the components, we simply used a cut-off of 0.5, that is, when the a posteriori probability for component one was higher than 0.5, the subject was categorized as belonging to the all-or-none learners, and otherwise the subject was categorized as a hypothesis tester. From developmental theory, it is expected that younger children are more likely to use an all-or-none strategy than are older children. This expectation is confirmed by a positive correlation between age and component membership $c = 0.353, t = 5.1, df = 183, p < .001$.

Assigning Subjects to Components

Assigning subjects to components in the manner used earlier is not completely satisfactory when trying to form subgroups. In particular, the mixture proportion for the all-or-none component was .483, but after assigning subjects in the previously described manner, only 52 out of 185 subjects were assigned to the all-or-none component. This corresponds to a proportion of .281. Similar problems occur in finite mixture distribution modeling, especially when one of two components has a much larger variance than the other. The a posteriori probabilities for assignment to the component with the smaller variance tend to be much higher. Something similar is happening in the case of our mixture of latent Markov models. This can be illustrated by a simple example. Subjects in the all-or-none component have a rather low learning rate. Even so, at least some of the subjects that use an all-or-none strategy in learning may master the task within the first three or four trials. Based on the learning rate $\alpha = 0.078$ in the all-or-none component, we can compute the number of all-or-none subjects that are expected to master the task within say three trials. First compute the number of subjects in the all-or-none component as $n_{AN} = 0.483 \times 185 = 89$. Of those, $0.078 \times 89 = 7$ are expected to learn at the first trial and so forth. At trial 3, already 19 of 89 all-or-none learners are expected to have mastered the task. These subjects are most likely assigned to the ci-component of the model because of their relatively fast learning. To remedy this, instead of using a simple cut-off at 0.5, we sample from the a posteriori distribution. That is, given an a posteriori probability of p_{AN} of belonging to the all-or-none component, we assign the subject this component based on a random draw from a uniform distribution between zero and one. This brings the proportion of subjects assigned to the all-or-none component closer to the fitted mixture proportion of 0.483. In the next two sections, the data are split into two components using this procedure.

Covariates

It has been suggested that in all-or-none learning, instead of having a stationary probability of learning, α, there should be an increasing probability of learning with trial number (Estes, 1950). This can be written as $\alpha_t = \alpha 0 + \beta t$, where t is the trial number. In the subgroup that corresponds to the all-or-none learners in our sample, we fitted a model with such a regression on the learning parameter. This is accomplished by introducing trial number as covariate in the data and fitting the all-or-none model with the described dependence between α and t. When this is done in the traditional all-or-none model, without error in the learned state, β is estimated at .001, and $\alpha_0 = .0517$, whereas, without the covariate, $\alpha = .0634$. The so-constrained model has an associated log-likelihood ratio of 1.7 ($p = .192$), indicating that adding the parameter does not result in significantly improved goodness-of-fit.

Combining Categorical and Continuous Data

In the subgroup of subjects that are hypothesis testing according to the ci model, there are also theoretical expectations about the response times (Erickson, Zajkowski, & Ehmann, 1966). In particular, we expect subjects to need more time to produce a response after they have made an error, because at such trials they have to select a new hypothesis based on their previous error. To test this hypothesis, we fitted a number of models that included the reaction times. The reaction time observed at trial t was included as indicator of the latent state at trial $t - 1$. The reason for introducing this lag in the reaction times is that these are hypothesized to depend on the feedback provided on the previous trial; that is, when a subject commits an error, the next trial is hypothesized to be slow, because the subject has to select a new hypothesis; conversely, when the current response is correct, the subject can retain his or her hypothesis, and hence, the response at the next trial will be relatively fast. The data hence consist of bivariate time series with the accuracy data and the lagged reaction time at each trial. We limited these analyses to the adult subjects, who follow a ci-model, only, because the variability in reaction times between the different age groups is very large.

The first model that was fitted had both accuracy and lagged reaction time as indicators for the three latent states. The log-likelihood for this model was

-1907.7, and its parameter values were $\alpha = 0.523$ and $e_l = .043$, the error probability in the learned state. In the mixture models, these parameters were 0.530 and 0.037 respectively. The estimated reaction times for the three states were 528.8 ms ($sd = 173$) in the learned state, 1150 ms ($sd = 1094$) in the correct state, and 1535 ms ($sd = 840$) in the error state, which is in agreement with our expectations.

To further improve the model, we included trial number as a covariate on the reaction times in each state, such that the reaction times were now modeled as $rt_t = rt_1 + \beta_{S_i} t_n$, where rt_t is the reaction time at trial t, and t_n is the trial number, and β_{S_i} are the regression coefficients for each state. The log-likelihood of the resulting model was -1896.4, and again the learning parameter and e_l parameter were virtually identical to the earlier model (0.524 and 0.044 respectively). The mean reaction times for each state were 638 ms ($sd = 163$) in the learned state, 1226 ms ($sd = 1095$) in the correct state, and 1640 ($sd = 830$) in the error state. The regression parameters for these states were estimated as -21.3 in the learned state, -17.0 in the correct state, and -73.5 in the error state. The log-likelihood ratio statistic for this model is 22.6, with $df = 3$, which has a $p-$value smaller then 0.001. Hence, adding the regression parameters to the model results in significantly better goodness-of-fit for the model. As can be seen from the parameter estimates, our hypothesis about the error and correct states was confirmed. That is, reaction times at trials after an error has been made are much slower than reaction times after a correct trial. Moreover, reaction times decrease sharply throughout the experiment. The regression parameters can be interpreted as the decrease in reaction times at each trial. So, after an error has been made, subjects respond relatively slowly at the start, 1640 ms, but their reaction times quickly decrease after errors, with steps of 73.5 ms.

14.7 SUMMARY AND DISCUSSION

In this chapter, we provide an illustration of the use of (mixtures of) latent Markov models in modeling (multivariate) longitudinal data. In particular, the results show that there are two qualitatively different modes of discrimination learning. This is shown by fitting a mixture of two latent Markov models to the accuracy data of subjects. To further characterize the component with slow learners, a model with covariates was used to test the hypothesis that these slow learners may be learning incrementally. The results indicated that that was not the case. Furthermore, we show an example of how reaction times can lend further support to the hypothesis that a subgroup of subjects learn by a process of hypothesis testing. A fuller treatment of the substantive issues in discrimination learning, and the interpretation of different components of the mixture models can be found in Schmittmann, Visser, and Raijmakers (2006).

Identifiability problems are pervasive in the application of latent class and latent Markov models (c.f. Wickens, 1982, chap. 7 for discussion). Using more than a single indicator may help identification of latent states by providing more information. In many psychological experiments, reaction times are measured alongside with accuracy data. However, in most cases, either the accuracy data or the reaction time data are analyzed, but they are seldom analyzed simultaneously. Using Markov models with multiple indicators can strengthen results based on accuracy data alone as we have shown in our example with reaction times. Similarly, covariates can be used to test specific hypothesis but also to possibly overcome identification issues of latent Markov models.

By presenting fitted models of time series up to lengths of 48 trials, we have shown the feasibility of fitting latent Markov models for relatively long time series. Former applications of latent Markov models usually involve a rather limited number of measurement occasions, with the exception of Böckenholt (1999), who modeled 21 measurement occasions. As Böckenholt (1999) pointed out, traditional goodness-of-fit measures, such as the χ^2 statistic break down in the face of long time series, and so alternatives have to be developed for the cases at hand. Together with the identifiability issues, this subject provides opportunities for further research.

ACKNOWLEDGMENTS

The research of Ingmar Visser was funded by a VENI grant from the Dutch Organization for Scientific Research (NWO). Funding for the work of Maartje Raijmakers was provided by EC Framework 6 project 516542 (NEST).

REFERENCES

Akaike, H. (1979). A Bayesian extension of the minimum AIC procedure of autoregressive models. *Biometrika*, *66*(2), 237–242.

Bijleveld, C. C. J., & Kamp, L. J. T. van der (1998). *Longitudinal data analysis.* Thousand Oaks, CA: Sage.

Böckenholt, U. (1999). Measuring change: Mixed Markov models for ordinal panel data. *British Journal of Mathematical and Statistical Psychology*, *52*, 125–136.

Bollen, K. A. (2002). Latent variables in psychology and the social sciences. *Annual Review of Psychology*, *53*, 605–634.

Bozdogan, H. (2000). Akaike's information criterion and recent developments in informational complexity. *Journal of Mathematical Psychology*, *44*(1), 62–91.

Erickson, J. R., Zajkowski, M., & Ehmann, E. D. (1966). All-or-none assumptions in concept identification: Analysis of latency data. *Journal of Experimental Psychology, 72*(5), 690-697.

Estes, W. K. (1950). Toward a statistical theory of learning. *Psychological Review, 57*, 94–107.

Ghysels, E. (1994). On the periodic structure of the business cycle. *Journal of Business and Economic Statistics, 12*(3), 289–298.

Golden, R. M. (2000). Statistical tests for comparing possibly misspecified and non-nested models. *Journal of Mathematical Psychology, 44*(1), 153–170.

Katsikopulos, K. V., & Fisher, D. L. (2001). Formal requirements of Markov state models for paired associate learning. *Journal of mathematical psychology, 45*, 324–333.

Kendler, T. S. (1979). The development of discrimination learning: a levels-of-functioning approach. *Advances in Child Development, 13*, 83–117.

Kim, C.-J. (1994). Dynamic linear models with Markov-switching. *Journal of Econometrics, 60*, 1–22.

Langeheine, R., Pannekoek, J., & Van de Pol, F. (1996). Bootstrapping goodness-of-fit measures in categorical data analysis. *Sociological methods and research, 24*(4), 492–516.

Langeheine, R., & Van de Pol, F. (1990). A unifying framework for Markov modeling in discrete space and discrete time. *Sociological Methods and Research, 18*(4), 416–441.

Langeheine, R., & Van de Pol, F. (2000). Fitting higher order Markov chains. *Methods of Psychological Research Online, 5*(1), 32–55.

Lystig, T. C., & Hughes, J. P. (2002). Exact computation of the observed information matrix for hidden markov models. *Journal of Computational and Graphical Statistics, 11*(3), 678–689.

Miller, G. A. (1952). Finite Markov processes in psychology. *Psychometrika, 17*, 149–167.

Miller, G. A., & Chomsky, N. (1963). Finitary models of language users. In R. Luce, R. R. Bush, & E. Galanter (Eds.), *Handbook of mathematical psychology* (pp. 419–491). New York: Wiley.

Neale, M. C., Boker, S. M., Xie, G., & Maes, H. H. (2003). *Mx: Statistical modeling*. Richmond, VA: Virginia Commonwealth University.

R Development Core Team. (2004). *R: A language and environment for statistical computing*. Vienna, Austria. (ISBN 3-900051-07-0)

Rabiner, L. R. (1989). A tutorial on hidden Markov models and selected applications in speech recognition. *Proceedings of IEEE, 77*(2), 267–295.

Raijmakers, M. E. J., Dolan, C. V., & Molenaar, P. C. M. (2001). Finite mixture distribution models of simple discrimination learning. *Memory & Cognition, 29*(5), 659–677.

Rainer, G., & Miller, E. K. (2000). Neural ensemble states in prefrontal cortex identified using a hidden Markov model with a modified em algorithm. *Neurocomputing, 32–33*, 961–966.

Rost, J. (2002). Mixed and latent Markov models as item response models. *Methods of Psychological Research Online, 2*, 53–72.

Schmittmann, V. D., Dolan, C. V., van der Maas, H. L. J., & Neale, M. C. (2005). Discrete latent Markov models for normally distributed response data. *Multivariate Behavioral Research, 40*(4), 461–488.

Schmittmann, V. D., Visser, I., & Raijmakers, M. E. J. (in press). Multiple learning modes in the development of rule-based category-learning task performance. *Neuropsychologia*.

Van de Pol, F., Langeheine, R., & Jong, W. D. (1996). *Panmark 3. Panel analysis using Markov chains: A latent class analysis program* [User manual]. Voorburg, The Netherlands: Statistics Netherlands.

Vermunt, J. K., Langeheine, R., & Böckenholt, U. (1999). Discrete-time discrete-state latent Markov modles with time-constant and time-varying covariates. *Journal of Educational and Behavioral Statistics, 24*(2), 179–207.

Vermunt, J. K., & Magidson, J. (2003). *Latent gold 3.0* [Computer program and user's guide]. Belmont, MA: Statistical Innovations.

Visser, I. (2005). Depmix: An R-package for fitting mixtures of latent Markov models on mixed data with covariates. Package on CRAN website: *http://cran.r-project.org/*.

Weingart, L. R., Prietula, M. J., Hyder, E. B., & Genovese, C. R. (1999). Knowledge and the sequential processes of negotiation: A Markov chain analysis of response-in-kind. *Journal of Experimental Social Psychology, 35*, 366–393.

White, D. J. (1993). A survey of applications of Markov decision processes. *Journal of the Operational Research Society, 44*(11), 1073–1096.

Wickens, T. D. (1982). *Models for behavior: Stochastic processes in psychology.* San Francisco: Freeman.

Chapter 15

The Use of Covariates in Distance Association Models for the Analysis of Change

Mark de Rooij

Leiden University, The Netherlands

15.1 INTRODUCTION TO CATEGORICAL REPEATED MEASUREMENTS

Many studies involve repeated measurements, that is, measurements on a number of time points. This longitudinal research is at the heart of understanding human development, both at the individual level as well as at the group level. Statistical methods for longitudinal data can be divided in two types: Methods for numerical variables where change is described in better versus worse or methods for categorical variables where change is described in terms of different versus the same.

The central assumption in this chapter is that people change step by step, making small moves. For example, when the length of a person is measured at repeated occasions, the growth will be gradually and in (relatively) small steps. The same thing is true for learning to speak or to read, children tend to change gradually in their development of such abilities. As an example, see the learning to read study (Jansen & Bus, 1982) and the analysis of the data in Timmerman and Kiers (2002). This gradual development should be taken into account when modeling repeated measurements. For interval type data, this is common; on a scale (in the first example, a length-scale) from small to long, people will make small steps from the left side (small) of this scale to the right side (long).

For categorical variables, however, this geometric framework of change is ignored in all common statistical methods for such data. Change is generally described by a number of transition probabilities, but no statistical method tries to recover the scale on which these changes occur. The terminology "scale" is often thought of as unidimensional. For categories of a variable like, for instance, political parties in the Netherlands, it is very plausible that they have a multidimensional nature (see Groenen, 2003). Therefore, the term scale is not very appropriate and "map" will be used instead. Distance association models (De Rooij, 2001a, 2001b, 2002, 2005a, 2005b; De Rooij & Heiser, 2003, 2005) assume such a map is present and people change gradually over this map, that is, categories that are close together on the map will have a high transition frequency, whereas categories that are far apart will have a low transition frequency. In other words, distance association models are the only models for longitudinal categorical data that take into account the geometric step by step aspect of change.

Distance association models (De Rooij, 2001a, 2001b, 2005a, 2005b; De Rooij & Heiser, 2003, 2005) are distance models for the analysis of contingency tables indexed by time. When there are measurements on two time points the table is square and the frequencies denote transitions between the categories of a variable. An example is political votes obtained from a sample of Dutch voters, where the categories are Dutch political parties, such as PvdA, CDA, VVD, D66, SP and so forth. The frequencies denote the number of voters that choose PvdA at the first time point and SP at the second. Similarly, when measurements are obtained at three time points, the frequencies denote the number of people voting PvdA at the first time point, SP at the second, and D66 at the third time point. This frequency (in case of two time points) is dependent on two things; the mass of each of the parties at the two time points and the distance between the two parties. The distances are estimated from the data and from these distances a map can be constructed that provides insight into the field of change, in this case the political field. In De Rooij and Heiser (2003, 2005), the theory is developed for two-way transition data. In De Rooij (2005a), distance association models are generalized to three time points using triadic distance models (De Rooij, 2002; De Rooij & Gower, 2003; De Rooij & Heiser, 2001; Gower & De Rooij, 2003), that define distances between three points. These triadic distances are easily generalized to distances between more points (see De Rooij, 2001, chap. 7). The geometry of such generalizations will not change compared to the triadic case. Not only do distance association models take into account the geometric aspect of change, because they are statistical models they can also be tested and statistical inference is possible. Other distance methods, often named multidimensional scaling, usually have an exploratory nature (see, for example, Borg & Groenen, 1997). The distance association models defined until this moment are suitable for change at the level of the whole group. It is, however, plausible that there are within group differences, for example between men and women. This chapter aims at

TABLE 15–1

Cross-Classification of Opinions on Clarence Thomas in September and October

			O	
P	S	F	U	N
L	f	18	4	7
L	u	4	43	7
L	n	43	32	54
M	f	77	7	31
M	u	12	36	12
M	n	108	41	127
C	f	99	3	21
C	u	8	11	4
C	n	55	24	59

Note. Favorable (F); Not Favorable (U); NO clear Opinion (N), differentiated by political orientation, Liberal (L); Moderate (M); Conservative (C). From Bergsma and Croon (2005).

extending distance association models for square contingency tables to include covariates, variables that represent differences between people.

To facilitate the discussion, we will use a small data set from Bergsma and Croon (2005). Bergsma and Croon (2005, p.84) describe this data set as follows:

> These data were obtained in a longitudinal survey in which a panel of respondents was interviewed in September and October of the same year on their opinion on the Supreme Court candidate Clarence Thomas (CT) who was nominated by President George Bush Senior. This nomination stimulated some public debate because of CT's Afro-American background and his allegedly extremely conservative views. Moreover, after the first survey was held on September 3-5, a charge for sexual harassment was brought against CT by his former aide Anita Hill on September 25. The second survey was then conducted on October 9. [...]. The variables S and O refer to the respondents' opinion in September and October, respectively. [...]. The variable P refers to Political orientation. We have grouped the original responses to this variable in three categories: Liberal, Moderate and Conservative.

The data is reproduced in Table 15–1, using codes F, U, N for Favorable, Unfavorable, No clear opinion. September opinions are in lower case, while October opinions are in upper case. For political orientation the codes Liberal (L), Moderate (M), and Conservative (C) are used.

The chapter is organized as follows. In the next section, we briefly outline the distance association models plus an analysis of the pooled data (Table
15–1). The third section discusses two ways of dealing with covariates: (1)
Using design matrices for a two-way table; (2) Using space transforming matrices. We describe both methods and show relationships to log-linear models.
In the fourth section we analyze Table 15–1 and we conclude with some discussion and possible extensions.

15.2 DISTANCE ASSOCIATION MODEL

15.2.1 The Model

Distance association models for the analysis of two-way contingency tables,
$\mathbf{F} = \{f_{ij}\}$, with $i = 1, \ldots, I$ and $j = 1, \ldots, J$, were proposed by De Rooij
and Heiser (2005). For longitudinal data, the i indicates categories at the first
time point, and j for the second, and typically $I = J$. The ingredients of distance association models are masses of the categories at the first and second
time point and distances between categories in a Euclidean space. This Euclidean space provides the map on which the transitions occur, that is, the multidimensional scale comparable to the one-dimensional length scale in the in-
troductory section. This map is of utmost importance to understand the change
process. The most general distance association model for a two-way table is
the two-mode distance association model, defined as

$$\pi_{ij} = \alpha_i \beta_j \exp\left(-d^2(\mathbf{x}_i, \mathbf{y}_j)\right) \tag{1}$$

where $d^2(\mathbf{x}_i, \mathbf{y}_j)$ is the squared Euclidean distance between two points defined
by the p-dimensional vectors $\mathbf{x}_i = [x_{i1}, \ldots, x_{ip}]^T$ and $\mathbf{y}_j = [y_{j1}, \ldots, y_{jp}]^T$.
The dimensionality cannot exceed $\min(I - 1, J - 1)$. When $p = \min(I -
1, J - 1)$ the model equals the saturated log-linear model for a two-way table;
when $p = 0$ the model equals the independence model for such a table.

In some cases the model where the row vectors and column vectors for a
specific category are constrained to be equal, that is, $\mathbf{x}_i = \mathbf{y}_i$, is of special
interest, leading to a symmetric association pattern. The model constrained in
that way is named the one-mode distance association model, defined by

$$\pi_{ij} = \alpha_i \beta_j \exp\left(-d^2(\mathbf{x}_i, \mathbf{x}_j)\right). \tag{2}$$

Again, the maximum dimensionality is $I - 1$, in which case the model equals
the quasi-symmetry model (Caussinus, 1965).

De Rooij and Heiser (2005) showed that the two-mode distance association model and the *RC(M)*-association model (Goodman, 1985) are equivalent in the expected frequencies. The interpretation of both models, however,
is quite different: The distance association model is interpreted in terms of

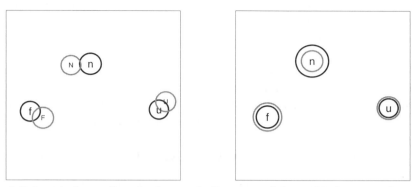

Note. Left frame is the two-dimensional two-mode distance association model. Lower case letters and black circles represent categories at September; Upper case letters and grey circles the categories at October. Right frame shows the two-dimensional one-mode distance association model, where black circles represent masses at September and grey circles masses at October.

Figure 15–1. Distance displays for the 3×3 table, ignoring political orientation.

distances whereas the *RC(M)*-association models should be interpreted using inner products. For a detailed discussion of the different interpretations and possible complications, see De Rooij and Heiser (2005) and De Rooij (2005a, 2005b).

15.2.2 Application to CT Data with Neglecting the Covariate

For sake of illustration of the distance association model, suppose we had not observed the respondents' political orientation. In that case, we have one table and one might be interested in whether the opinion about CT changed or not. The 3×3 table obtained by summing over political orientation is therefore analyzed. The two-dimensional two-mode distance association model is equal to the saturated log-linear model. Looking at its graphical display gives much insight into the structure (see left frame of Figure 15–1). The masses (main effects) are represented by the area of circles, like is discussed in De Rooij (2005a).

We see that there is a large continuity in the opinion of CT, that is, the favorable categories at September and October are close together, as well as for the other two categories, unfavorable and no clear opinion. Furthermore, we see that the distance from unfavorable at September to favorable in October $(d(u, F))$ is smaller than the other way around $(d(f, U))$, indicating that given the masses there are more transitions from unfavorable to favorable than reverse. Some more minor asymmetries are detectable from the left frame, but one might ask whether these asymmetries are due to sampling error or not. Therefore, the two-dimensional one-mode model is fitted, and this model indeed fits the data well ($X^2 = 2.84$; $G^2 = 2.89$; $df = 1$), and the solution is shown in the right frame of Figure 15–1. There we see that the masses of favorable and unfavorable increase whereas the mass of no clear opinion declined. Furthermore we see that the distance between no clear opinion and favorable is smallest, indicating relatively many transitions, whereas the distance between favorable and unfavorable is large, indicating relatively few transitions.

15.3 COVARIATES IN DISTANCE ASSOCIATIONS MODELS

In many cases of research involving longitudinal categorical data covariates are present and of utmost importance. Consider cases like pretest posttest designs, where in between the two measurements, subgroups get different treatments. Another case is where the subjects can be divided into natural groups, like boys/girls. In the CT example we have an intermediate case, where the covariate is not an experimental condition or a natural grouping, but distinguishes the respondents on a presumed important characteristic.

   In this section, we discuss two approaches to incorporate such covariates into our distance association model. The first way is to reorganize the table as a two-way table and use the two-mode distance association model on that table. Design matrices for the row coordinates might be used to obtain simpler models. The second way is to define a three-way table where the third way corresponds to the covariate mode and uses three-way distance models. We discuss both approaches and link them to hierarchical log-linear models like the saturated model and the no three-factor association model (see, for example, Agresti, 1990, p. 148).

   Before we start the discussion some notation is needed: The measurements at the two time points are denoted by T_1 and T_2 and the covariate by Z. The categories of the variable at T_1 are indexed by $i = 1, \ldots, I$, those at T_2 with $j = 1, \ldots, J$ and the categories of the covariate with $k = 1, \ldots, K$.

15.3.1 Approach I: Design Matrices

The way to take covariates into account as discussed in this section is based on methods proposed by Takane (1998). Basically, the table is reordered to be a two-way table and the two-mode distance association can be applied to this table. Because the table is in fact three-way, we label the model as follows:

$$\pi_{ijk} = \alpha_{ik}\beta_j \exp\left(-d^2(\mathbf{x}_{ik}, \mathbf{y}_j)\right). \tag{3}$$

For the CT example, the data is reordered to be of size 9×3. Without constraints on the row coordinates and in two dimensions, the distance association model equals the saturated model for such a table, and thus also for the original three-way table. By imposing a dimensionality constraint (i.e., a one-dimensional solution), the number of parameters is reduced and we obtain a testable model.

If we write $\mathbf{X} = [\mathbf{x}_{11}^T, \ldots, \mathbf{x}_{ik}^T, \ldots, \mathbf{x}_{IK}^T]^T$ then restrictions on these coordinates can be imposed by using design matrices $\mathbf{A}$, i.e. $\mathbf{X} = \mathbf{AX}^*$. These design matrices are equal to the design matrices used in regression analysis with categorical predictors. Without restrictions the matrix $\mathbf{A}$ might be written as

$$\mathbf{A} = [\mathbf{a}_1, \mathbf{A}_{M_1}, \mathbf{A}_{M_2}, \mathbf{A}_A] = \begin{pmatrix} 1 & 1 & 0 & 1 & 0 & 1 & 0 & 0 & 0 \\ 1 & 1 & 0 & 0 & 1 & 0 & 1 & 0 & 0 \\ 1 & 1 & 0 & -1 & -1 & -1 & -1 & 0 & 0 \\ 1 & 0 & 1 & 1 & 0 & 0 & 0 & 1 & 0 \\ 1 & 0 & 1 & 0 & 1 & 0 & 0 & 0 & 1 \\ 1 & 0 & 1 & -1 & -1 & 0 & 0 & -1 & -1 \\ 1 & -1 & -1 & 1 & 0 & -1 & 0 & -1 & 0 \\ 1 & -1 & -1 & 0 & 1 & 0 & -1 & 0 & -1 \\ 1 & -1 & -1 & -1 & -1 & 1 & 1 & 1 & 1 \end{pmatrix}.$$

The vertical lines correspond to different parts, the constant, the main effects and the association effect all of the association: $\mathbf{A} = [\mathbf{a}_1, \mathbf{A}_{M_1}, \mathbf{A}_{M_2}, \mathbf{A}_A]$. The main effect of the association indicates a two variable association, where the association of the association indicates a three variable association. Because the coordinates for the rows and columns are usually centered, the constant term ($\mathbf{a}_1$) is not necessary for fitting. However, to obtain the correct number of degrees of freedom, it is necessary. To obtain simpler models we could, for example, leave the $\mathbf{A}_A$ out of $\mathbf{A}$. In that case, the distances represent an association between the covariate(s) and the measurement on the second time point and an association between the two time points, that is, in that case the model in maximum dimensionality equals the no three-factor association log-linear model ($[ZT_1][ZT_2][T_1T_2]$).

We could also apply the matrix $\mathbf{A}$ to the main effect vector $\boldsymbol{\alpha}$, with $\boldsymbol{\alpha} = \{\alpha_{ik}\}$. Then instead of an interaction between the covariates and the measurement at the first time point, the $\boldsymbol{\alpha}$ represents the two main effects. The model using the design matrix on both the main effect as well as the row coordinates in full dimensionality equals the log-linear model $[ZT_2][T_1T_2]$.

It should be noted that in this modeling approach, the one-mode distance association model is not possible, or put otherwise, is equal to the model for the 3×3 table with symmetry restrictions.

15.3.2 Approach II: Space Transforming Matrices

The second way of treating covariates has its roots in articles of Carroll and Chang (1970) and Carroll and Wish (1974) where they discuss individual difference models in multidimensional scaling. The table to be analyzed in these proposals is three-way where two of its ways represent the same mode. The mentioned papers only discuss one-mode models, but the ideas can easily be generalized to two-mode models. The idea of this approach is that for each $k = 1, \ldots, K$ a different distance model can be fitted, but that these distance models can be related to each other in a functional way. The function is then defined by a space transforming matrix ($\mathbf{B}_k$). Without the functional constraints the model is

$$\pi_{ijk} = \alpha_{ik}\beta_{jk} \exp\left(-d^2(\mathbf{x}_{ik}, \mathbf{y}_{jk})\right) \tag{4}$$

Let us define the matrices $\mathbf{X}_k$ and $\mathbf{Y}_k$ as $\mathbf{X}_k = [\mathbf{x}_{1k}, \ldots, \mathbf{x}_{ik}, \ldots, \mathbf{x}_{Ik}]^T$, and $\mathbf{Y}_k = [\mathbf{y}_{1k}, \ldots, \mathbf{y}_{jk}, \ldots, \mathbf{y}_{Jk}]^T$. Now, in order to obtain simpler models the $\mathbf{X}_k$'s ($\mathbf{Y}_k$'s) can be constrained for $k = 1, \ldots, K$ to be related to each other in a number of ways, where always the following equality holds: $\mathbf{X}_k = \mathbf{X}\mathbf{B}_k$. The different possibilities are that $\mathbf{B}_k$ is nonsingular, is diagonal, or is equal to the identity matrix. Furthermore, one-mode restrictions, $\mathbf{X}_k = \mathbf{Y}_k$, are possible.

The model defined in Equation 4 in its most general form is equal to the saturated log-linear model ($[ZT_1T_2]$); without the distance part the model equals the log-linear model ($[ZT_1][ZT_2]$). So, the distances represent the two-way association between T_1 and T_2, but also the three-way association ZT_1T_2. When the matrices $\mathbf{B}_k$ do not depend on the index k, no three-way association is represented by the distances.

15.4 APPLICATION TO CT DATA

In this section, we apply the described approaches to the data in Table 15–1. The two approaches are dealt with in the two subsections.

15.4.1 Approach I

In Table 15–2 the results for some models are summarized, where we use the subscript $i + k$ to indicate that a design matrix with $\mathbf{A}_A$ removed was used, that is, $\mathbf{A} = [\mathbf{a}_1, \mathbf{A}_{M_1}, \mathbf{A}_{M_2}]$, and the subscript ik for the unrestricted case.

In Table 15–2 we see that all one-dimensional models give a bad fit. For the two-dimensional models, we see that only the saturated (i.e., without constraints) and the model with restrictions on the row coordinates fit well. The latter model equals the model with all pairwise associations.

The solution is shown in Figure 15–2. In this graphical representation, the masses of row points are difficult to compare to the masses of the column points. We can, however, easily compare them within the row or column categories. Concerning the distances, like in the analysis without covariate, a clear consistency in opinion is visible, that is, the favorable categories at Septem-

TABLE 15–2

Fit Statistics for Distance Association Models Using Design Matrices

model	dimensionality	
	$p = 1$	$p = 2$
$\alpha_{ik}\beta_j \exp\left(-d^2(x_{ik}, y_j)\right)$	21.19/20.99 (7)	0/0 (0)
$\alpha_{ik}\beta_j \exp\left(-d^2(x_{i+k}, y_j)\right)$	33.93/32.47 (11)	7.67/7.80 (8)
$\alpha_{i+k}\beta_j \exp\left(-d^2(x_{i+k}, y_j)\right)$	67.39/68.12 (15)	41.73/42.41 (12)
$\alpha_{ik}\beta_j \exp\left(-d^2(x_i, y_j)\right)$	57.45/49.46 (13)	28.15/27.15 (12)

Note. The numbers refer to X^2/G^2 (*df*).

ber are close to the favorable category of October, and similarly for the other opinion categories. Furthermore, there are little differences between political orientations. The liberals are generally somewhat closer to the unfavorable

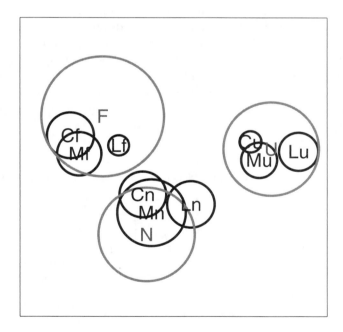

Note. Double letters with black circles refer to combinations of political orientation and opinion about CT at September. Upper case letters with grey circles refer to opinion at October.

Figure 15–2. Distance display in two dimensions with a design matrix on the row categories for the 9 × 3 table.

opinion; The conservatives somewhat closer to the favorable condition; The moderates are closer to the no clear opinion category. Are these differences important? On the last line of Table 15–2 the fit statistics of the model in which these points are constrained to be equal shows that they are indeed important, that is, the model does not fit the data.

15.4.2 Approach II

In this section, we discuss the second approach to dealing with covariates for the data represented in Table 15–1. Fit statistics are given in Table 15–3. Again, one-dimensional models do not fit the data adequately. From the two-dimensional models, the most simple one, the two-dimensional one-mode with restriction $\mathbf{B}_k = \mathbf{I}$ fits the data well and is shown in Figure 15–3. The association is the same for each group of subjects and is symmetric. Thus for each of the tables we have a quasi-symmetric form, where the margins may differ but the association structure is symmetric. In Figure 15–3 the masses are represented by the radius of the circle, where black circles are used for T_1 and grey circles for T_2. We see that the frames of Figure 15–3, corresponding to the three groups of political orientation, hardly differ. Some minor noticeable differences are that for the conservative group (right frame), the masses for unfavorable are relatively small, whereas for the liberal group (left frame), the masses of the favorable group are relatively small. Moreover, it seems that in the moderate group (middle frame) the masses of no clear opinion is relatively large. The pattern of masses is the same in all three groups; favorable and unfavorable gain mass where no clear opinion loses mass.

TABLE 15–3

Fit Statistics for Distance Association Models Using Space Transforming Matrices

Distance defined by	dimensionality	
	$p = 1$	$p = 2$
$\mathbf{X}_k, \mathbf{Y}_k$	18.66/18.98 (3)	0/0 (0)
$\mathbf{XB}_k, \mathbf{YB}_k$ with $\mathbf{B}_k$ diagonal	31.11/28.96 (7)	0.47/0.47 (2)
$\mathbf{X}, \mathbf{Y}$	31.35/29.53 (9)	7.67/7.80 (8)
$\mathbf{X}_k$	21.97/22.19 (6)	5.10/5.34 (3)
$\mathbf{XB}_k$ with $\mathbf{B}_k$ diagonal	32.73/30.76 (8)	5.13/5.37 (4)
$\mathbf{X}$	33.30/31.42 (10)	10.16/10.23 (9)

Note. The numbers refer to $X^2/G^2(df)$.

15.5 STABILITY

To obtain stability estimates of parameters, data reuse methods can be used, like the bootstrap and the jackknife. Here the jackknife procedure is exploited,

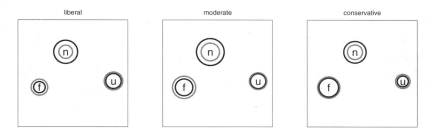

Note. Left plot for the 'liberals', middle plot for the 'moderates', and right plot for the 'conservatives'. Masses are represented by the area of the circles: Black circles for September; Grey for October.

Figure 15–3. The two-dimensional one-mode solution with restriction $\mathbf{B}_k = \mathbf{I}$.

because for contingency tables, it is computationally very cheap (Clogg & Shidadeh, 1994, pp. 34-38; Dayton, 1998, pp. 22-23). Let ξ be any parameter of interest and $\hat{\xi}$ be its estimator. For a data set with n observations an estimate of ξ is obtained for n samples where the i-th observation is deleted, $i = 1, \ldots, n$. Let $\hat{\xi}_i$ be the estimate with the i-th observation deleted. The estimated standard error using the jackknife is defined as (see Dayton, 1998, pp. 22-23)

$$SE_J(\hat{\xi}) = \sqrt{\frac{n}{n-1} \sum_{i=1}^{n} (\hat{\xi}_i - \hat{\xi})^2}. \tag{5}$$

TABLE 15–4

Coordinates and Standard Errors for Solution Shown in Figure 15–2

Category	Coordinate-1	SE	Coordinate-2	SE
Lf	-0.4289	0.1056	0.1697	0.0953
Lu	0.9777	0.0676	0.1202	0.0587
Ln	0.1361	0.0779	-0.3013	0.0921
Mf	-0.7373	0.0922	0.1022	0.0692
Mu	0.6693	0.0740	0.0527	0.0726
Mn	-0.1723	0.0788	-0.3689	0.0635
Cf	-0.8053	0.0804	0.2487	0.0633
Cu	0.6012	0.0941	0.1991	0.0823
Cn	-0.2403	0.0948	-0.2224	0.0843
F	-0.5529	0.0510	0.4021	0.0467
U	0.7634	0.0250	0.1414	0.0464
N	-0.2105	0.0679	-0.5435	0.0252

There is some evidence that the standard errors obtained from the jackknife procedure are somewhat too large (see Dayton, 1998, p. 37). In general the number of computations to be done is equal to the sample size. However, for contingency tables each observation in a given cell produces the same calculation as other observations in this cell. Therefore the number of calculations reduces from the sample size (n) to the number of cells of the contingency table. Confidence intervals can be obtained from these estimated standard errors by $\hat{\xi} \pm 1.96 \times SE_J(\hat{\xi})$.

We do not show the standard errors of all solutions, but use the solution shown in Figure 15–2 as an exemplar. Table 15–4 gives the coordinates of all categories on the two dimensions plus the standard errors. It can be seen that the solution is quite stable.[1] This is probably due to the fact that the data contain few small frequencies.

15.6 CONCLUSIONS AND DISCUSSION

Distance association models are discussed for longitudinal categorical data. These models provide a map or scale on which the transitions occur. The incorporation of categorical covariate variables was introduced. Two approaches to incorporate covariates into the distance association models are treated: The first approach has the advantage that the final model can be represented in a single display, whereas two displays are needed for the representation of the model in the second approach. The second approach has the advantage that the strength of the association between the measurements of the two time points in different groups can be compared: The larger the distances the stronger the association.

We only discuss models for a single covariate. In practical situations it is most likely that more information about the subjects is available. In that case both approaches can still be used. In the first approach, the design matrices just become larger with more main effects and more interaction effects. In the second approach, more displays are obtained, but the space transforming matrices itself might be subjected to design matrices itself.

In the case of measurements at three time points, *triadic distance models* might be used. Triadic distance association models were discussed in De Rooij (2005a). The incorporation of covariates in such a framework can follow the lines suggested here. However, with increasing time points and an increasing number of covariates, the number of cells in the table also increases rapidly and one has to be careful not to obtain very sparse tables. Moreover, in that case, there is also risk of loosing subjects over time. How to deal with such patterns of missing data in the current framework is still a subject of research.

---

[1] This is also true for the other solutions shown in this chapter.

REFERENCES

Agresti, A. (1990). *Categorical data analysis.* New York: Wiley.

Bergsma, W. P., & Croon, M. A. (2003). Analyzing categorical data by marginal models. In L. A. van der Ark, M. A. Croon, & K. Sijtsma (Eds.), *New developments in categorical data analysis for the social and behavioral sciences* (p. 83-101). Mahwah, NJ: Lawrence Erlbaum Associates.

Borg, I., & Groenen, P. (1997). *Modern multidimensional scaling: Theory and applications.* New York: Springer.

Carroll, J. D., & Chang, J. J. (1970). Analysis of individual differences in multidimensional scaling via an N-way generalization of 'Eckart-Young' decomposition. *Psychometrika, 35,* 283-319.

Carroll, J. D., & Wish, M. (1974). Models and methods for three-way multidimensional scaling. In D. H. Krant, R. C. Atkinson, R. D. Luce, & P. Suppes (Eds.), *Contemporary developments in mathematical psychology* (p. 57-105). San Francisco: Freeman.

Caussinus, H. (1965). Contribution à l'analyse statistique des tableaux de corrélation [Contributions to the statistical analysis of correlation matrices]. *Annals of the Faculty of Science, University of Toulouse, 29,* 715-720.

Clogg, C. C., & Shidadeh, E. S. (1994). *Statistical models for ordinal variables.* Thousand Oaks, CA: Sage.

Dayton, C. M. (1998). *Latent class scaling analysis.* Thousand Oaks, CA: Sage.

De Rooij, M. (2001a). Distance association models for the analysis of repeated transition frequency data. *Statistica Neerlandica, 55,* 157–181.

De Rooij, M. (2001b). *Distance models for the analysis of transition frequencies.* Unpublished doctoral dissertation, Leiden University.

De Rooij, M. (2002). Distance models for three-way tables and three-way association. *Journal of Classification, 19,* 161–178.

De Rooij, M. (2005a). *The analysis of change, Newton's law of gravity, and association models.* Manuscript submitted for publication.

De Rooij, M. (2005b). *The geometry of generalized biadditive models.* Manuscript submitted for publication.

De Rooij, M., & Gower, J. C. (2003). The geometry of triadic distance models. *Journal of Classification, 20,* 181–220.

De Rooij, M., & Heiser, W. J. (2000). Triadic distance models for the analysis of asymmetric three-way proximity data. *British Journal of Mathematical and Statistical Psychology, 53,* 99–119.

De Rooij, M., & Heiser, W. J. (2003). A distance representation of the quasi-symmetry model and related distance models. In H. Yanai, A. Okada,

K. Shigemasu, Y. Kano, & J. J. Meulman (Eds.), *New developments on psychometrics: Proceedings of the international meeting of the psychometric society* (pp. 487–494). Tokyo: Springer.

De Rooij, M., & Heiser, W. J. (2005). Graphical representations and odds ratios in a distance-association model for the analysis of cross-classified data. *Psychometrika, 70*, 99-122.

Goodman, L. A. (1985). The analysis of cross-classified data having ordered and/or unordered categories: Association models, correlation models, and asymmetric models for contingency tables with or without missing entries. *The Annals of Statistics, 13*, 10-69.

Gower, J. C., & De Rooij, M. (2003). A comparison of the multidimensional scaling of triadic and dyadic distances. *Journal of Classification, 20*, 115–136.

Groenen, P. J. F. (2003). *Dynamische meerdimensionele schaling: Statistiek op de kaart [Dynamic multidimensional scaling: Statistics on the map].* Rotterdam, The Netherlands: Inaugural address Erasmus Research Institute of Management.

Jansen, G. G. H., & Bus, A. G. (1982). *An application of a logistic bio-assay model to achievement test data* (Tech. Rep.). Groningen University: Department of Education.

Takane, Y. (1998). Visualization in ideal point discriminant analysis. In J. Blasius & M. J. Greenacre (Eds.), *Visualization of categorical data* (pp. 441–459). New York: Academic Press.

Timmerman, M. E., & Kiers, H. A. L. (2002). Three-mode principal component analysis with smoothness constraints. *Computational Statistics & Data Analysis, 40*, 447-470.

Chapter 16

Multitrait-Multimethod Models for Longitudinal Research

A. Scherpenzeel and W.E. Saris

University of Amsterdam, The Netherlands

16.1 INTRODUCTION

Campbell and Fiske introduced the multitrait-multimethod (MTMM) design at the end of the 1950s. The design involves the use of different methods to make repeated measurements of various traits. The covariances or correlations between the resulting measurements are then ordered in a matrix that is analyzed with a confirmatory factor model. The purpose of this analysis is to obtain estimates of measurement quality: validity, method effects, and reliability. De Wit and Billiet (1995) wrote an historical review of the development of the MTMM design and the conceptualization of validity, method effects, and reliability, which we summarize briefly. Campbell and Fiske (1959) spoke of "convergent validity" if measurements of the same traits, using different methods, correlated strongly. Although this convergence was considered to be a necessary part of the validation process, it was not considered, by itself, to be sufficient. Campbell and Fiske thus proposed a supplementary criterion, "discriminant validity," which applied if measures of different traits, using the same method, did not correlate strongly. The overall analysis technique used by Campbell and Fiske was largely qualitative and provided a rough indication of the convergent and discriminant validity of the MTMM measures. A decade later, confirmatory factor analysis using structural equation models became the main method for analyzing MTMM data. CFA offered the possibility to test different model specifications for MTMM data, for example correlated uniqueness models versus models with latent method factors, models with correlated versus models with uncorrelated trait and method factors, single-indicor versus multiple-indicator models. Eid et al. (2003) gave a comprehensive overview of the main models and discussed their properties and limitations.

The MTMM design and the CFA models were used mainly in psychometrics for a long time, until Andrews (1984) demonstrated how they could also be used to evaluate the measurement quality of survey questions. Since then, several large methodological research projects based on the MTMM model have been carried out to evaluate the quality of survey data (Andrews, 1984; Corten et al., 2002; Költringer, 1995; Saris & Münnich, 1995; Scherpenzeel & Saris, 1997).

In all of these projects, the repetition of survey questions required by the MTMM design presents a critical problem in both a theoretical and a practical sense. When repetitions of the same questions are presented within a single interview, respondents may recall their previous answers and their responses may be based on attempts to maintain consistency. Van Meurs and Saris (1990) have shown that, due to such memory effects, measures in MTMM studies that involve less than 20 minutes between repeated observations may not be considered independent, and may result in overestimation of the validity and reliability. On the practical side too, such repetitions can lead to irritation of the respondents, possibly increasing nonresponse or lowering the reliability of responses given later in the survey. In addition, a questionnaire design including repetitions of the same questions frequently provokes resistance from fellow researchers, research directors, and fieldwork institutes who all fear higher dropout rates and longer interviews.

To reduce the problems that can be caused by repeating questions, various adaptations to the MTMM design have recently been conceived. Saris, Satorra, and Coenders (2004) have proposed the split ballot MTMM experiment in which repetitions of the questions are spread over two identical subsamples from the same population. Scherpenzeel (2001) used an incomplete, balanced block MTMM design for the combination of the traits and the methods.

In the present chapter, we propose a panel MTMM design in which the repetitions of questions are spread temporally, over different waves of interviewing, in combination with an adapted MTMM model. We consider this to be a design perfectly suited to longitudinal studies.

16.2 THE CLASSICAL MTMM DESIGN AND MODEL SPECIFICATION

Saris and Andrews (1991) proposed the true score MTMM model for classical MTMM experiments. Here we give a brief summary of this model. For more detail, Saris & Andrews (1991) and Scherpenzeel & Saris (1997) may be referenced.

The response y on item i can be decomposed into a random component, e_i, and a stable component T_i, which is called the "true score" in classical test theory (Heise & Bohrnstedt, 1970; Lord & Novick, 1968). If the response variable and the variable representing the stable component are standardized, Equation 1 results:

$$y_i = h_i T_i + e_i \tag{1}$$

Here h_i represents the strength of the relationship between the stable component, or true score, and the response. The true score can be further decomposed into a component representing the score on the variable of interest, F_j, and a component, M_k, due to the method used. After standardization, this leads to the formulation of Equation 2:

$$T_i = b_{ij} F_j + g_{ik} M_k \tag{2}$$

Here b_{ij} represents the strength of the relationship between the latent variable of interest and the true score, and g_{ik} indicates the effect of the method on the true score. All three variables are standardized so the three coefficients mentioned are also standardized. Furthermore, we assume, as is normally done, that the correlations between the disturbance variables and the explanatory variables in each equation and across equations is zero, and that the trait factors are correlated but that the method factors are not correlated with each other nor with the trait factors. If all variables except the disturbance terms are standardized, the coefficients of the model have a special interpretation. In this case, h_i is called the "reliability coefficient" and its square is an estimate of test-retest reliability in the sense of the classical test theory; b_{ij} is called the "true score validity coefficient" because the square of this coefficient is the variance in the true score explained by the variable of interest; g_{ik} is called the "method effect" because the square of this coefficient is the variance in the true score explained by the method used.

For identification purposes the study should include at least three traits and three methods. Equation 2 represents the basic equation of the classical MTMM model and generates the factor structure presented in Table 16-1. The model is illustrated in Figure 16-1.

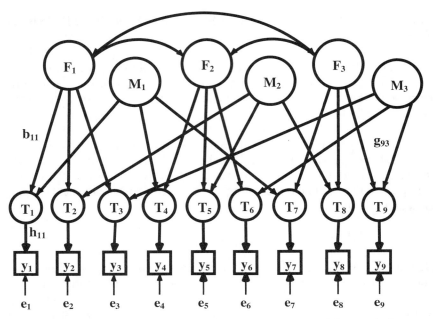

Figure 16-1. The standard true-score MTMM model for three traits and three methods.

TABLE 16-1
Factor Structure for the Standard 3x3 MTMM Design

	F_1	F_2	F_3	M_1	M_2	M_3
T_1	b_{11}			g_{11}		
T_2	b_{21}				g_{22}	
T_3	b_{31}					g_{33}
T_4		b_{42}		g_{41}		
T_5		b_{52}			g_{52}	
T_6		b_{62}				g_{63}
T_7			b_{73}	g_{71}		
T_8			b_{83}		g_{82}	
T_9			b_{93}			g_{93}

NOTE. T_i is the true score, F_j is the trait factor, M_k is the method factor

Because the CFA analysis of this factor structure often leads to problems of identification and convergence, many different assumptions and restrictions have been made in the past, each leading to a slightly different model specification and interpretation of the parameters. Saris and Andrews (1991) suggested making the assumption that the method effects are the same for all traits affected by the same method. If this assumption is made, all parameters of this model are identified and no convergence problems occur in estimation, as has been shown by Corten et al. (2002).

The major problem of this design is that the respondents have to answer the same questions approximately three times.

16.3 THE PANEL MTMM DESIGN AND MODEL

The panel MTMM design reduces the problems associated with question repetition. In this design, the repetitions are spread temporally over different waves. Given this time lapse, the model should allow for changes in the traits over time. Two repetitions of the same questions within the same interview are still required to separate the method effects from change in traits over time, but this is easier to carry out than three repetitions. Van Meurs and Saris (1990) showed that memory effects disappear if intervals between repetitions are greater than 20 minutes and are filled with questions of similar form and content to the repeated questions. This requirement is easier to meet when only two repetitions of the questions are needed instead of three.

In each wave, two measurements of the same traits are needed. The time between the two waves should be two or more weeks, because in their study of memory effects Van Meurs and Saris (1990) found that after two weeks, nearly all respondents had forgotten the answers they had given in the previous interview. Given this time lapse, the model should allow for changes in the traits over time.

In principle the model is specified as in Equations 1 and 2. However, the factor structure of Equation 2 can also have a different form. We will indicate two possibilities.

The first possibility follows directly from the specification of the true score model. When we use four methods to measure three traits in two waves, we observe 12 variables. Each question is repeated once in each wave. For this design, we suggest the factor structure shown in Table 16-2, with the same three latent trait variables in the first and second waves and with two methods in each wave.

TABLE 16-2
Factor Structure for the Two-Wave Panel MTMM Model.

	Wave 1			Wave 2			Method			
	F_1W_1	F_2W_1	F_3W_1	F_1W_2	F_2W_2	F_3W_2	M_1	M_2	M_3	M_4
T_1	$b_{1,11}$						g_{11}			
T_2	$b_{2,11}$							g_{22}		
T_3		$b_{3,21}$					g_{31}			
T_4		$b_{4,21}$						g_{42}		
T_5			$B_{5,31}$				g_{51}			
T_6			$B_{6,31}$					g_{62}		
T_7				$b_{7,12}$					g_{73}	
T_8				$b_{8,12}$						g_{84}
T_9					$b_{9,22}$				g_{93}	
T_{10}					$b_{10,22}$					$g_{10,4}$
T_{11}						$b_{11,32}$			$g_{11,3}$	
T_{12}						$b_{12,32}$				$g_{12,4}$

Note. T_i is the true score, F_jW_r is the trait factor j in wave r, M_k the method factor.

In this design, F_1W_2 represents in the second wave the same trait that F_1W_1 represents in the first wave. The same relationship exists between F_2W_2 and F_2W_1, and F_3W_2 and F_3W_1. The assumptions are the same as before: The traits can be correlated within and across waves but they are not correlated with the methods. In addition, the methods are not correlated with each other. The model is shown in Figure 16-2.

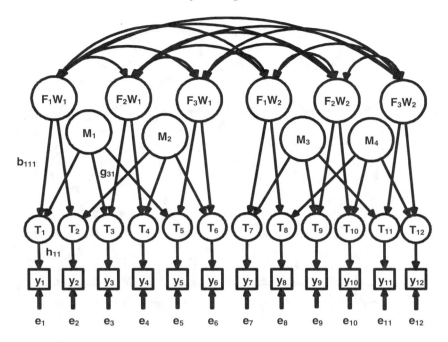

Figure 16-2. The two-wave panel MTMM model for three traits and four methods.

Again, we need to assume that method effects are equal across affected traits to identify the model with two indicators per trait. Because the correlations between traits are essential in the identification of the model, serious problems would arise if these correlations were found to be zero. Fortunately, because the same traits are measured in the two waves, this possibility can be excluded.

An interesting new aspect of this design is that it also provides estimates of the correlations between the traits over time. The structure of these relationships can again be analyzed by a factor model, but with an added, time-specific component. This can be formulated as written in Equation 3:

$$F_j W_r = c_{jr,n} F_n + S_{jr} \qquad (3)$$

Here, as usual, the unique component, S_{jr}, is supposed to be independent of the explanatory variables, that is, the stable trait factors, F_n. The latent traits, F_n, are correlated.

Assuming two time points and three traits, the third order factor model shown in Table 16-3 follows from Equation 3.

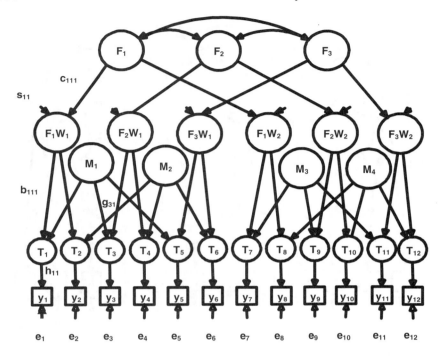

Figure 16-3. Third order factor model for three traits, four methods and two waves.

TABLE 16-3
Third order factor model for three traits and two waves.

	F_1	F_2	F_3
F_1W_1	$c_{11,1}$		
F_2W_1		$c_{21,2}$	
F_3W_1			$c_{31,3}$
F_1W_2	$c_{12,1}$		
F_2W_2		$c_{22,2}$	
F_3W_2			$c_{32,3}$

Note. F_jW_r is the time-specific trait factor j in wave r, F_n is the third order stable trait factor.

The coefficients $c_{jr,n}$ indicate the strength of relationships between stable trait factors and time-specific opinion j in wave r. The model formulated in Equations 1, 2 and 3 is shown in Figure 16-3. This formulation is in line with the latent state-trait models as described, for example, by Steyer and Schmitt (1990), Steyer, Schmitt, and Eid (1999) and Steyer, Krambeer, and Hannöver. (2004). In terms of a latent state-trait model, our time-specific, second order trait factors $F_{jr}W_r$ can also be called latent *state* factors, and our stable, third order trait factors can be called latent *trait* factors. The unique components S_j can be considered to represent the latent state residual or situational effect. Steyer, Krambeer, and Hannöver (2004) modeled true trait-change, as a result of therapy, in a similar way as we did earlier. In general, state-trait models have been used widely in psychological research. In this chapter, comparable concepts and models are applied to socio-economical survey data. However, the "state-trait" terminology is strongly associated with psychological research, aiming to measure (change in) true personality traits, as distinguised from person-situation specific psychological states. In the context of socio-economical survey research, we consider the terms stable traits or crystallized attitudes versus time-specific opinions as more appropriate. In this sense, the model presented is also in line with debates in political science about non-attitudes (Converse, 1964; Saris & Sniderman, 2004; Van der Veld & Saris, 2004) or opinion strength and crystallisation (Billiet et al.., 1986; Bizer et al.., 2004).

The second possibility to specify the factor structure for the true scores is an alternative but equivalent specification of the same model. If Equation 3 is substituted into Equation 2 the following model is obtained:

$$T_i = f_{in}F_n + g_{ik}M_k + b_{ir}S_{jr} \qquad (4)$$

Where the new coefficient f_{in} is equal to the product of the coefficients b_{ij} and $c_{jr,n}$. The model characterized by Equations 1 and 4 clearly defines the observed score, y_i, to be the sum of the stable trait score, method effects, time-specific thoughts, and random errors. We see that the errors and the method effects remain the same and, consequently, so do the reliability and validity coefficients in these two specifications. At the same time, the other parameters can be shown to be functions of each other.

Both models described earlier can be estimated using programs for structural equation models. Although these models are equivalent, we prefer to use the first one, specified in Equations 1 - 3, because it is more flexible with respect to the relationships between the traits over time. In this formulation, different alternative models can be specified, whereas the formulation in Equations 1 and 4 allows for the specification of only a single model. This advantage is illustrated later.

An Example: A Panel Study of Satisfaction

We now illustrate the panel MTMM design with an example that considers the traits of satisfaction with life in general, satisfaction with financial situation, and satisfaction with social contacts. The different methods used in this study are types of response scales. In a first interview, respondents indicated their degree of satisfaction two times for each of the three items listed above: One time they did so on a line drawing scale and one time they used a 10-point scale. In a second interview, two weeks later, the same items were again judged twice, this time once on a 100-point number scale and once on a five-point category scale. Special care was taken to formulate the satisfaction questions in exactly the same way each time they were presented, with the only variation existing in the response scale in order to satisfy the assumption of zero unique variance (see equation 2). To prevent memory effects, the questions were included in questionnaires filled with similar requests about living situation and well-being in such a way as to allow for at least 20 minutes between the first and the second presentations of the repeated questions. The complete design of the study is presented in Table 16-4.

TABLE 16-4
Design of the Satisfaction Study.

Measure	Trait	Method	
1	Satisfaction with life	line scale	
2	Satisfaction with finances	line scale	
3	Satisfaction with contacts	line scale	
	>20 minutes of other questions		Interview 1
4	Satisfaction with life	10-point scale	
5	Satisfaction with finances	10-point scale	
6	Satisfaction with contacts	10-point scale	
	2 weeks		
7	Satisfaction with life	100-point scale	
8	Satisfaction with finances	100-point scale	
9	Satisfaction with contacts	100-point scale	
	>20 minutes of other questions		Interview 2
10	Satisfaction with life	5-category scale	
11	Satisfaction with finances	5-category scale	
12	Satisfaction with contacts	5-category scale	

It can be seen that this design results in 12 measures (three traits x four methods). Polychoric / polyserial correlations[1] were calculated between all 12 measures. The correlation matrix obtained can be found in Appendix 1.

Table 16-5 shows the three "heterotrait-monomethod" triangles of this correlation matrix, containing the correlations between different traits as measured by the same method. It can be seen that, for the same respondents, very different correlations between the same traits can be obtained, depending on the response scale used. However, it is not clear which of the correlation matrices best approximates the real situation. The correlations obtained with the 100-point number scale are, for example, much larger than the correlations obtained with any of the other scales. This could mean that the 100-point measures contain less random error *or* that they contain more correlated error, due to method effects, than the other measures.

TABLE 16-5

Heterotrait-monomethod correlations

	Sat life	Sat fin	Sat life	Sat fin
	Line		**10 point**	
Sat fin	.37		.46	
Sat cont	.45	.30	.49	.33
	100 point		**5 category**	
Sat fin	.54		.44	
Sat cont	.64	.52	.46	27

Note. The correlations in the table are polychoric / polyserial correlations, estimated with Prelis (Jöreskog & Sörbom, 1998; see footnote 1).

The results of the panel MTMM model indicate which explanation is correct. At the same time, by distinguishing different forms of measurement error, it clarifies why the correlation patterns differ so much between the various scales. Finally, the model also provides an estimate of the change or stability over time of the traits, corrected for measurement error.

Using the first panel model formulation, the trait factors are the satisfaction domains at two different points in time and the method factors are the response scales. For example, the domain "satisfaction with life in general" is split into

[1] The five-point and 10-point scales used in this study can be considered categorical scales. Költringer (1995) showed that the quality estimates obtained with the true score MTMM model are affected by categorization, but that this effect can be avoided by using polychoric / polyserial correlations (see also Coenders & Saris, 1995).

two different traits: satisfaction with life in general at time 1, measured with the line and the 10-point number scales, and satisfaction with life in general at time 2, measured with the 100-point number and the 5-category scales. This applies to the other domains as well.

On the basis of the correlation matrix presented in Appendix 1, the parameters of the panel model, formulated in Equations 1 - 3, have been estimated. The overall fit of the model was acceptable (SRMR = .037)[2]. The reliability coefficient, h_i, and method effects, g_{ik}, obtained from this solution for each satisfaction measure are presented in Table 16-6. It can be seen that the reliability coefficients are rather stable across methods, but vary somewhat between the traits: *satisfaction with life in general* had, in all cases, a slightly lower reliability than *satisfaction with finances* or *satisfaction with social contacts*. The method effects are clearly dependent on the response scale used: The 100-point measures have much stronger method effects than the other measures for all three traits. The method variance in the true score MTMM model is the complement of the valid variance, and the validity coefficients thus support the same conclusions as the method effects. The 100-point measures suffer much more from lack of validity than any of the other measures.

TABLE 16-6

Quality estimates for the satisfaction measures

	Reliability coefficients h_i			Validity coefficients b_{ij}			Method effects g_{ik}		
	Sat life	Sat fin	Sat cont	Sat life	Sat fin	Sat cont	Sat life	Sat fin	Sat cont
line scale	.85	.92	.92	.94	.95	.95	.35	.32	.32
10-point scale	.89	.99	.92	.96	.97	.97	.27	.24	.26
100-point scale	.81	.92	.92	.70	.78	.78	.72	.62	.62
5-category scale	.88	.97	.92	.95	.96	.95	.32	.29	.31

[2] We have chosen the Standardised Root Mean-square Residual, which has a value of zero if the model perfectly describes the data, as statistic to evaluate the fit of the model because it is less sensitive to violations of the assumption of normal distribution of observed variables and to the size of the parameter values than other fit statistics (see also p. 396).

As the reliability of the 100-point measures is not higher than that of the other measures, it can be concluded that the high correlations between the 100-point measures shown in Table 16-5 were not caused by the absence of random error but by a high degree of correlated error. The panel model has thus clarified the source of the differences in correlation in Table 16-5.

As we mentioned earlier, the first panel model formulation also provides information about correlations between the two series of latent traits. These estimations are presented in Table 16-7.

TABLE 16-7
Stability and Correlations Between the Traits.

		Time 1			Time 2		
		Sat life	Sat fin	Sat con	Sat life	Sat fin	Sat con
Time 1	Sat life						
	Sat fin	.473					
	Sat con	.555	.321				
Time 2	Sat life	.739	.435	.451			
	Sat fin	.386	.817	.240	.467		
	Sat con	.421	.237	.751	.568	.237	

At both time points, the highest correlation was between satisfaction with life and satisfaction with social contacts (about .55), followed by the correlation between satisfaction with life and satisfaction with financial situation (.47 for both waves). The lowest correlation was between satisfaction with financial situation and satisfaction with social contacts (about .3). The stability of these correlations over time suggests that, in this case, the factor model formulated in Equation 3 may provide an appropriate description of the relationships between these latent variables over time. Table 16-8 summarizes the results of this analysis[3].

---

[3] This analysis was done simultaneously with the analysis of the other parts of the model.

TABLE 16-8

The Relationships $c_{jr,n}$ Between Time-Specific Opinions and Stable Trait Factors

	F_1	F_2	F_3
F_1W_1	.90		
F_2W_1		.98	
F_3W_1			.94
F_1W_2	.91		
F_2W_2		.87	
F_3W_2			.87

Note. F_jW_r is the time-specific trait factor j in wave r, F_n is the third order stable trait factor.

The correlations between the stable trait factors are: .52 between F_1 and F_2, .61 between F_1 and F_3, and .30 between F_2 and F_3. This model closely approximates the correlations presented in Table 16-4. The largest residual is smaller than .02.

The analysis yields crystallization coefficients, $c_{jr,n}$, that are rather high, indicating that the opinions are fairly strong. It seems that incidental effects may only slightly disturb results at the different points in time.

We can also formulate alternative models for the correlations between the time-specific opinions. Table 16-7 shows the overall correlation coefficients across both waves: .74 for satisfaction with life, .82 for satisfaction with finances, and .75 for satisfaction with social contacts. This across-wave structure may also be formulated in a different way. Let us suppose that the level of satisfaction at the second wave (W_2) depends on the level at the first wave (W_1). This yields:

$$F_1W_2 = v_{12,11} F_1W_1 + u_{12}$$
$$F_2W_2 = v_{22,21} F_2W_1 + u_{22} \tag{5}$$
$$F_3W_2 = v_{32,31} F_3W_1 + u_{32}$$

With $E(F_iW_r u_{jr}) = 0$ for all i,j,r and $E(u_{ir}u_{jr}) = 0$ if i is not equal to j.

The bases for this model are the correlations between the latent traits at W_1; the correlations between the traits at W_2 depend on the stability of the opinions. This model predicts that the correlations between the traits at W_2 will be smaller than the correlations at W_1 unless the standardized stability coefficients, $v_{ir,jr}$, are very close to 1. However, as Table 16-7 shows, the correlations at W_1 and W_2 are rather similar and, consequently, the model does not fit the data very well when we estimate it. However, even though application of the model of Equation 5 is not plausible in this example, it might still be useful for other data. If the model specified by Equation 1 and (4) would have been used the model of Equations 5 could not have been specified. This shows the flexibility of the model specified by Equations 1 and 2.

16.4 EVALUATION OF THE MODEL IN PRACTICE

Between 1989 and 1993, 12 different surveys using the multitrait-multimethod model were carried out in the Netherlands (Scherpenzeel & Saris, 1997). This study was intended as an extension of the large evaluation study done by Andrews (1984). The panel MTMM design with two waves was used in six of the 12 surveys and an extended panel MTMM design with three waves was used in one of the 12. The total sample size in these studies varied between 486 and 3,491 persons and experimental subgroups varied in size between 199 and 631 persons. As Saris (1990) has shown, a total sample of about 400 persons or more or subgroups of more than 200 persons give sufficiently precise parameter values in a CFA analysis of MTMM data. We may examine this project to determine the adequacy and utility of the panel model in practice.

The adequacy of a model can be evaluated on the basis of three criteria (Andrews, 1984). First, the model should be theoretically reasonable. In general, the arguments behind the true score MTMM model that have been discussed and that are grounded in classic measurement theory satisfy this criterion. More recent extensions of classical test theory are the latent state-trait models. The panel MTMM model presented here combines the classic MTMM model and the model of state-trait theory: It is an extension of the MTMM model with the possibility of separating time-specific opinions from stable traits and estimated true trait change, and at the same time an extension of the state-trait model with different method factors and estimates of validity and reliability.

Second, a proper solution should be found, which means the parameter estimates should have acceptable values. Unacceptable parameter estimates are estimates that have values that deviate far from expectation, such as a negative correlation where a positive one is expected, or estimates that are improper such as negative variances. In MTMM models, these improper solutions are very often due to overfactoring (Eid et al, 2003; Rindskopf, 1984), in which case they can easily be solved by restricting the non-significant loadings of one trait or one method factor to zero. For about half of the 40 panel MTMM matrices[4] the solution indeed contained some small, nonsignificant negative estimates of random error variance or method variance. However, these improper solutions seemed to be related more to categorization effects than to

[4] Each of the 12 surveys included two or three MTMM designs and various subgroups.

the panel design. The same problems appeared in the 18 one-wave MTMM matrices of the project. Moreover, for both the panel MTMM and the one-wave MTMM model, the problems arose only for matrices including two- or three-point scales. Restricting the error variances to zero could usually solve the problem[5]. A proper solution was found for each panel MTMM design including only scales with five or more categories

Third, the model should fit the survey data, which means it should predict relationships close to the observed relationships. Many statistics are available for evaluating the fit of these kind of models, and we have chosen to use the Standardised Root Mean-square Residual (SRMR, for RMR see Jöreskog & Sörbom, 1989), because this statistic is less sensitive to violations of the assumption of normal distribution of observed variables and to the size of the parameter values (Saris, Satorra, & Sörbom, 1987) than other fit statistics. The SRMR, which has a value of zero if the model perfectly describes the data, had a mean value of .041 across the panel MTMM analyses for this project. Hence, the fit of the model can be considered acceptable in general.

On the basis of these three evaluation criteria, it can be concluded that the adequacy of the panel MTMM model is fairly good.

16.5 CONCLUSION

We have discussed that the major drawback of the multitrait-multimethod model, in both a theoretical and practical sense, is the required repetitions of the same questions. When such repetitions are included in a single survey interview, memory effects may lead to overestimation of validity and reliability. On the practical side as well, such repetitions can irritate the respondents and yield longer interviews and higher dropout rates. We have proposed in this chapter a MTMM design specifically appropriate for longitudinal studies, which spreads the repetitions of the questions over different waves and estimates the changes in traits over time. In this design, each trait is split into two separate traits, one at each point in time. The correlation between these two traits indicates how much the opinion or attitude has changed over time. This model is identified when the same assumptions are made as for the usual MTMM model, and it can be formulated in the same way. Eid et al (2003) have proposed an alternative MTMM model that, in contrast to our model, allows the estimation of trait-specific method effects. However, for this model and for the whole class of multiple-indicator MTMM models that

---

[5] The small negative method variances seemed to indicate that one method factor had no effect. This is probably due to the correction for categorization effects created by using polychoric/polyserial correlations. Due to this correction, the method effects of the most severely categorized scales, the two- and three-point scales, were more or less filtered out. See also Saris, Van Wijk, & Scherpenzeel (1998).

they discuss, even more indicators are needed at each point in time in the classical MTMM design. This type of model requires three observed indicators for each of the 3x3 trait-method units. Eid et al used three different parts of a psychological scale as the different indicators and different raters (self, friend, acquintance) as the methods in a psychological study. However, in a socio-economical survey, the multiple indicator MTMM design would require an even greater number of repetitions of questions for the same respondents. It is exactly the burden caused by too many repeated measures that we wanted to the diminish with the panel MTMM model presented here.

The definition of the quality estimates in the panel MTMM model is the same as in the usual model. In addition, the panel MTMM model can provide estimates of the true relationships between traits of interest, corrected for different forms of measurement error. The importance of this correction is made obvious in our satisfaction example in which the correlation patterns between the traits of interest differed for the same respondents, depending on the type of response scale used. When only one method is used, as is usually the case in surveys, it is impossible to see any method effects that may be present. The panel MTMM model can clarify why correlation patterns may differ between scales by distinguishing different forms of measurement error present in the data. At the same time, it can correct the relationships between traits for each form of measurement error and can give an estimation of the true relationships. Likewise, the model also provides an estimation of true change or stability over time in traits, corrected for measurement error.

The Panel MTMM design also has one more advantage. We have shown that it provides information about strength of opinions by analyzing relationships between traits over time. For this analysis, we can formulate different models. In our example study, the factor model fit the data better than the alternative model, but that does not exclude the possibility of using other models for different data sets.

In general, the model formulated in Equations 1 and 2, which explicitly uses two sets of trait factors, is preferred above the decomposition model formulated in Equations 1 and 4 because it allows for the specification of alternative models of the stability of traits over time.

REFERENCES

Andrews, F. M. (1984). Construct validity and error components of survey measures: A structural modelling approach. *Public Opinion Quarterly, 48*, 409–422.

Billiet J., Loosveldt, G. & Waterplas, L. (1986). *Het survey-interview onderzocht: Effecten van het onderwerp en gebruik van vragenlijsten op de*

kwaliteit van antwoorden. Leuven: Sociologisch Onderzoeksinstituut
  K.U.Leuven.
Bizer, G. Y., Visser, P. S., Berent, M. K., & Krosnick, J. (2004). Importance,
  knowledge and accessobility: Exploring the dimensionality of
  strength-related attitude properties. In W. E. Saris & P. S. Sniderman
  (Eds.), *Studies in public opinion* (pp. 215–242). Princeton, NJ:
  Princeton University Press.
Campbell, D. T., & Fiske, D. W. (1959). Convergent and discriminant valida-
  tion by the multimethod-multitrait matrix. *Psychological Bulletin,
  56,* 833–853.
Coenders, G., & Saris, W. E. (1995). Categorization and measurement quality.
  The choice between Pearson and Polychoric correlations. In W. E.
  Saris & A. Münnich (Eds.), *The multitrait-multimethod approach to
  evaluate measurement instruments* (pp. 125–144). Budapest: Eötvös
  University Press.
Converse P. (1964), The nature of belief systems in mass publics. In D. A. Ap-
  ter (Ed.) *Ideology and dicontent* (pp. 206–261). New York, Free
  Press.
Corten I., Saris, W.E., Coenders, G., Van der Veld, W., Aalbers, W., & Kor-
  nelis, C. (2002). Fit of different models for multitrait-multimethod
  experiments. *Structural Equation models, 9,* 213–233.
De Wit, H., & Billiet, J. (1995). The MTMM design: back to the Founding
  Fathers. In W.E. Saris & A. Münnich (Eds.) *The multitrait-
  multimethod approach to evaluate measurement instruments* (pp.
  39–59). Budapest: Eötvös University Press.
Eid, M., Lischetzke, T., Nussbeck, F. W., & Trierweiler, L. I. (2003). Separating trait effects from trait-specific method effects in multitrait-
  multimethod models: A multiple indicator CTC(M-1) model. *Psy-
  chological Methods, 8,* 38–60.
Heise, D. R., & Bohrnstedt, G. W. (1970). Validity, invalidity and reliability. In
  E. F. Borgatta & G. W. Bohrnstedt (Eds.). *Sociological methodology*
  (pp. 104–129). San Francisco, CA: Jossey-Bass.
Jöreskog, K.G., & Sörbom, D. (1988). *Prelis: a program for multivariate data
  screening and data summarization* (2nd ed.). Mooresville: Scientific
  Software.
Jöreskog, K.G., & Sörbom, D. (1989). *Lisrel VII: Users reference guide.*
  Mooresville: Scientific Software.
Költringer, R. (1995a). Categorization and measurement quality: A population study using artificial multitrait-multimethod data. In W. E. Saris & A. Münnich (Eds.), *The multitrait-multimethods approach to
  evaluate measurement instruments* (pp. 103–124). Budapest: Eötvös University Press.

Költringer, R. (1995b). Measurement quality in Austrian personal interview surveys. In W. E. Saris & A. Münnich (Eds.) *The multitrait-multimethods approach to evaluate measurement instruments* (pp. 207–225). Budapest: Eötvös University Press.

Lord, F., & Novick, M. R. (1968). *Statistical theories of mental test scores.* Reading, MA: Addison-Wesley.

Rindskopf, D. (1984). Structural equation models: Empirical identification, Heywood cases, and related problems. *Sociological Methods and Research, 13,* 109–119.

Saris, W.E. (1990). The choice of a research design for MTMM studies. In W. E. Saris and A. van Meurs (Eds.), *Evaluation of measurement instruments by meta-analysis of multitrait-multimethod studies* (pp. 160–167). Amsterdam: North Holland.

Saris, W. E., & Andrews, F. M. (1991). Evaluation of measurement instruments using a structural modelling approach. In P. P. Biemer. R. M. Groves, L. E. Lyberg, N. Mathiowetz & S. Sudman, (Eds.). *Measurement errors in surveys* (pp. 575–597). New York: Wiley.

Saris, W. E. and Münnich, A. (1995) *The multitrait-multimethod approach to evaluate measurement instruments.* Budapest: Eötvös University Press.

Saris, W. E., Satorra, A., & Coenders, G. (2004) A new approach to evaluating the quality of measurment instruments: The split ballot MTMM design. *Sociological Methodology, 4,* 311–347.

Saris, W. E., Satorra, A., & Sörbom, D. (1987). The detection and correction of specification errors in structural equation models. In C. C. Clogg (Ed.). *Sociological methodology* (pp. 105–129). Washington, DC: American Sociological Association.

Saris, W. E., & Sniderman, P. S. (2004). *Studies in public opinion.* Princeton, NJ: Princeton University Press.

Saris W.E., Van Wijk, T., & Scherpenzeel, A. (1998). Validity and reliability of subjective social indicators: The effect of different measures of association. *Social Indicators Research, 45,* 173–199.

Scherpenzeel, A. (2001). Mode effects in panel surveys: A comparison of CAPI and CATI. *Actualités OFS,* order no. 448-0100, Neuchatel: Swiss Federal Statistical Office.

Scherpenzeel, A., & Saris, W. E. (1997). The validity and reliability of survey questions: A meta-analysis of MTMM studies. *Sociological Methods and Research, 25,* 341–383.

Steyer R, & Schmitt, M. J. (1990). Latent state- trait models in attitude research. *Quality and Quantity, 24,* 427–445

Steyer, R., Schmitt, M. & Eid, M. (1999). Latent state-trait theory and research in personality and individual differences. *European Journal of Personality, 13,* 389–408.

Steyer, R., Krambeer, S. & Hannöver, W. (2004). Modeling Latent Trait-Change. In K. Van Montfort, H. Oud & A. Satorra (eds.), *Recent developments on structural equation modeling: Theory and applications* (pp. 337–357). Amsterdam: Kluwer Academic Publishers.

Van Meurs, A., & Saris, W. E. (1990). Memory effects in MTMM studies. In W. E. Saris & A. van Meurs (Eds.), *Evaluation of measurement instruments by meta-analysis of multitrait-multimethod studies* (pp. 134–146). Amsterdam: North Holland.

Van der Veld, W., & Saris, W. E. (2004). Separation of error, method effect instability and attitude strength. In W. E. Saris & P. S. Sniderman (eds.), *Studies in public opinion* (pp. 37–63). Princeton, NJ: Princeton University Press.

Appendix 1. The correlation matrix between observed variables obtained from STP, March + April 1991.

	satlin1	satlin3	satlin4	sat10p1	sat10p3	sat10p4
atlin1	1.00					
satlin3	0.37	1.00				
tlin4	0.45	0.30	1.00			
at10p1	0.68	0.34	0.43	1.00		
at10p3	0.36	0.83	0.30	0.46	1.00	
sat10p4	0.35	0.19	0.76	0.49	0.33	1.00
sat1001	0.38	0.20	0.29	0.42	0.24	0.29
at1003	0.28	0.57	0.23	0.29	0.59	0.18
sat1004	0.27	0.19	0.51	0.32	0.24	0.52
at5p1	0.48	0.29	0.27	0.51	0.37	0.34
sat5p3	0.25	0.66	0.19	0.31	0.72	0.18
sat5p4	0.26	0.09	0.51	0.32	0.17	0.61

Correlation Matrix

	sat1001	sat1003	sat1004	sat5p1	sat5p3	sat5p4
sat1001	1.00					
sat1003	0.54	1.00				
sat1004	0.64	0.52	1.00			
sat5p1	0.53	0.37	0.40	1.00		
sat5p3	0.22	0.69	0.23	0.45	1.00	
sat5p4	0.27	0.15	0.63	0.46	0.27	1.00

Chapter 17

Patterns of House-Price Inflation in New-Zealand

Nicholas T. Longford

Universitat Pompeu Fabra, Spain

Iona McCarthy and Garry Dowse

Massey University, New Zealand

17.1 INTRODUCTION

The prices of residential properties are closely watched by prospective buyers, sellers, estate agencies, mortgage lending institutions, government agencies with economic and welfare remits and the construction industry. Media in the United Kingdom and other industrialized countries have periodically reported annual increases in house prices far in excess of or well below the retail price index or the inflation rate based on components of household expenditure that do not include housing costs. House prices tend to rise at unequal rates, more so than other elements of household expenditure, and so the house-price inflation has to be evaluated in and reported for regions or districts of the country.

Despite its generally appreciated importance, the house-price inflation is evaluated by elementary methods and without clearly conveying the assumptions made. The inflation rate is derived by comparing the sale prices of properties in two nonoverlapping time periods (years, or the same months of two consecutive years). The intended interpretation of the inflation rate is the increase in the sale price of two identical properties sold a given period (a year, quarter or month) apart. This would be appropriate if the properties sold were a noninformative subsample of the housing stock and the housing stock were subject to no development or deterioration — if the properties sold in the two periods were comparable. This is an unrealistic assumption that could, in principle, be addressed by adjusting for all the relevant factors. However, these factors include not only attributes of the dwelling (rooms and their decoration, fixtures and fittings, state of repairs, garden, garage, and the like), but all the "commodities" purchased with the property; the neighborhood profile, employment opportunities, and the quality of the local services (education, health, retail, police) and their reputation, and these are changing constantly.

To avoid any concerns about the distinctly nonnormal distribution of the sale prices, the medians of the prices are compared. Although this is effective, it is difficult to derive any meaningful measures of precision of the comparisons of interest, and impossible to extend the analysis to an adjustment for covariates. The outcome of the established analysis is the ratio of the median sale prices in the compared periods for the country and each region or district, expressed as a percentage. The results for the many districts are difficult to summarize and relate to comparisons in other pairs of periods. Some phenomena, such as the growing differentiation (prices rising faster in areas where the prices are already higher), are often described by pointing to areas that represent the extremes; there are no established ways of summarizing them in terms of graphs or parameter estimates.

We address the outlined problems by applying a log-normal multilevel model to the relevant data for several years. In this approach, the variance-matrix components provide an effective description for the course of inflation over the years. With the log-transformation, inflation compounded over several years converts to the total of annual log-inflations, so the related calculations generate no difficulties. By borrowing strength across the areas and over time (years), empirical Bayes methods convey an important advantage over methods based on the median price. The methods are illustrated on the register of all sales of freehold single-unit residential properties in New Zealand in the period 1996–2002.

The analysis is extended by an adjustment for rating valuation (RV), the local government's assessment of the value of each property within a local authority district. The valuation is conducted once every three years in most, and annually in some districts, at dates that differ from district to district (usually on 1st September of a year), and is updated when the property undergoes substantial changes, such as extension, alteration of use, or plot-splitting. The outcome of the valuation of a property is a monetary value of the property, comprising the value of the building and its immediate surroundings, such as fence and paving, and of the land that is part of the property. Their total is referred to as the *capital value* (CV). Throughout, we emphasize the advantage of simultaneous modelling of data for several years, without any detriment to the desired inferences about the recent inflation.

Mixture models that attempt to split the districts into a small number of groups with distinct patterns of inflation over the studied period are fitted. Their purpose is to find a more detailed description of the patterns of inflation and to identify any districts or valuation rolls (subdivisions of districts) with outlying patterns. Because any absolutely continuous multivariate distribution can be approximated with arbitrary precision by a mixture of multivariate normal distributions, mixtures can be regarded as a nonparametric generalization of the (log-)normal models.

17.2 THE DATABASE

The database comprises over 1.25 million records of transactions involving residential and related properties in New Zealand in years 1996–2003. A record comprises the location and identification of the property (district, valuation roll, street address and assessment number, a unique identification of the property in its valuation roll), surnames of the seller and purchaser, attributes of the property (the decade of its construction, its type and condition, floor area of the property's principal building and area of the land around the property), dates of the last RV and sale, tenure of the property, and the financial details; sale price and RV (CV and land value) in force at the date of the sale and on 1st January 2003. For some properties, the land value is a substantial fraction of CV, and so their sales are more appropriately regarded as sales of land. Our analysis makes use only of the monetary values and the dates of RV and sale and of the district and valuation roll identification. Other variables related to the price, such as the type and condition of the building, and the floor and land areas, are coded inconsistently and are missing for many properties. They are bound to be much poorer predictors than the valuation that incorporates them as factors.

The database contains duplicates; these are relatively easy to identify by the address, assessment code, transaction date, and the names of the seller and purchaser, although typos and inconsistencies present some problems. Some properties are recorded as sold for unrealistically small amounts (NZ\$1, NZ\$20, NZ\$100, and the like), and cannot be regarded as genuine sales. In other instances, the sale price is several times higher than the valuation, and cannot be regarded as genuine either. For instance, a sale of several single-household properties is recorded once for each property, but their total sale price is quoted in each record.

Properties are excluded from the analysis when the recorded sale price is lower than NZ\$10 000 (NZ\$1 was equivalent to approximately UK£0.36 and US\$0.68 in mid-2003), the land value exceeds 50% of CV, or the land area

TABLE 17–1

Numbers of Transactions of Freehold Single-Unit Residential Properties in New Zealand in 1996–2002

	Year							
	1996	1997	1998	1999	2000	2001	2002	Total
Transactions	93 457	83 562	64 580	60 514	53 742	59 189	70 224	485 268

is in excess of one hectare. The latter are deemed to be principally sales of land or of properties not solely for residence. So called "life-style" properties, which combine residence and small-scale (not necessarily commercial) agricultural production and related activities, are also excluded. Only properties that comprise a single unit (for one household) and their tenure is freehold (not leasehold, cross-lease or other) are retained. As a result of this selection and removal of duplicates, the analyzed data comprise 485 356 records (38% of the database); Table 17–1 gives their distribution across the years. For orientation, the population of New Zealand is about 4.0 million and its residential housing stock is about 1.5 million single-household units.

New Zealand is administratively divided into 74 local authorities (districts); 49 of them are on the North Island, 24 on the South Island, and the remaining district, Chatham Islands, is several hundreds of miles east of either Island in the Pacific Ocean. It is sparsely populated and there are only a handful of transactions annually — these are not included in the database. Of the 73 districts, 15 are city districts, four of them on the South Island. The Auckland metropolitan area comprises four districts, and the area around Wellington, the capital, another three city districts in addition to Wellington City. The districts and the basic information about them are listed in the left-hand part of Table 17–6 in the concluding Section 17.6, together with a summary of the results. A map of New Zealand, with all the districts mentioned in this chapter, is drawn in Figure 17–1. The valuation rolls have been defined as divisions of districts specifically for the purpose of RV.

The districts vary a great deal in their population sizes and numbers of transactions. Eleven districts have fewer than 1000 transactions each and six districts have over 20 000 transactions each over the period of seven years. The latter include all four districts that comprise the Auckland metropolitan area; these four districts account for over 125 000 transactions, more than a quarter of the total. A few rural districts have only a few valuation rolls (12 districts have 6–11 rolls each), and six districts have over 80 rolls each. In total, there are 2495 rolls represented in the data, but 549 of them have no transactions in at least one year. These rolls account for only 12 332 transactions (2.5%). Just

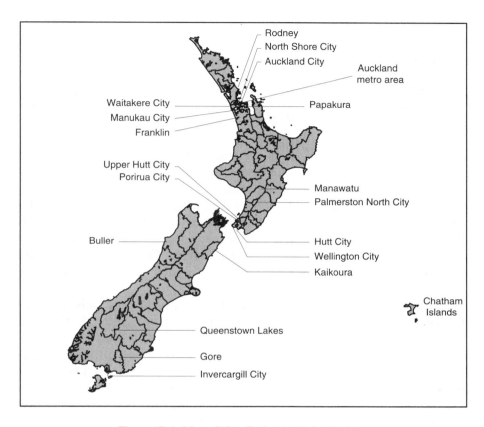

Figure 17–1. Map of New Zealand with its districts.

over a thousand rolls (41%) have fewer than 100 transactions each. The rolls in a part of Auckland City were redrawn in 1999. The rolls for all the earlier transactions in this district were recoded to agree with the current boundaries.

The next section describes the analysis of the sale prices by a random-effects analysis of covariance with years, rolls, and districts as factors. The analogue of the year-by-district and year-by-roll interactions that would be considered in a fixed-effects analysis is the pattern of variation, described by a variance matrix for the districts and one for the rolls. In Section 17.4, multi-level regression is applied to adjust for CV, and to regard time as a continuous variable. The analysis in Section 17.3 aims to describe the annual inflation in districts and valuation rolls, whereas the results of Section 17.4 can be used for prediction and, in principle, even for setting of the sale prices of individual properties, based on CV. Section 17.5 derives and compares estimates of the inflation rates based on the models fitted in Sections 17.3 and 17.4. Section 17.6 contains a discussion and a summary of the results.

17.3 ANALYSIS

Because the database is so large, it is practical to carry out as many of the computations as possible separately for the districts. This is facilitated by organizing all the computations so that the required sufficient statistics for each analysis are evaluated first, immediately after data input and selection of the records for the analysis. A set of minimal sufficient statistics for the most complex multilevel model considered are the year-by-roll means and totals of squares and crossproducts of all the variables involved; log-prices and log-valuations, and the numbers of transactions on which they are based. A similar principle is applied in the software VARCL (Longford, 1993a), although it has only rudimentary data handling and no graphics facilities. All the computing described here was carried out in R (R Development Core Team, 2004), after extracting the relevant data for each district using the grep command in the Unix operating system.

For modelling, it is attractive to associate the districts and rolls with random effects, by referring to a superpopulation, even though the districts and rolls are fixed, in that a hypothetical replication of the data-generating process would yield the same "effects" for each district, roll, and year, but a different set of properties sold. The replicate prices of any given property might also vary. An advantage of applying linear models with random coefficients to the logarithms of the sale prices over using medians is that a connection is maintained between the raw averages and the corresponding model-based estimators.

17.3.1 District-Level Analysis

Most districts have so many transactions each year that the underlying annual means and variances of the log-sale prices are estimated by their sample counterparts with high precision. The log-means are presented more effectively graphically than by a table. In Figure 17–2, the lines connect the seven annual log-means for a district. We refer to them as *inflation trajectories*. If the districts had identical inflation rates and their log-mean prices were increasing or decreasing by the same rate in each year, the trajectories would be parallel; in the absence of any inflation, they would be horizontal lines. The graph shows that the log-means have become more dispersed over the years, but their relative ordering has changed only slightly — districts with the highest (geometric or log-) means in the earlier years tend to have the highest log-means also in the more recent years. A notable exception is Queenstown Lakes District on the South Island (highlighted and marked in the margins of the left-hand panel by

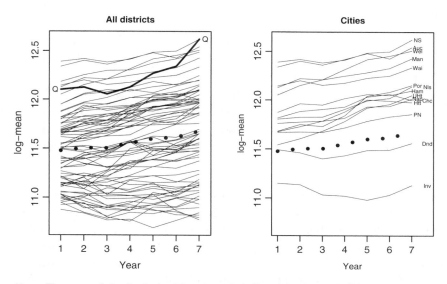

Note. The mean of the district-level log-means is indicated by dots. The fifteen cities plotted in the right-hand panel are, from top to bottom: North Shore, Auckland, Wellington, Manukau, Waitakere, Porirua, Nelson, Hamilton, Upper Hutt, Napier, Christchurch, Hutt, Palmerston North, Dunedin and Invercargill. The labels of the cities on the South Island are indented.

Figure 17–2. The inflation trajectories for the districts of New Zealand, from 1996 (year 1) to 2002 (year 7).

"Q"), which has undergone extensive development as a holiday resort. In 1996 (year 1) it had the sixth highest log-mean and by 2002 (year 7) its log-mean has matched North Shore City, the district with the highest log-mean in every year except for year 4 (1999). The city districts tend to have higher means; the right-hand panel of Figure 17–2 is an extract of the left-hand panel containing only the trajectories for the 15 city districts.

Log-normality of the sale prices is strongly corroborated by the relevant histograms and test statistics. Also, the district-level medians differ very little from the corresponding geometric means. (Details are omitted.) For orientation, log-prices of 11.5 and 12.0 correspond to NZ\$98 700 and NZ\$162 750, respectively.

The pattern of the inflation trajectories in Figure 17–2 can be described by the means of the district-level vectors of annual log-means, equal to

$$(11.466, \quad 11.505, \quad 11.504, \quad 11.555, \quad 11.600, \quad 11.615, \quad 11.677),$$

marked in Figure 17–2 by large dots, variances

$$(0.140, \quad 0.171, \quad 0.188, \quad 0.198, \quad 0.214, \quad 0.224, \quad 0.243), \qquad (1)$$

and the correlation matrix

$$\frac{1}{1000}\begin{pmatrix} 1000 & 990 & 979 & 966 & 966 & 965 & 958 \\ 990 & 1000 & 990 & 979 & 976 & 973 & 964 \\ 979 & 990 & 1000 & 993 & 988 & 983 & 971 \\ 966 & 979 & 993 & 1000 & 991 & 988 & 978 \\ 966 & 976 & 988 & 991 & 1000 & 995 & 986 \\ 965 & 973 & 983 & 988 & 995 & 1000 & 993 \\ 958 & 964 & 971 & 978 & 986 & 993 & 1000 \end{pmatrix}. \tag{2}$$

Except for 1997–1998, the log-means are increasing, by up to 0.062. Such small differences on the log-scale are readily translated to differences in percentages by multiplying them by 100, as the approximation $\exp(x) \doteq 1 + x$ is quite precise. For instance, the increase by 0.062 on the log-scale corresponds to the increase by $100(e^{0.062} - 1) = 6.4\%$. The variances are increasing, by 22% in 1996–1997 and by between 5% and 10% in the following years. Although dropping with the time elapsed, at an uneven rate, the correlation is very high even between years 1996 and 2002. Perfect correlations and increasing variances would correspond to the lines in Figure 17–2 fanning out in a regular pattern, without any criss-crossing.

An apparent deficiency of this analysis is that it ignores the within-district variation. Account of this can be taken by fitting the two-level model

$$y_{tda} = \mu_a + \gamma_{da} + \varepsilon_{tda}, \tag{3}$$

where y_{tda} is the log-price in transaction t in district d in year a and $\gamma_d = (\gamma_{d1}, \ldots, \gamma_{d7})^\top$ and ε_{tda} are the respective district- and transaction-level deviations, assumed to be independent random samples from centred normal distributions; $\gamma_d \sim \mathcal{N}_7(\mathbf{0}, \Sigma_D)$ and $\varepsilon_{tda} \sim \mathcal{N}(0, \sigma_a^2)$. (By $\mathbf{0}$ we denote the zero vector or matrix with dimensions implied by the context, or given in its subscript. Similarly, we use the symbol $\mathbf{1}$ for a vector of ones.) We use a separate residual variance σ_a^2 for each year, as the within-district variances of the log-prices are not constant over the years. These variances are

$$\hat{\sigma}_A^2 = (0.201, \ 0.200, \ 0.220, \ 0.232, \ 0.244, \ 0.249, \ 0.249);$$

being estimated with degrees of freedom in the vicinity of the numbers in Table 17–1, their sampling variation is negligible. Note that the national means of log-prices differ from the means of the district-level log-means because the more populous districts, and cities in particular, tend to have more expensive housing. The national log-means,

$$\hat{\mu}^\dagger = (11.840, \ 11.887, \ 11.851, \ 11.887, \ 11.914, \ 11.932, \ 11.983), \tag{4}$$

increase over the years, except for a reversal between years 2 and 3 that is recovered in year 4. The fitted district-level variances and covariances are only about 2% smaller than their counterparts in (1); most of this reduction, about 1/72, can be attributed to the difference between full and restricted maximum likelihood. The heuristic reasoning for this is that the variance matrix given by (1) and (2) is derived with the denominator 72, whereas the maximum likelihood estimator, if each district had infinitely many transactions and the within-district variances were known, would have the denominator 73. See Longford (2000) for the related derivations.

Multivariate normality of the district-level log-means can be assessed by simulating from the fitted seven-variate distribution; see Longford (2001) for details. Mixture models can be regarded as an alternative, assuming that the 73 districts originate from a specified small number of subpopulations of districts with distinct distributions. The subpopulations have different distributions of their district-level log-means, and therefore different patterns of trajectories. One of these subpopulations may comprise outliers. Note that multivariate outliers need not be outliers in any particular year. For example, a district that had its log-mean well below the national mean in 1996 and 2002, but well above the mean in 1999, is a case in point. In the EM algorithm used for fitting these models, each district's group is regarded as the missing information. In the iterations comprising E- and M-steps (Dempster, Laird, & Rubin, 1977; and McLachlan & Peel, 2000), the conditional probabilities of belonging to each group are estimated for every district.

The model fit for two components is summarized in Table 17–2. To conserve space, information about the fitted 7×7 variance matrices is condensed to the variances and the ranges of the correlations. The E-step (multinomial) conditional probabilities can be regarded as evidence of a district belonging to either component. The two components differ in the sets of annual log-means by between 0.456 (57%) in year 1 and 0.605 (83%) in year 7. The districts are assigned to components with high level of certainty; 43 districts are assigned to component 1 and 29 to component 2 with E-step probabilities exceeding 0.99, and the remaining district is assigned to component 2 with probability 0.98. Note, however, that these probabilities are conditional on the estimates of all the model parameters, so the probabilities overstate the level of certainty.

Most of the districts with higher log-means are assigned to component 2, but Auckland City and Queenstown Lakes are two notable exceptions. Apart from the mean of log-means, the two components differ also in their patterns of district-level variation and magnitudes of the transaction-level variances. In component 1, the estimated district-level variance increases steadily to end up in year 7 twice as high as it was in year 1, whereas in component 2 the estimated variance is low, in the range 0.070–0.087, throughout the seven years. Thus, trajectories of the districts in component 1 fan out over the years, and

TABLE 17–2

Summary of the Two-Component Mixture Model Fit to the Log-Sale Prices

				Year				
Component	1	2	3	4	5	6	7	
log-mean								
1	11.289	11.297	11.271	11.322	11.359	11.369	11.429	
2	11.745	11.809	11.836	11.888	11.950	11.973	12.034	
Transaction-level (within-district) variances								
1	0.249	0.249	0.280	0.293	0.319	0.328	0.323	
2	0.173	0.170	0.180	0.186	0.185	0.183	0.191	
District-level variances								*Correlations*
1	0.099	0.119	0.133	0.150	0.171	0.175	0.201	0.947–0.996
2	0.077	0.087	0.077	0.072	0.070	0.072	0.079	0.955–0.999

trajectories of the districts in component 2 are much closer to being parallel. Auckland City and Queenstown Lakes are assigned to component 1 because their trajectories differ from the relatively tight pattern in component 2. The district-level standard deviations are of the same order of magnitude as the differences of the log-means between the two components, so the trajectories of the two groups of districts are by no means well separated.

A finer division of the districts is derived by fitting the three-component mixture model. It splits the districts to groups of 31, 25 and 17. In the E-step, trinomial conditional probabilities are evaluated; in the concluding iteration, they are in excess of 0.99 for a component for every district. The results are summarized in Table 17–3 using the same layout as in Table 17–2. The group assigned to each district is given in the column headed "Grp" in the middle of Table 17–6. The three components can be interpreted as follows. The first and third components retain the most typical districts of the first and second component of the two-component mixture fit (Table 17–2), and component 2 is formed from the districts that, relatively speaking, did not fit well in either group of the two-component solution. The "new" component 2 comprises 12 districts (including Queenstown Lakes) from the "old" component 1 and 13 from the "old" component 2.

The assignment of the districts to components in the two mixture model fits is summarized in Figure 17–3. The same trajectories, derived from the three-component solution, are drawn in each panel, with the districts that have the assignments indicated in the titles highlighted. Despite the ordering of the estimated log-means, the three components cannot be interpreted as "cheap", "medium" and "expensive" because of the substantial district-level variation in relation to the differences in the log-means, and because the pattern of inflation trajectories also has an impact on the assignment, as do the within-district variances. As an extreme example, Auckland City is assigned to component 1 in both two- and three-component solutions. In the latter, component 1 appears to be best suited for Auckland City because it has the highest within-district variances. The diagram confirms the observations based on the fitted variance matrices: The inflation trajectories of districts in component 1 fan out; the trajectories of districts in component 3 are nearly parallel; and the trajectories in component 2 are halfway between the other two components. There are some

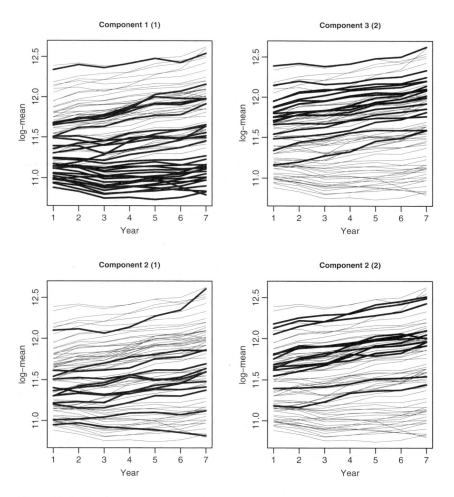

Figure 17–3. The fitted district-level inflation trajectories for the districts assigned to the groups in the two- and three-component mixture models. The group in the two-component solution is indicated in the titles in parentheses.

TABLE 17–3

Summary of the Three-Component Mixture Model Fit to the Log-Sale Prices

Component	Year							
	1	2	3	4	5	6	7	
log-mean								
1	11.256	11.256	11.223	11.270	11.307	11.312	11.366	
2	11.558	11.603	11.621	11.681	11.733	11.757	11.822	
3	11.760	11.823	11.841	11.885	11.946	11.965	12.032	
Transaction-level (within-district) variances								
1	0.259	0.261	0.295	0.313	0.341	0.351	0.345	
2	0.205	0.197	0.209	0.215	0.224	0.218	0.228	
3	0.144	0.144	0.158	0.167	0.164	0.168	0.169	
District-level variances								*Correlations*
1	0.097	0.120	0.138	0.157	0.180	0.177	0.193	0.942–0.996
2	0.112	0.133	0.136	0.137	0.154	0.169	0.187	0.958–0.997
3	0.078	0.080	0.070	0.066	0.059	0.058	0.066	0.962–0.998

exceptions, because the assignment to the components is also affected by the log-means and the within-district variances. Arguably, the status of Auckland City as an outlier can be judged more clearly among the districts in the same mixture component. We point out that the numbers of transactions in the districts vary a great deal, but each district is represented "equally" in the diagram.

More detailed division of the districts can be obtained by fitting mixture models with four or more components. Judging by conventional goodness-of-fit criteria, more components provide a better fit, but the advantage of an appealing interpretation is lost.

17.3.2 Roll-Level Analysis

The valuation rolls are represented as a source of variation in the three-level model

$$y_{trda} = \mu_a + \gamma_{da} + \delta_{rda} + \varepsilon_{trda}, \qquad (5)$$

in which the indices t, r, d, and a represent the transaction (sale), roll, district, and year, respectively. The vectors of district-level deviations $\boldsymbol{\gamma}_d = (\gamma_{d1}, \ldots, \gamma_{d7})$ and roll-level deviations $\boldsymbol{\delta}_{rd} = (\delta_{d1}, \ldots, \delta_{d7})$ are mutually independent random samples from respective centered normal distributions $\mathcal{N}(\mathbf{0}_7, \boldsymbol{\Sigma}_D)$ and $\mathcal{N}(\mathbf{0}_7, \boldsymbol{\Sigma}_R)$, independent of the within-roll deviations $\varepsilon_{trda} \sim \mathcal{N}(0, \sigma_a^2)$, which have variances specific to each year. No structure is imposed on the variance matrices $\boldsymbol{\Sigma}_D$ and $\boldsymbol{\Sigma}_R$ in this application, although constraints can in general be imposed on them.

The model fit comprises the same objects as the fit in the district-level analysis, supplemented by the estimate of the roll-level variance matrix:

$$\hat{\mu} = (11.439,\ 11.470,\ 11.465,\ 11.510,\ 11.549,\ 11.564,\ 11.633)$$

$$\hat{\sigma}_A^2 = (0.132,\ 0.136,\ 0.151,\ 0.160,\ 0.161,\ 0.150,\ 0.152)$$

$$\mathrm{diag}(\hat{\Sigma}_R) = (0.100,\ 0.093,\ 0.095,\ 0.102,\ 0.115,\ 0.132,\ 0.139)$$

$$\widehat{\mathrm{cor}}(\delta_{rd}) = \frac{1}{1000} \begin{pmatrix} 1000 & 984 & 976 & 968 & 951 & 933 & 931 \\ 984 & 1000 & 991 & 983 & 966 & 952 & 948 \\ 976 & 991 & 1000 & 989 & 972 & 963 & 959 \\ 968 & 983 & 989 & 1000 & 985 & 975 & 973 \\ 951 & 966 & 972 & 985 & 1000 & 988 & 982 \\ 933 & 952 & 963 & 975 & 988 & 1000 & 993 \\ 931 & 948 & 959 & 973 & 982 & 993 & 1000 \end{pmatrix}$$

$$\mathrm{diag}(\hat{\Sigma}_D) = (0.145,\ 0.172,\ 0.187,\ 0.197,\ 0.215,\ 0.223,\ 0.240)$$

$$\widehat{\mathrm{cor}}(\gamma_d) = \frac{1}{1000} \begin{pmatrix} 1000 & 994 & 982 & 975 & 972 & 969 & 966 \\ 994 & 1000 & 996 & 990 & 983 & 978 & 969 \\ 982 & 996 & 1000 & 998 & 992 & 987 & 975 \\ 975 & 990 & 998 & 1000 & 997 & 992 & 981 \\ 972 & 983 & 992 & 997 & 1000 & 998 & 989 \\ 969 & 978 & 987 & 992 & 998 & 1000 & 995 \\ 966 & 969 & 975 & 981 & 989 & 995 & 1000 \end{pmatrix}.$$

The estimate of the log-means, $\hat{\mu}$, differs from its counterpart in the district-level analysis because the roll-level deviations δ_{rd} are weighed equally within districts in the roll-level analysis, whereas the numbers of transactions are the effective weights in the district-level analysis. The differences between the two sets of log-means are in the range 2.3–4.7% (in favor of the district-level analysis), increasing over the seven years. The estimated transaction-level variances $\hat{\sigma}_A^2$ in the two analyses differ substantially because the elementary-level variation in the district-level analysis is now represented by within- and between-roll variation. The within-roll variances σ_A^2 increase up to year 5 and then decrease. Apart from a dip in year 2, the roll-level variances $\mathrm{diag}(\hat{\Sigma}_R)$ increase, but do so at a much slower rate than the district-level variances $\mathrm{diag}(\hat{\Sigma}_D)$. The correlations in $\hat{\Sigma}_R$ are somewhat lower than their counterparts in $\hat{\Sigma}_D$, but are very high none-the-less. Thus, inflation trajectories of the rolls within a typical district fan out much less and their pattern of fanning out over the seven years is slightly "noisier" than for the trajectories of the districts. Note that this statement is about the roll-level log-means underlying the model in (5), $\mu_a + \gamma_{da} + \delta_{rda}$, not about the realized log-means $y_{\cdot rda}$ that are much more dispersed because many of them are based on very few transactions.

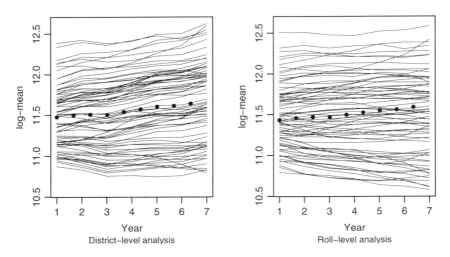

Figure 17–4. Estimates of the district-level log-means based on the district- and roll-level analyses.

The district- and roll-level deviations are estimated by their conditional expectations given the model fit. The district-level deviations, after the adjustment for the overall log-mean $\hat{\mu}$, closely resemble the sample log-means because most districts are represented by a lot of data. Figure 17–4 presents the estimated district-level log-means $\hat{\mu} + \hat{\gamma}_d$ based on the district- and roll-level analyses. Some differences among the two sets of estimates are perceptible, even for the most populous districts (cities) because the roll-level analysis aims to recover a superpopulation version of the mean of the annual roll-level log-means, $\mu_a + \gamma_{da}$ in (5), whereas the district-level analysis estimates the log-means of the sale prices, disregarding the location of the transactions in the rolls. However, the relative positions of the districts differ across the analyses only slightly.

The estimates of the log-means for the rolls in the city of Palmerston North and the adjacent (rural) district of Manawatu are drawn in Figure 17–5. Thinner lines are used for the rolls with fewer than 100 transactions each in the period of seven years; there are five such rolls in Palmerston North (out of 33) and 17 (out of 24) in Manawatu. Over the studied period, there were 10 007 transactions in Palmerston North and 3227 in Manawatu.

The estimates suggest that the roll-level deviations are substantially skewed in opposite directions. Two rolls in Palmerston North have much more expensive properties on average than the rest, whereas Manawatu has a few rolls where properties tend to be much cheaper than elsewhere. Such skewness is not a contradiction with the model assumptions because they require nor-

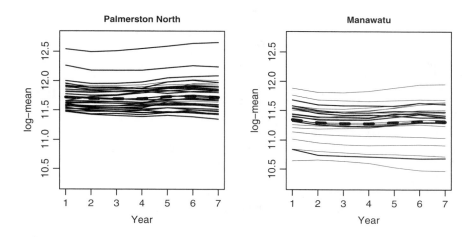

Figure 17–5. Estimates of the log-means in the valuation rolls of Palmerston North City and Manawatu districts. The estimated log-mean for the district is drawn by thick dashes.

mality only of the nation's *all* vectors of roll-level deviations δ_{rd}. The plots of the estimates of these 2495 log-means and histograms of their components are much closer to normality. However, in view of the vast variation of the population sizes of the rolls, and hence in the shrinkage applied in the estimation of δ_{rd}, such graphs are not a good guide. See Shen and Louis (1998) for ways of addressing this problem, and Gelman and Price (1999) for a principled solution. However, its application requires a resolution of the contradiction between the fixed-effects setting (see beginning of Section 17.3) and the random-effects assumptions on the model in (5).

As in Section 17.3.1, more detailed description of the district- (and roll-)level log-means is obtained by finite mixture models. We are concerned only with grouping of the districts. In principle, mixture models can be applied also to rolls, but it is not meaningful to split the rolls of a district among the mixture components.

The estimates for the two-component model are displayed in Table 17–4. The fit divides the country into groups of 36 and 37 districts. Group 1 has much smaller district-level variances and slightly higher correlations at both roll and district levels. The roll-level variances increase faster for group 1 than for group 2, after both groups' variances have a dip in year 2. The differences of the log-means (0.05–0.14) are small in relation to the district-level variation.

TABLE 17–4

Summary of the Two-Component Mixture Model Fit to the Log-Sale Prices; Roll-Level
Models

				Year				
Component	1	2	3	4	5	6	7	
log-mean								
1	11.403	11.432	11.416	11.454	11.477	11.502	11.579	
2	11.457	11.504	11.514	11.563	11.617	11.623	11.683	
Transaction-level (within-roll) variances								
1	0.128	0.132	0.156	0.161	0.167	0.164	0.156	
2	0.134	0.138	0.149	0.159	0.158	0.149	0.148	
Roll-level variances								*Correlations*
1	0.104	0.096	0.098	0.107	0.123	0.143	0.153	0.938–0.996
2	0.097	0.089	0.092	0.098	0.108	0.124	0.129	0.925–0.993
District-level variances								
1	0.120	0.156	0.175	0.184	0.197	0.197	0.206	0.972–0.999
2	0.198	0.216	0.224	0.238	0.264	0.279	0.302	0.963–0.998

The assignment of the districts to groups, 37 in group 1 and 36 in group 2, is with a great deal of certainty; all the E-step probabilities are either greater than 0.999 or smaller than 0.001. However, the division is not related in any obvious way to the two- or three-component solutions in the district-level analysis. Fitting the three-component model resulted in a singularity in several attempts, assigning no weight to one component and reproducing the two-component solution.

17.4 ADJUSTMENT FOR RATING VALUATION

The analysis in the previous section lacks any adjustment for the systematic differences among the sets of properties sold in the compared time periods (years). The RV, performed for every residential property in New Zealand once every three years (in a few districts annually), provides an effective way of adjusting for such differences. Of course, it is far from perfect because such a large-scale exercise is bound to involve elements of subjective judgment and convention, as well as some minor systematic differences in the procedures applied. The CVs, the key outcome of the valuation, are issued on the same day for every property in a district, but the date differs from district to district (see Table 17–6). The valuation aims to establish, or estimate, the market value of the property on the day of the valuation, and so, despite its imperfections, it is without a competitor as an adjustment variable. With an adjustment, we assume that two properties with the same CV on a given day are alike. Although somewhat problematic for properties in different districts, it is reasonable for properties within a district, and probably even more so within a roll. Therefore, in our regression model we adjust for CV of the property and for the time elapsed between the dates of valuation and sale. For greater flexibility, we fit a quadratic regression on the time elapsed. The time is represented by the number of days divided by 1000 (denoted by u), so that three years correspond to about 1.1 units.

We consider the three-level model

$$y_{trd} = \mathbf{x}_{trd}(\boldsymbol{\beta} + \boldsymbol{\gamma}_d + \boldsymbol{\delta}_{rd}) + \varepsilon_{trd}, \tag{6}$$

where y is the logarithm of the sale price, $\mathbf{x}$ the (row) vector of regressors, comprising the logarithm of CV in force on 1st January 2003, v, the scaled number of days between valuation and sale, u, its squared distance from $\frac{1}{2}$, $(u - \frac{1}{2})^2$, and the intercept. Each regressor is associated with variation at both roll and district levels.

Instead of the variance matrices $\boldsymbol{\Sigma}_R = \text{var}(\boldsymbol{\gamma}_d)$ and $\boldsymbol{\Sigma}_D = \text{var}(\boldsymbol{\delta}_d)$, their scaled versions $\boldsymbol{\Omega}_R = \sigma^{-2}\boldsymbol{\Sigma}_R$ and $\boldsymbol{\Omega}_D = \sigma^{-2}\boldsymbol{\Sigma}_D$ are estimated; σ^2 is the transaction-level variance $\text{var}(\varepsilon_{trd})$. The model fitting algorithm is simplified as the information about σ^2 on the one hand and $\boldsymbol{\Omega}_R$ and $\boldsymbol{\Omega}_D$ on the other are orthogonal. We consider the submodel with $\boldsymbol{\Omega}_R = \mathbf{0}$, in parallel with the analysis in Section 17.3.1. The purpose of this is not model parsimony but setting aside the impact of the rolls on the analysis, so that the contribution of a district's transaction to the analysis would depend only on its vector $\mathbf{x}_{trd}$, unaffected by the composition of its valuation roll rd.

The district-level analysis yields the model fit

$$\hat{\text{E}}(y) = 0.9364v - 0.0883u - 0.0570\left(u - \tfrac{1}{2}\right)^2 + 0.7053$$

$$\hat{\sigma}^2 = 0.0705$$

$$\hat{\boldsymbol{\Omega}}_D = \begin{pmatrix} 0.0983 & -0.0476 & 0.0039 & -0.0509 \\ -0.0476 & 0.1164 & -0.0006 & 0.0014 \\ 0.0039 & -0.0006 & 0.3778 & -0.0686 \\ -0.0509 & 0.0014 & -0.0686 & 0.0915 \end{pmatrix}$$

(the order of the variables in $\hat{\boldsymbol{\Omega}}_D$ is the same as in the regression equation). Thus, the fitted regression slope of the log-sale price on log-valuation is smaller than unity, suggesting that the valuation is associated with a discrepancy akin to measurement error. However, the *average* regression slope, 0.936 (the associated standard error is 0.010), should be interpreted together with the variation of the within-district regressions. Their standard deviation is $\sqrt{0.0705 \times 0.0983} = 0.0832$, so a slope on log-valuation in excess of unity is not unusual.

Because the inflation is modelled by a quadratic function with unrestricted pattern of variation, it is more practical to represent it graphically. In Figure 17–6, the estimated within-district regressions are plotted for a set of four CVs indicated in the panels by titles and horizontal dashes. The fitted average (national) regression is drawn by thick dots, and the districts' fitted inflation trajectories $\mathbf{x}(\hat{\beta} + \hat{\gamma}_d)$, functions of the time elapsed since valuation, are drawn by thin solid lines. The trajectories are drawn only for districts in which the reference CV lies between the 5th and 95th percentiles of the CVs in the district, so that all the predictions implied by the trajectories are well within the range of the data. Although on different scales, the vertical axes of the four panels have identical widths (about 0.8 on the log-scale, that is, the top is $\exp(0.8) \doteq 2.25$-multiple of the bottom), so that the variation of the predictions can be compared across the panels.

The fitted curves for the urban areas of the North Island tend to be above and for the sparsely populated districts of the South Island below the national regression line. For instance, the highest log-sale prices for a property with capital value NZ\$100 000 throughout the period of 1000 days after valuation are predicted for Papakura and Franklin districts (southern neighbors of the Auckland metropolitan area), and the predictions after 1000 days are lowest for Gore and Buller, both sparsely populated districts on the South Island. The regressions for most city districts are not drawn in the panels for NZ\$60 000 or NZ\$100 000 because such values fall below the 5th percentile in them. For CV of NZ\$160 000, the predictions between 200 and 600 days after valuation are highest for Waitakere City and Rodney District (the neighbor of Auckland metropolitan area to the north), with distinctly concave trajectories, followed by Auckland and North Shore Cities, the latter two having the highest predictions by the end of the period of 1000 days. At the other extreme, Invercargill City has a distinctly convex (bathtub shape) fitted trajectory, with the lowest prediction between 250 and 750 days after valuation.

The two-component mixture model fit is summarized in Table 17–5. All districts are assigned to a component with near certainty; 29 districts to group 1 and 44 to group 2. Two features of the results are easy to interpret in Table 17–5. Group 2 has much greater fitted within-district variance $\hat{\sigma}^2$ and its variation in the curvature of the inflation trajectories is also much greater. (The absolute variances, $\hat{\sigma}^2\hat{\Omega}_{D,33}$, estimated by $0.3953 \times 0.0843 = 0.0333$ and $0.2632 \times 0.0590 = 0.0155$, should be compared, not the scaled variances $\hat{\Omega}_{D,33}$.) Graphs similar to those in Figure 17–6 confirm this conclusion. For instance, Auckland City, Rodney and Manawatu districts are assigned to group 2. The three-component mixture model fit splits the districts to almost the same groups as its roll-level counterpart discussed later, and so we omit all details.

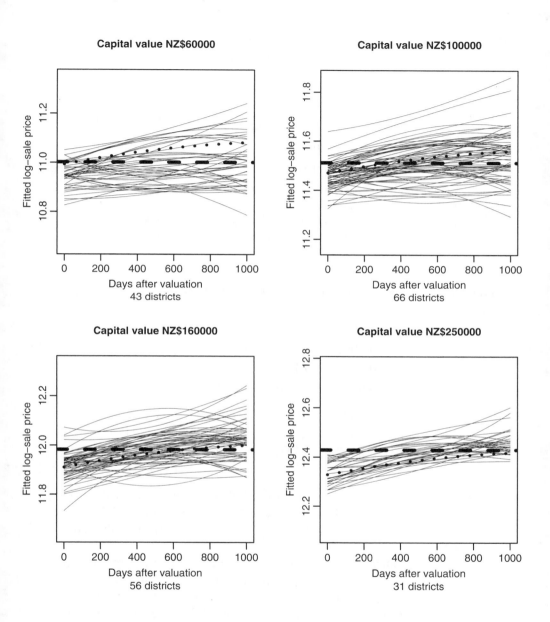

Figure 17–6. The estimated inflation trajectories for specific capital values in districts in which the reference capital value lies between the 5th and 95th percentiles.

The fit to the model in (6) without any restriction on Ω_R involves the average (national) regression

$$\hat{E}(y) = 0.9048v + 0.0865u - 0.0740 \left(u - \tfrac{1}{2}\right)^2 + 1.0832,$$

TABLE 17–5

The Two-Component Mixture Model Fit for Regression on Capital Value and Time Elapsed
Since Valuation; District-Level Models

	Group 1 (29 districts)				Group 2 (44 districts)			
	Capital value	$u = \frac{\text{Days}}{1000}$	$\left(u - \frac{1}{2}\right)^2$	Int-cpt	Capital value	$u = \frac{\text{Days}}{1000}$	$\left(u - \frac{1}{2}\right)^2$	Int-cpt
$\hat{\beta}$	0.9429	0.0847	−0.0746	0.6311	0.9312	0.0908	−0.0449	0.7456
$\hat{\sigma}^2$				0.0590				0.0843
$\hat{\Omega}_\text{D}$	$\begin{pmatrix} 0.1053 & -0.0502 & 0.0201 & -0.0604 \\ -0.0502 & 0.0967 & 0.0160 & 0.0021 \\ 0.0201 & 0.0160 & 0.2632 & -0.0380 \\ -0.0604 & 0.0021 & -0.0580 & 0.0697 \end{pmatrix}$				$\begin{pmatrix} 0.0855 & -0.0424 & -0.0029 & -0.0452 \\ -0.0424 & 0.1164 & -0.0091 & 0.0022 \\ -0.0029 & -0.0091 & 0.3953 & -0.0618 \\ -0.0452 & 0.0022 & -0.0618 & 0.0860 \end{pmatrix}$			

with residual variance $\hat{\sigma}^2 = 0.0666$ and roll- and district-level scaled variance matrices

$$\hat{\Omega}_\text{R} = \begin{pmatrix} 0.1648 & -0.0093 & 0.0541 & -0.0368 \\ -0.0093 & 0.0635 & -0.1102 & -0.0115 \\ 0.0541 & -0.1102 & 0.6523 & -0.0062 \\ -0.0368 & -0.0115 & -0.0062 & 0.0464 \end{pmatrix}$$

$$\hat{\Omega}_\text{D} = \begin{pmatrix} 0.1396 & -0.0384 & -0.0266 & -0.0870 \\ -0.0384 & 0.1001 & 0.0241 & 0.0014 \\ -0.0266 & 0.2415 & 0.4110 & -0.0586 \\ -0.0870 & 0.0014 & -0.0586 & 0.1279 \end{pmatrix},$$

respectively. The two-component version of this model fit splits the districts into the same groups as the district-level two-component model fit, with slightly less certainty. The fitted variances $\hat{\sigma}^2$ and matrices $\hat{\Omega}_\text{D}$ have the same features as observed earlier.

The three-component mixture model fit "discards" 14 districts from group 1 and 15 from group 2 of the two-component fit, and these 29 districts form the new group 3. The group assignment of the districts is given in the right-most column of Table 17–6. The three groups have the following fitted national regressions:

$$\mathbf{x}\hat{\beta}^{(1)} = 0.932v + 0.084u - 0.052\left(u - \tfrac{1}{2}\right)^2 + 0.799$$

$$\mathbf{x}\hat{\beta}^{(2)} = 0.904v + 0.102u - 0.048\left(u - \tfrac{1}{2}\right)^2 + 1.036$$

$$\mathbf{x}\hat{\beta}^{(3)} = 0.892v + 0.076u - 0.111\left(u - \tfrac{1}{2}\right)^2 + 1.245.$$

Their differences are difficult to assess because they have to be related to the fitted variance matrices $\hat{\Sigma}_D$ and $\hat{\Sigma}_R$. Inspecting the inflation trajectories may be more constructive, although this has to be done for a range of CVs. The fitted inflation trajectories for the districts are presented in Figure 17–7 for CV of NZ\$100 000. In the panels at the top, the districts assigned to the indicated group are highlighted; in the bottom panels the districts in the intersections of the groups defined by the two- and three-component solutions are highlighted. Seven districts are not represented in either of the panels because NZ\$100 000 is outside the 5%–95% range of their CVs.

The fitted variance matrices $\hat{\Sigma}_R^{(m)} = \hat{\sigma}_{(m)}^2 \hat{\Omega}_R^{(m)}$ for the components $m = 1, 2, 3$ are

$$\hat{\Sigma}_R^{(1)} = \frac{1}{10^4} \begin{pmatrix} 82.79 & 2.38 & 7.61 & -14.15 \\ 2.38 & 19.78 & -9.82 & -4.92 \\ 7.61 & -9.82 & 210.44 & -0.46 \\ -14.15 & -4.92 & -0.46 & 22.28 \end{pmatrix}$$

$$\hat{\Sigma}_R^{(2)} = \frac{1}{10^4} \begin{pmatrix} 161.51 & -31.38 & 80.11 & -6.91 \\ -31.38 & 83.82 & -105.11 & -21.36 \\ 80.11 & -105.11 & 447.92 & 13.45 \\ -6.91 & -21.36 & 13.45 & 60.57 \end{pmatrix}$$

$$\hat{\Sigma}_R^{(3)} = \frac{1}{10^4} \begin{pmatrix} 100.92 & -1.54 & 31.88 & -28.56 \\ -1.54 & 40.38 & -103.38 & -7.96 \\ 31.88 & -103.38 & 538.60 & -6.71 \\ -28.56 & -7.96 & -6.71 & 24.33 \end{pmatrix} .$$

Group 1 has much smaller roll-level variation of the regression than the other two groups on all three covariates. We illustrate this in Figure 17–8 by comparing the fitted trajectories for the rolls in Palmerston North City, assigned to group 1, and Manawatu, assigned to group 2. The fitted trajectories are in a narrower band and have much more uniform curvatures for Palmerston North, even though they are subject to less shrinkage, as most of its rolls have more transactions than the rolls in Manawatu. One roll in Palmerston North has a substantial estimated curvature, but most of the other rolls' trajectories are nearly linear and parallel to one another. In contrast, Manawatu has several rolls with convex and concave fitted trajectories.

Table 17–6 lists the predicted log-means for properties with CVs equal to NZ\$100 000, NZ\$200 000 and NZ\$300 000, based on the district-level model (with $\Sigma_R = 0$) and the group assigned by the three-component mixture model. All the predictions are in NZ\$, obtained by exponentiation. The exponentiated figures are not adjusted for variation, according to the identity

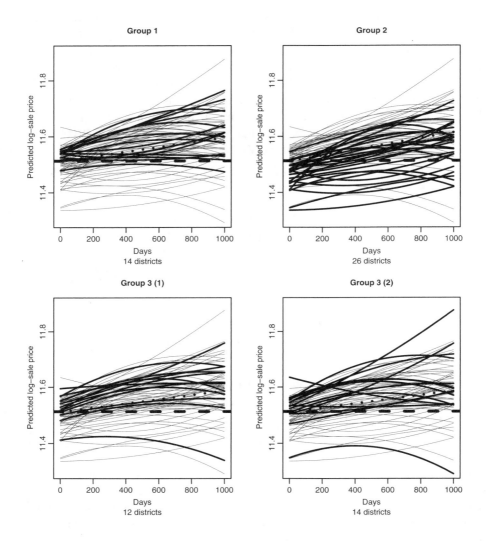

Figure 17–7. Estimated inflation trajectories for the districts assigned to the components of the two- and three-component mixture models for capital value of NZ$100 000.

$E(e^X) = \exp\{E(X) + \frac{1}{2}\mathrm{var}(X)\}$ for a normally distributed random variable X, because the predictions are for geometric means. We prefer this target over the arithmetic mean because of its affinity with the median.

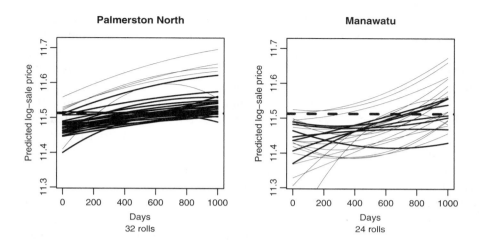

Figure 17–8. Estimated inflation trajectories for the rolls of Palmerston North City and Manawatu for the capital value of NZ$100 000. The trajectories are drawn by thicker lines for rolls with at least 100 transactions in 1996–2002.

17.5 HOUSE-PRICE INFLATION RATES

The main purpose and interpretation of an index of house-price inflation is a comparison of sale prices across time periods. Care is required to ensure that any comparison made is of like with like, motivating the adjustment by regression or, more generally, model-based estimation. Although a better fitting model, with smaller residual variation, is in general preferred for such comparisons, the adopted model has to reflect the definition of the inflation rate (index). For instance, estimates from a district-level analysis are not comparable with the corresponding estimates from a roll-level analysis, as illustrated by Figure 17–4, because their underlying quantities differ.

The annual log-means of sale prices are estimated with high precision for most districts even directly by their sample log-means. For these districts, only slight shrinkage is induced by the fit of any multilevel model, and so the estimates based on alternative models differ very little. For example, the geometric mean of the 1183 sale prices in year 2002 in Rodney District is estimated by NZ$265 524, NZ$265 335, NZ$265 550 and NZ$265 487 using the sample log-mean (enumeration), single-, two- and three-component district-level mixture models, respectively. The corresponding figures for Kaikoura District, which had only 103 transactions in 2002, NZ$131 258, NZ$136 049, NZ$134 833 and NZ$135 599, differ much more because more shrinkage is applied. The shrinkage estimates conform more closely with the pattern (correlation structure) implied by the model fit, and are affected by the log-means in the previous years. However, the dominant component of the shrinkage is an increment toward the national log-mean because Kaikoura's transactions in the previous years contain relatively little information. In the enumeration perspective, the sample mean is precise, whereas in the superpopulation perspective, the estimates derived from model fits, and among them those from the three-component mixture, are superior.

Figure 17–9 presents the estimated inflation rates for the districts in 2001–2002. They are derived by exponentiating the differences of the estimated log-means in 2002 and 2001 based on enumeration and the three district-level models. Different symbols are used for the four sets of estimates and the smallest and largest of the estimates for each district are connected by vertical dashes. The districts are presented in the descending order of their numbers of transactions in 2001 and 2002. The diagram illustrates that more smoothing takes place for the less populous districts, although there are several exceptions to this trend. For example, the sample estimate for Queenstown Lakes (marked as "Q"), in excess of 30%, is adjusted downward to an extent that is out of proportion with its number of transactions, as are the estimates for a few other districts with above average estimates. It remains a contention whether the substantial increase is a "blip" or reflects of a (long-term) trend. For most districts, the three sets of model-based estimates differ less from one another than they do from the estimates based on the sample log-means.

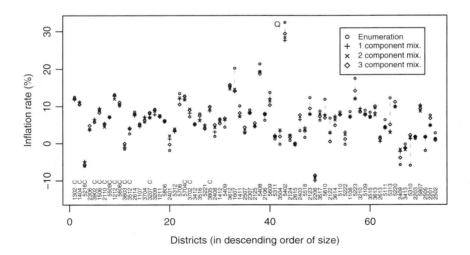

Figure 17–9. Estimated house-price inflation rates for years 2001–2002 based on the enumeration and on single-, two- and three-component mixtures of district-level models. The district codes are indicated at the bottom of the diagram, with the codes for districts on the South Island indented. Cities are marked with symbol "C". See Table 17–6 to identify the districts.

With the adjustment for CV, the inflation rates can be estimated with higher precision because CV is *prima facie* a powerful predictor of the sale price. Further advantage is gained by using exact dates, as opposed to merely the year of the sale. However, the meaning of inflation rate is no longer straightforward — that is the price for its flexible modelling. The inflation rates may be compared for "typical" CVs, chosen for each district as the geometric mean of its CVs, either of the entire housing stock or of the values of the properties sold in the period concerned. The different dates of RV are another confounding factor; they have to be taken into account when calculating the estimated inflation rates as the model fit is a nonlinear function of the days elapsed since RV.

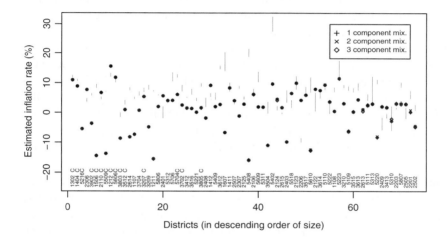

Figure 17–10. Estimated house-price inflation rates for years 2001–2002 based on the enumeration and on single- two- and three-component mixtures of district-level models with adjustment for rating valuation.

Figure 17-10 displays the estimated inflation rates between 1st July of 2001 and 2002, evaluated for the districts' typical capital values, based on the single-, two- and three-component district-level mixture models with adjustment for CV. The range of the inflation rates plotted in Figure 17–9 by vertical dashes is copied in this diagram and drawn by vertical solid lines. The three sets of estimated inflation rates are in very close agreement, but for several districts they differ a great deal from the rates derived without adjustment for CV. Notably, the "adjusted" estimates for Queenstown Lakes, although still among the highest in the country, are no longer remarkable. There are some large differences even for a few populous cities; the "adjusted" rates are lower for a majority of the districts. These differences arise because the distribution of the CVs of the properties sold changes over time. With the available data we cannot separate the effects of improvements made to the existing properties, changes of the housing stock due to new construction and demolition and drift in the demand toward the more expensive properties in the districts. The seasonal distribution of the properties sold in a district may also exert some influence.

17.6 DISCUSSION

The variance-matrix component models applied in Sections 17.3 and 17.4 provide a compact description of the house-price trends in the country and its districts, avoiding the largely episodic description of variation in terms of observed extremes. Data from several years are analyzed, so that the consistency of the pattern of inflation can be assessed.

After the log-transformation, linear mixed models can be applied. Although useful, the adjustment for CV entails several problems that can be overcome only when the process that establishes them is highly standardized across the districts. Substantial roll-level variation (within districts) suggests that the inconsistencies in the valuation process have an element associated with both districts and rolls. The variation due to such inconsistencies cannot be separated from the genuine differences in the inflation trajectories of the rolls of a district.

The CVs of the residential properties are publicly available. When they are published they are likely to exert a nontrivial influence on both the asking and agreed prices, at least in the short term, and this influence may be uneven across the districts. Such a "feedback" effect is difficult to model without an intimate understanding of the property market. Also, owners are bound to influence the process by delayed or earlier reporting of salient changes to their properties, in pursuit of advantages, such as lower local taxes (or delay of their increases) and improved prospects of a higher sales price for their property. Notwithstanding these problems, CV is a key covariate that is recorded more consistently, and with much greater credence, than other potential covariates, such as the age of the property, quality of its construction, floor area, and the like.

Most districts have sufficient numbers of transactions for an analysis on their own. Indeed, the multilevel analysis yields estimates for the districts that differ only slightly from the results of separate analyses. However, the variance matrix of the district-level log-means provides an easy way to interpret description of the house-price trends in the districts. We have confirmed the opinion, generally held in New Zealand, of continuing differentiation of the districts; the increases of average prices in the "expensive" districts have consistently outstripped the increases in the "cheaper" districts. A similar, although somewhat weaker trend is present for the rolls within districts. Apart from defining more general models and seeking a better model fit for the data, finite mixture models have the same attractions as cluster analysis, especially when the division entails very little uncertainty. However, the division is governed by the model assumptions (of log-normality and homoscedasticity), and so mixture models pay more attention to patterns of variation and heterogeneity as opposed to (relatively small) systematic differences. Mixture models have the potential to identify outliers as a group, but our analysis failed to identify Auckland City (high prices and high inflation rate) or Queenstown Lakes (sudden rise in the house prices in 2001–2002) as outlying.

The assignment of districts to groups would entail much more uncertainty in a univariate setting because the district-level distribution of the log-means (with or without adjustment) does not comprise well separated normal components. With several dimensions (years or covariates), not only is there more data, but also more scope for a good separation along one of the numerous subspaces. That is why the assignment to groups in Sections 17.3 and 17.4 is with such high degree of certainty, conditional on the model parameters.

The model fitting algorithm combines Fisher scoring with EM, so that the M-step is itself iterative. Nesting M-step iterations within EM iterations is discussed by Meng and Rubin (1993) and acceleration of convergence by Meng and van Dyk (1998). The issues of organizing the iterations optimally or adapting them in any way are not important in our context because no convergence problems arise. For details of the Fisher scoring algorithm, see Longford (1993b & 2005), and Pinheiro and Bates (2000) for a suite of `Splus` functions implementing it. McLachlan and Peel (2000) is a recognized reference for mixture models. See Longford and Pittau (2003) for an application closely related to the one presented here.

The regressions on CV and time fitted for districts and rolls in Section 17.4 can be used for prediction. The sampling variance of the prediction is quite small, especially for the districts. However, the prediction for any particular property is subject to much more uncertainty because of the substantial transaction-level (residual) variation. For instance, the residual variance of 0.0625 (see Table 17–5) corresponds to the multiplicative standard error of prediction $100(e^{0.25} - 1) = 28\%$. Apart from the imperfection of CV, which cannot take account of some details of the property, this uncertainty includes the process bargaining between the buyer and seller.

Our results can be presented by graphs of the inflation trajectories, with interactive highlighting of the district (or roll) of interest. All the graphs we present are on the log scale. They can be converted to the linear scale, although linearity, and constant difference in particular, of the trajectories (and associations) is more natural on the log scale.

TABLE 17–6

Estimates of Geometric Means of House Prices for the Districts of New Zealand and
Predictions of Mean Sale Prices on 1st July 2005 for Properties with Capital Values of
NZ$100000, NZ$200000 and NZ$300000.

City?	District	Code	Rolls	Sales	Geometric mean 2001	Geometric mean 2002	Grp	Valuat'n date	NZ$100K	NZ$200K	NZ$300K	Grp
North Island												
	Whangarei	1107	32	9248	149 500	157 100	3	1/09/01	104 300	189 300	268 200	3
	Kaipara	1108	28	1861	108 200	115 900	2	1/09/02	110 900	212 700	311 300	1
	Rodney	1211	57	8244	247 700	265 500	1	1/09/01	100 800	177 300	246 800	1
C	North Shore	1212	86	21323	268 700	303 500	1	1/09/02	146 100	246 200	334 200	3
C	Auckland	1302	96	46979	250 100	280 300	1	1/09/02	139 300	247 300	346 000	1
C	Manukau	1404	100	34200	225 900	249 800	2	1/09/02	128 800	226 700	315 500	3
	Papakura	1411	14	4955	192 100	207 800	1	1/09/00	192 900	310 000	409 000	3
	Franklin	1412	24	4399	169 000	178 100	2	1/09/00	153 200	256 500	346 900	3
C	Waitakere	1506	129	23357	209 400	226 800	1	1/09/01	107 200	180 700	245 100	3
	Far North	1607	97	4275	131 300	149 800	3	1/09/01	100 600	194 800	286 700	1
	Thames Corom.	2106	33	3959	183 700	198 000	1	1/09/00	104 000	191 500	273 700	2
C	Hamilton	2110	59	19408	170 600	179 700	1	1/09/00	138 400	245 800	343 900	2
	Hauraki	2122	25	2267	107 700	108 200	1	1/09/00	140 100	241 700		1
	Waikato	2123	31	2801	99 500	108 900	1	1/09/00	161 300	302 000		1
	Matamata P.	2124	22	3350	126 600	128 700	1	1/09/00	121 900	233 500		2
	Waipa	2125	29	4789	153 300	161 700	2	1/09/02	111 900	203 500	288 800	3
	Otorohanga	2201	11	575	87 100	93 000	1	1/09/01	112 100	219 900		3
	Waitomo	2203	11	726	63 900	65 100	1	1/09/00	102 200	213 100		1
	South Waikato	2206	18	2783	53 300	48 800	1	1/09/00	129 000	269 900		1
	Tauranga	2306	63	18433	189 500	198 600	1	1/09/00	122 500	227 600	326 900	3
	Western BOP	2307	33	3523	166 100	179 900	1	1/09/02	115 800	209 300	295 900	1
	Rotorua	2401	46	8249	141 100	140 700	2	1/09/02	112 100	204 900	291 600	3
	Whakatane	2403	25	2860	148 100	159 400	1	1/09/01	94 600	182 100	267 100	3
	Taupo	2408	34	5344	151 600	159 200	2	1/07/02	100 700	202 600	304 800	3
	Kawerau	2409	6	974	51 700	49 700	3	1/09/00	137 600	289 800		2
	Opotiki	2502	9	695	97 400	98 300	1	1/09/01	99 300	181 500		1
	Wairoa	2505	10	603	59 600	60 500	1	1/09/00	98 500	207 200		1
	Gisborne	2507	37	4029	96 400	100 500	1	1/09/02	98 000	193 500		1
	Stratford	2613	9	1001	67 100	68 000	1	1/09/02	89 600	181 200		3
	New Plymouth	2614	40	8951	111 300	120 100	2	1/09/01	84 400	167 800	250 800	2
	S. Taranaki	2615	29	2949	70 600	70 600	1	1/09/00	97 200	193 600		1
C	Napier	3207	28	7687	152 900	165 600	1	1/09/02	105 400	205 100	302 700	3
	Hastings	3209	41	7504	130 100	141 800	2	1/09/01	92 600	184 100	275 300	3
	C. Hawkes Bay	3210	14	1430	87 100	94 500	3	1/09/00	93 500	177 700		1
	Wanganui	3412	27	5744	75 000	79 000	2	1/07/02	93 700	194 700		3
	Rangitikei	3413	19	944	51 600	51 000	2	1/09/00	93 000	197 000		1
	Manawatu	3504	24	3227	94 900	96 600	1	1/09/01	82 400	163 800		1
C	Palmerston N.	3512	32	10007	135 800	141 300	2	1/09/00	98 300	191 700	283 400	2
	Ruapehu	3515	24	1288	47 300	50 600	3	1/07/02	87 800	171 400		1
	Horowhenua	3516	22	4956	80 900	86 900	1	1/09/02	98 500	198 000		3

TABLE 17–6 (Continued)

City? District	Code	Rolls	Sales	Geometric mean 2001	2002	Grp	Valuat'n date	Prediction for capital value NZ$100K	NZ$200K	NZ$300K	Grp
North Island (Continued)											
Tararua	3517	28	1862	58 900	63 200	2	1/09/02	89 600	*168 900*		1
Masterton	3612	20	3658	94 400	109 200	2	1/09/02	104 800	*210 400*		3
Carterton	3613	7	969	97 800	107 600	2	1/09/00	130 500	*258 900*		2
S. Wairarapa	3614	14	1604	108 100	113 300	3	1/09/00	80 500	152 600		1
C Porirua	3702	32	6378	174 700	190 400	2	1/09/01	120 000	236 100	*350 700*	2
Kapiti Coast	3704	31	8509	168 800	179 300	3	1/09/02	108 900	206 200	*299 600*	3
C Hutt	3803	61	13114	159 900	159 800	3	1/09/01	98 200	192 000	284 300	2
C Upper Hutt	3805	16	5476	155 200	170 600	3	1/09/01	108 600	218 900	*329 800*	3
C Wellington	3902	80	23918	256 400	271 200	1	1/09/02	106 000	202 200	295 100	3
South Island											
Buller	5109	17	1207	54 100	58 300	1	1/09/01	79 000	*148 300*		1
Grey	5110	13	1683	70 300	75 800	2	1/09/00	139 800	*279 400*		1
Westland	5111	11	981	66 300	69 200	1	1/09/02	89 700	*174 700*		1
C Christchurch	5216	182	37714	172 800	162 900	3	1/09/01	101 500	190 300	274 700	2
Hurunui	5220	19	1133	102 000	113 400	2	1/09/01	91 000	*177 300*		3
Waimakariri	5221	31	4999	144 600	150 400	1	1/09/02	105 100	191 600		3
Banks Pen.	5222	15	1392	162 400	164 300	3	1/09/00	119 300	217 700	*309 500*	1
Selwyn	5223	26	1524	136 500	155 800	3	1/09/00	85 800	156 500		1
Waimate	5310	10	624	57 000	58 200	2	1/09/01	92 000	*186 200*		2
Ashburton	5311	20	3021	101 100	103 000	2	1/09/00	93 500	177 600		3
Timaru	5312	33	5744	87 400	90 500	2	1/09/02	98 600	*196 800*		2
MacKenzie	5313	7	693	64 500	67 700	2	1/09/00	112 000	*213 400*		1
Queenstown L.	5402	27	3158	230 600	298 300	2	1/09/02	119 000	223 000	322 000	1
Central Otago	5408	30	2757	95 500	113 400	3	1/09/01	75 900	150 700		1
Waitaki	5409	27	3350	62 800	67 100	1	1/09/00	90 400	*175 400*		1
C Dunedin	5509	74	16076	97 900	104 800	1	1/09/01	76 700	155 300	*234 500*	3
Clutha	5518	31	2050	52 500	54 300	3	1/09/02	94 500	*184 100*		1
C Invercargill	5606	27	8978	61 300	68 100	3	1/09/02	100 800	*189 300*		1
Southland	5609	40	2833	64 400	71 100	3	1/09/00	74 600	*136 500*		1
Gore	5610	9	1711	56 100	60 000	3	1/09/01	70 200	*140 000*		3
C Nelson	5704	21	6416	165 500	186 500	2	1/09/00	86 500	170 700	*254 000*	3
Tasman	5706	23	5070	159 300	176 100	2	1/09/02	105 900	207 700	*307 900*	3
Marlborough	5806	32	6287	140 700	149 300	2	1/09/02	103 700	202 400	*299 400*	3
Kaikoura	5807	7	482	123 900	135 600	1	1/09/00	84 600	167 600		2

To conclude, Table 17–6 gives the basic information about the districts of New Zealand and lists the estimates of the geometric means of the sale prices in 2001 and 2002, based on the district-level models fitted in Section 17.3.1, and predictions of the sale prices on 1st July 2005 for properties with CVs of NZ$100 000, NZ$200 000 and NZ$300 000. The predictions are based on the RV that was in force on 1st January 2003. The columns headed "Grp" give the group to which the district is assigned by the three-component mixture of district-level models fitted in Section 17.3 (middle of the table) and in Section 17.4 (the extreme right-hand side column). The predictions that amount to extrapolation (where the reference CV is below the 5th or above the 95th percentile) are given in italics. No prediction is given for CV of NZ$300 000 for districts in which even the 99th percentile falls short of NZ$300 000. Even though only 17 districts have CV of NZ$300 000 between their 5th and 95th percentiles, these districts account for a substantial fraction of the transactions. The group given in the extreme right column is based on the three-component mixture of roll-level regression models.

ACKNOWLEDGMENTS

The data for the presented analysis were provided by Headway Systems Ltd. of Christchurch, New Zealand. We thank Mrs. O'Donoghue from Quotable NZ, Auckland, for information about the realignment of the valuation rolls in Auckland City in 1999. Mr. Sisk of Valuation Consultants NZ introduced the first author (NTL) to the background to the residential property market in New Zealand. Hospitality of the Institute of Information Sciences and Technology, Massey University, New Zealand, where NTL was an Academic Visitor when the project described in this paper was initiated in October 2003, is acknowledged. Ross Ihaka helped us with drawing the map of New Zealand in Figure 17. Steve Haslett's constructive comments on an earlier version of the paper are acknowledged.

REFERENCES

Dempster, A. P., Laird, N. M., & Rubin, D. B. (1977). Maximum likelihood from incomplete data via the EM algorithm. *Journal of the Royal Statistical Society (Ser. B), 39*, 1–38.

Gelman, A., & Price, P. N. (1999). All maps of parameter estimates are misleading. *Statistics in Medicine, 18*, 3221–3234.

Longford, N. T. (1993a). *Software for variance component analysis of data with nested random effects (maximum likelihood).* Groningen, The Netherlands: iec ProGamma.

Longford, N. T. (1993b). *Random coefficient models.* Oxford, UK: Oxford University Press.

Longford, N. T. (2000). On estimating standard errors in multilevel analysis. *The Statistician, 49*, 389–398.

Longford, N. T. (2001). Simulation-based diagnostics in random coefficient models. *Journal of the Royal Statistical Society (Ser. A), 164*, 259–273.

Longford, N. T. (2005). *Missing data and small area estimation: Modern analytical equipment for the survey statistician.* New York: Springer.

Longford, N. T., & Pittau, M. G. (2003). *Stability of household income in European countries in the 1990's* [IRISS Working Paper Series No. 2003–08]. Differdange, Luxembourg: CEPS/INSTEAD.

McLachlan, G., & Peel, D. (2000). *Finite mixture models.* New York: Wiley.

Meng, X.-L., & Rubin, D. B. (1993). Maximum likelihood estimation via the ECM algorithm: A general framework. *Biometrika, 80,* 267–278.

Meng, X.-L., & van Dyk, D. A. (1998). Fast EM-type implementations for mixed effects models. *Journal of the Royal Statistical Society (Ser. B), 60,* 559–578.

Pinheiro, J. C., & Bates, D. M. (2000). *Mixed-effects models in S and S-PLUS.* New York: Springer.

R Development Core Team. (2004). *R: A language and environment for statistical computing.* Vienna, Austria: R Foundation for Statistical Computing.

Shen, W., & Louis, T. A. (1998) Triple-goal estimates in two-stage hierarchical models. *Journal of the Royal Statistical Society (Ser. B), 60,* 455–471.

Author index

Subject index

444   *Subject index*